THE ENCYCLOPEDIA OF

CHILDREN'S HEALTH AND WELLNESS

Volume I

Carol Turkington
and
Albert Tzeel, M.D., F.A.A.P.

☑®
Facts On File, Inc.

The Encyclopedia of Children's Health and Wellness

Copyright © 2004 by Carol Turkington

Facts On File, Inc.
132 West 31st Street
New York NY 10001

Library of Congress Cataloging-in-Publication Data

Turkington, Carol.
The encyclopedia of children's health and wellness / Carol Turkington ; foreword by Albert Tzeel
p. cm.
Includes bibliographical references and index.
ISBN 0-8160-4821-5 (hc. ; alk. paper)
1. Pediatrics—Encyclopedias. 2. Children—Diseases—Encyclopedias. I. Title.
[DNLM: 1. Pediatrics—Encyclopedias—English. WS 13 T939e 2004]
RJ45.T9465 2004
618.92—dc22   2004043251

Facts On File books are available at special discounts when purchased in bulk quantities for businesses, associations, institutions, or sales promotions. Please call our Special Sales Department in New York at (212) 967-8800 or (800) 322-8755.

You can find Facts On File on the World Wide Web at http://www.factsonfile.com

Text and cover design by Cathy Rincon

Printed in the United States of America

VB Hermitage 10 9 8 7 6 5 4 3 2 1

This book is printed on acid-free paper.

CONTENTS

FOREWORD

When I graduated from medical school, I was told that the half-life of medical knowledge was about five years—in other words, about half of what we graduating physicians were taught as the "truth" of medical care would be updated, disproved, or found irrelevant within five years. At such a rate of change, physicians require rigorous attention to the advances made in both medicine and in medical care.

What we were never taught, however, was that the prime focus within medical care—the doctor-patient relationship—would also undergo dramatic advances. In the middle of the 20th century, the doctor-patient relationship was rather one-sided and paternalistic—the doctor gave the patient options and recommendations for treatment, and the patient almost always accepted the doctor's sage counsel. But by the mid-1980s, that reality gave way to a new catchphrase: *shared decision making.*

The idea of shared decision making includes three key tenets: sharing uncertainty, sharing potential foibles, and sharing responsibility for the decision.[1] However, given the asymmetry found within this health-care information exchange (that is, the doctor had the majority of the medical knowledge while the patient depended on the physician for this knowledge), this process invari-

ably resulted in little more than an affirmation of consent for the doctor's recommendation.

Yet within the last 10 years, a new and powerful force has emerged within health care: the informed consumer. Between the information-sharing opportunities of the Internet and the movement to empower patients to take control of their own health, consumerism has found a place within health care. While many physicians remain undecided about the ultimate impact of giving health-care consumers access to medical information, the genie is out of the bottle. Although more and more Americans go online when they need health information,[2] one can never be sure about the quality of the information obtained.[3]

That's where this book comes in. We know that readers want to know more about children's health. (If you did not, you would not be looking at this book!) That being the case, we have gone out of our way to provide you with a reference that is accessible, readable, understandable, and current (within the limitations and constraints of the publishing industry). We want you to be both an empowered consumer who can find the information you are looking for and an active and knowledgeable partner in the care of your child. If, in providing you this credible information, we can

[1] Katz, J. *The Silent World of Doctor and Patient.* New York: Free Press, 1984. p. 166.
[2] Vuong, M. "Online health sites a key resource." *Seattle Post-Intelligencer.* July 17, 2003. Available online. URL: http://seattlepi.nwsource.com/health/131213_onlinehealth17.html. Accessed July 17, 2003.
[3] Mettle, M. "The Healthwise Communities Project: Where Healthcare is Practiced by All." In *Connecting with the New Healthcare Consumer Defining Your Strategy,* edited by D. B. Nash et al. New York: McGraw-Hill Health Education Group, 2000. pp. 375–396.

ease your fears, allay your anxieties or point out pertinent facts, then we will have accomplished what we set out to do.

Since my graduation from medical school nearly 18 years ago, I've seen a lot of changes. I sincerely hope that the information found in this book provides you with the ability to change your child's health for the better.

I wish you and your child good health, positive parenting, and effective empowerment.

—Albert Tzeel, M.D., F.A.A.P.
Milwaukee, Wisconsin

ACKNOWLEDGMENTS

The creation of a two-volume encyclopedia involves the help and guidance of a wide range of experts, without whom this book could not have been possible. Thanks to the staffs of the National Institutes of Health; the American Academy of Pediatrics; Adoptive Families of America; Alexander Graham Bell Association for the Deaf; American Academy of Allergy, Asthma & Immunology; American Academy of Child and Adolescent Psychiatry; American Academy of Dermatology; American Academy of Pediatric Dentistry; American Academy of Sleep Medicine; American Association of Kidney Patients; American Association of People with Disabilities; American Association of Suicidology; American Association on Mental Retardation; American Brain Tumor Association; American Cleft Palate-Craniofacial Association; American College of Obstetricians and Gynecologists; American Council of the Blind; and the American Dental Association.

Thanks also to the American Epilepsy Society, American Heart Association, American Library Association, American Liver Foundation, American Lung Association, American Lyme Disease Foundation, American Medical Association, American Occupational Therapy Association, American Physical Therapy Association, American Psychiatric Association, American Psychological Association, American Red Cross, American SIDS Institute, American Sleep Apnea Association, American Social Health Association, American Society for Deaf Children, American Society of Hematology, American Speech-Language-Hearing Association, Anxiety Disorders Association of America, Arthritis Foundation, Association of Birth Defect Children, Asthma and Allergy Foundation of America, Autism Network International, Autism Research Institute, Autism Society of America, Boys Town, Brady Center to Prevent Gun Violence, Brain Injury Association, Brain Trauma Foundation, Cancer Information Service, Center for Study of Multiple Birth, Center for the Prevention of School Violence, Centers for Disease Control and Prevention, Child Abuse Prevention Network, Child Welfare League, Childhelp USA National Headquarters, Childhood Apraxia of Speech Association of North America, Childhood Brain Tumor Foundation, Children and Adults with Attention Deficit Disorder, Children's Brain Tumor Foundation, Children's Defense Fund, and the Children's Craniofacial Association.

Also helpful were the Children's Health Information Network; Children's Hospice International; Children's Oncology Camps of America; Christopher Reeve Paralysis Association; Cleft Palate Foundation; Council for Exceptional Children; Council for Learning Disabilities; Crohn's Colitis Foundation of America; Cystic Fibrosis Foundation; Dana Alliance for Brain Initiatives; Depression and Bipolar Support Alliance; Elizabeth Glaser Pediatric AIDS Foundation; Environmental Protection Agency; Epilepsy Foundation; ERIC Clearinghouse on Disabilities and Gifted Education; Family Center for Technology and Disabilities; Family Education Network; Federal Trade Commission; Federation for Children with Special Needs; Federation of Families for Children's Mental Health; the Food and Drug Administration; Learning Disabilities Association; Leukemia & Lymphoma Society;

Lupus Foundation of America; March of Dimes Birth Defects Foundation; Maternal Child and Health Bureau; Muscular Dystrophy Association; National ADD Association; National Adoption Center; National Alliance for Autism Research; National Alliance for the Mentally Ill; National Aphasia Association; National Association for the Education of Young Children; National Association for the Visually Handicapped; National Association of Anorexia Nervosa; National Association of the Deaf; National Ataxia Foundation; National Brain Tumor Foundation; National Cancer Institute; National Center for Injury Prevention and Control; National Center for Lead-Safe Housing; National Center for Learning Disabilities; National Center for Missing and Exploited Children; National Childhood Cancer Foundation; National Children's Leukemia Foundation; National Clearinghouse on Child Abuse and Neglect Information; National Committee for the Prevention of Child Abuse; National Down Syndrome Congress; National Down Syndrome Society; National Easter Seal Society; National Eating Disorders Association; National Foster Parent Association; National Foundation for Children's Pediatric Brain Tumors; National Head Start Association; National Headache Foundation; National Health Information Center; National Heart, Lung, and Blood Institute; National Hemophilia Foundation; National Information Center for Children and Youth with Disabilities; National Institute of Allergy and Infectious Diseases; National Institute of Arthritis and Musculoskeletal and Skin Diseases; National Institute of Child Health and Human Development; National Institute of Diabetes and Digestive and Kidney Diseases; National Institute of Mental Health; National Institute of Neurological Disorders and Stroke; National Institute on Deafness and Other Communication Disorders; National Kidney Foundation; National Lead Information Center.

In addition the National Multiple Sclerosis Society, National Neurofibromatosis Foundation, National Organization for Rare Disorders, National Organization of Fetal Alcohol Syndrome, National Psoriasis Foundation, National Reye's Syndrome Foundation, National Safe Kids Campaign, National Safety Council, National Scoliosis Foundation, National Tay Sachs and Allied Diseases Association, National Vaccine Information Center, Nation's Missing Children Organization, Nonverbal Learning Disorders Association, Obsessive-Compulsive Foundation, Pediatric Brain Tumor Foundation, Progeria Research Foundation, Rett Syndrome Research Foundation, Self Help for Hard of Hearing People, Sickle Cell Disease Association of America, Spina Bifida Association of America, Stepfamily Association of America, Tourette's Syndrome Association, U.S. Consumer Product Safety Commission, United Cerebral Palsy Association, Voice of the Retarded, and Zero to Three provided useful information.

Finally, thanks to my agent Gene Brissie of James Peter Associates; to Bert Holtje; to my editor, James Chambers; to Sarah Fogarty, Grace Persico, and Vanessa Nittoli at Facts On File; and to Kara and Michael.

INTRODUCTION

The fast-paced world that children face today is both a more challenging and dangerous one than the world their parents knew. While the risk of many diseases is lower today than ever before, children's health-care needs are nevertheless complex because of their rapid growth and development during a period when their body systems are immature and, therefore, vulnerable.

It is important to remember that children are not just tiny adults; they are unique biological beings who may be affected quite differently than adults by germs, toxins, and medications. With new and more virulent infections that threaten worldwide pandemics, new risks of terrorism, more serious safety issues, and ever-evolving new vaccinations and medications, the child-care health scene is constantly changing.

Nevertheless, the United States today is a fairly healthy place for children to grow up. As the years pass, the chances that children in America will die in childhood is lessening. Specifically, children today are also less likely to smoke and less likely to give birth during adolescence than they were in earlier years, according to the 2003 government report: *America's Children: Key National Indicators of Well-Being.* The report, compiled by the Federal Interagency Forum on Child and Family Statistics, presents a comprehensive look at critical areas of child well-being, including economic security, health status, behavior, social environment, and education.

The report also noted that adolescents are more likely to take honors courses, children overall are less likely to die in childhood or in adolescence, and young women have continued the downward trend of giving birth in adolescence. Moreover, children from ages three to five are more likely to be read to daily by a family member.

On the other hand, U.S. infant mortality in 2002 rose for the first time in more than 40 years, climbing from 6.8 deaths per 1,000 live births in 2001 to 7.0 deaths per 1,000 in 2002. Experts believe the rise in infant mortality might reflect the long trend among American women toward delaying motherhood; women who put off motherhood until their 30s or 40s are more likely to have babies with birth defects or other potentially deadly complications. In addition, older women are more likely to use fertility drugs to get pregnant, and such drugs often lead to twins, triplets, or other multiple births. Multiple births carry a higher risk of premature labor and low birth weight—conditions that can endanger babies' lives. Recent birth rates for women ages 35 to 44 were the highest levels for those age groups in three decades, according to the U.S. Centers for Disease Control and Prevention, and more than half of the multiple births in 2002 were born preterm or had low birth weight.

The Encyclopedia of Children's Health and Wellness includes the most up-to-date information on all the physical, emotional, and intellectual conditions that influence a child's life from infancy through adolescence. It has been designed as a guide and reference to a wide range of subjects important to the understanding of children's health and includes a wide variety of contact information for organizations and government agencies affiliated with pediatric issues, including current Web site addresses and telephone numbers. However, the book is not designed as a substitute for prompt assessment and treatment by pediatric experts in the diagnosis and treatment of children's diseases and health issues.

In this encyclopedia, we have tried to prevent the latest information in the field, based on the newest research. Although information in this book comes from the most up-to-date medical journals and research sources, readers should keep in mind that changes occur very quickly in pediatric health. A bibliography has been included for those who seek additional sources of information.

ENTRIES A–L

ability test   Tests of ability, such as intelligence tests, measure an individual's ability to perform a task, manipulate information, or solve problems. Typically, tests of ability are used to assess specific performance abilities or potential for future learning, rather than stored information. Among the most commonly used ability tests are the Wechsler Intelligence Scale for Children, either revised or third edition (WISC-R or WISC-III), the Scholastic Aptitude Test (SAT), which is widely used in college admissions processes, and the Woodcock-Johnson-III cognitive battery, which is commonly used in public school settings to define a baseline of aptitude against which achievement can be measured in determining whether a learning disability is present.

Ability tests can be physical or mental. They can test verbal or nonverbal areas, and are also frequently used to assess potential employees for specific tasks. Depending on the nature of the test, a wide spectrum of individuals may be involved in administration. Specific clinical training in psychology is required in order to administer the Wechsler or other intelligence tests, while the Woodcock-Johnson may be administered by school guidance counselors with appropriate training. Standardized tests such as the SAT must be administered in specific contexts according to specific testing procedures, but overseeing such tests requires no formal professional training.

Ability tests have particular importance in relation to the Americans with Disabilities Act, which protects individuals with disabilities from discrimination, especially in the workplace. Ability tests designed to assess mechanical abilities, clerical abilities, and other job-related abilities can prevent equal access. Individuals can request alternative assessment of their abilities if they can provide doc-umentation of a disability and they are otherwise qualified for a position.

abrasion   A superficial rubbing off of the uppermost layers of the skin, usually caused by a scrape or a brush burn. Abrasions are usually minor injuries that can be treated at home. The skin may bleed or drain small amounts of pus at the time of the injury. A physician should be contacted if the abrasion is located close to the eye or on the face, if there is embedded dirt, stones, or gravel, if there are signs of infection (increased warmth, redness, swelling, or drainage), or if the abrasion covers a large area of the body (such as the chest or back or an entire limb).

Treatment
The abraded area should be washed well with soap and water (but not scrubbed). Any dirt should be removed by running water over the area for several minutes. A dirty abrasion that is not well cleaned can cause scarring. An antiseptic lotion or cream should be applied, and then covered with an adhesive bandage or gauze pad if the area is on the hands or feet, or if it is likely to drain onto clothing. The dressing should be changed often and be checked each day. Blowing on the abrasion is not recommended, since this can cause germs to grow.

academic skills disorders   Students with academic skills disorders often lag far behind their classmates in developing reading, writing, or arithmetic skills. These disorders can be divided into *developmental reading disorders, developmental writing disorders,* and *developmental arithmetic disorders.*

Developmental reading disorder (also known as DYSLEXIA) is quite widespread, affecting from two percent to eight percent of elementary school children. The ability to read requires a rich, intact network of nerve cells that connect the brain's centers of vision, language, and memory. While a person can have problems in any of the tasks involved in reading, scientists have found that a significant number of people with dyslexia share an inability to distinguish or separate the sounds in spoken words. For example, a child might not be able to identify the word "cat" by sounding out the individual letters, "c-a-t," or to play rhyming games.

Fortunately, remedial reading specialists have developed techniques that can help many children with dyslexia acquire these skills. However, there is more to reading than recognizing words. If the brain cannot form images or relate new ideas to those stored in memory, the reader will not be able to understand or remember the new concepts. This is why other types of reading disabilities can appear in the upper grades when the focus of reading shifts from word identification to comprehension.

Writing also involves several brain areas and functions. The brain networks for vocabulary, grammar, hand movement, and memory must all work well if the child is to be able to write well. A developmental writing disorder may be caused by problems in any of these areas. A child with a writing disability, particularly an expressive language disorder, might be unable to compose complete, grammatical sentences.

Arithmetic involves recognizing numbers and symbols, memorizing facts such as the multiplication table, aligning numbers, and understanding abstract concepts like place value and fractions. Any of these may be difficult for children with developmental arithmetic disorders. Problems with numbers or basic concepts are likely to show up early, whereas problems that appear in the later grades are more often tied to problems in reasoning.

Many aspects of speaking, listening, reading, writing, and arithmetic overlap and build on the same brain capabilities, so it is not surprising that people can be diagnosed as having more than one area of learning disability. For example, the ability to understand language underlies the ability to learn to speak. Therefore, any disorder that interferes with the ability to understand language will also interfere with the development of speech,

which in turn hinders learning to read and write. A single problem in the brain's operation can disrupt many types of activity.

Acanthamoeba infection *Acanthamoeba* are microscopic amoeba commonly found in the environment. They can cause a serious infection in the brain, the lungs, or the eyes. The amoeba can enter a child's skin through a cut or wound, or through the child's nostrils. Once inside the body, the amoeba can travel to the lungs and other parts of the body, especially the central nervous system (brain and spinal cord), through the bloodstream. Through improper storage, handling, and disinfection of contact lenses, the amoeba can enter the eye and cause a serious infection.

The species of *Acanthamoeba* that infect humans include: *A. culbertsoni, A. polyphaga, A. castellanii, A. healyi, A. astronyxis, A. hatchetti,* and *A. rhysodes.*

Acanthamoeba species (spp.) are found worldwide in the soil and dust, in freshwater sources such as lakes, rivers, and hot springs, and in hot tubs, or in brackish water and seawater. Amoeba can also be found in heating, venting, and air conditioner units, humidifiers, dialysis units, and contact lens equipment. The microbes have been found in the nose and throat of healthy people as well as those with compromised immune systems.

Cause

Eye infections may be caused by a contaminated contact lenses as a result of improper cleaning and handling. The risk of infection is higher for those who make their own contact lens cleaning solution. Acanthamoeba enter the eye via contact lenses or through a corneal cut or sore, triggering infection or a corneal ulcer.

Symptoms

Acanthamoeba spp. can cause skin lesions or a body-wide infection. In addition, the amoeba can lead to a serious, often deadly infection called granulomatous amoebic encephalitis (GAE). Once infected, a person may suffer headaches, stiff neck, nausea and vomiting, tiredness, confusion, lack of attention to people and surroundings, loss of balance and bodily control, seizures, and hallucinations. This condition is usually fatal.

Treatment

Eye and skin infections are generally treatable with proper medication. Although most cases of brain infection with *Acanthamoeba* have been fatal, a few patients have recovered from the infection with proper treatment.

Prevention

Eye infections may be prevented by using commercially prepared contact lens cleaning solution rather than making homemade solutions. There is little that can be done to prevent skin and body infection.

accidents   Injury from an accident is one of the major reasons for a childhood emergency room visit, and trauma is the leading cause of death in children over one year of age, according to the National Safety Council and the National Center for Injury Prevention and Control. Each year, more than 28,000 deaths and almost seven million injuries occur from accidents in the home. This means that a death occurs every 19 minutes from a home accident, and a disabling injury every five seconds.

The types of trauma that cause death in children (in order of frequency) are:

1. motor-vehicle accidents
2. drowning
3. burns
4. poisonings
5. firearms
6. falls

Accutane   See ISOTRETINOIN.

acetaminophen (Tylenol)   A nonprescription medication found in many over-the-counter pain relievers that is effective for pain relief but not for inflammation. It is often prescribed as a fever reducer. Easier on the stomach than either ASPIRIN or IBUPROFEN, it does not significantly prolong bleeding. Therefore, children who are about to have a medical procedure that may cause bleeding (such as tooth extractions) or children who have frequent nosebleeds or other bleeding problems can safely take acetaminophen for pain relief.

On the other hand, some pediatricians worry that parents are overmedicating their children and risking an overdose by giving their children acetaminophen whenever they run a fever. In fact, even fever of 102°F may not be dangerous to a small child, since fever is a normal response to an infection and no cause for alarm. A typical dose of acetaminophen for a child is 10 to 15 mg per kg to a maximum of 1 gram (two 500 mg tablets).

Adverse Effects

While most parents believe that children's acetaminophen is perfectly safe because it is a nonprescription medication, it does pose a special risk in children. An overdose—or even a normal dose combined with other medications, or when a child has not eaten—can overwhelm the child's liver. In extreme cases, the liver may be damaged beyond repair.

An overdose typically causes nausea, vomiting, and loss of appetite, all of which usually disappear in a day or two. However, it is during this time that liver failure may be occurring. Liver damage can be reversed with intravenous administration of an antidote, if given in time.

achievement test   Achievement tests are standardized measures of knowledge, information, or procedural learning (such as how to do something). This type of assessment is used to measure student learning in comparison to a norm.

Achievement tests may assess general academic skill areas, such as reading, writing, or mathematics, or they may test for content knowledge in a specific academic subject such as biology or American history. Achievement tests are used by school systems to provide a standard measure of individual student performance and to provide an aggregated measure of performance that enables school systems to evaluate their effectiveness. Achievement tests are also used as part of the diagnostic assessment of individuals to determine whether they have a learning disability and therefore qualify for special education services.

acne   The most common skin disease in the United States, this very common inflammatory reaction in oil-producing follicles usually appears on the face, shoulders, and back. While most common during the teenage years, it may also affect newborns. Because it can lead to permanent scarring on the face, acne can have profound and long-lasting psychological effects.

In boys, acne usually begins in early adolescence, tends to be more severe than in girls, and improves in the early to mid-twenties. In girls, acne usually begins in the mid-teens and is often less severe. In some individuals, the problem can continue into adulthood.

Cause

Acne is not caused by diet (chocolate or fats), dirt, or surface oil. Normally, oil is produced in glands in the skin, traveling up to the hair follicles and flowing out onto the surface of the skin. When oil glands within the hair follicles are stimulated and begin to enlarge, usually as a result of hormonal changes at puberty, they begin to produce more oil. Acne bacteria (*Propionibacterium* acnes) inside the follicles multiply and produce fatty acids, which irritate the lining of the pores. At the same time, the number of thicker cells in the lining of the pores increases and they clump together, narrowing and clogging the pore openings with oil, skin cells, and debris.

As the pressure builds within these clogged pores, the constant production of oil together with irritation from bacteria ruptures the pore walls. When the oil pathway gets blocked and the plug pushes up to the surface, it causes a blackhead (comedo). When the opening is very tightly closed, the material behind it causes a whitehead.

While there are many factors behind the inflammatory changes seen in acne, one of the most important is the different levels of bacteria found on the skin. While acne is not a bacterial infection, experts believe that inflammation results from the by-products released by the bacterium *Propionibacterium acnes* found deep in the follicle.

Emotional stress, cosmetics, genetics, and certain drugs (such as birth control pills) may worsen the condition. Estrogen, however, will improve acne.

Acne is hereditary, and the tendency to develop it runs in families. If both parents have acne, then three out of four of their children will also have acne. Oil in cosmetics also can contribute to acne, which is why makeup should be washed off each night.

Treatment

There are excellent types of therapy for all kinds of acne, including topical treatment, antibiotics, and hormonal manipulation. Most teenagers benefit from a combination of peeling the skin, destroying bacteria, and applying products that affect whiteheads and blackheads.

Treatments should begin with soap and water cleansing every night, with a good diet, and regular exercise. For milder cases, medications containing benzoyl peroxide (5 percent) or those containing sulfur or a combination of sulfur and resorcinol or salicylic acid are effective.

Since oil buildup attracts bacteria, and the bacteria's fatty acids irritate the skin, one of the best ways to fight acne is to kill the bacteria. Those products that are effective in treating acne actually cut down the oil production of the glands slightly and destroy bacteria in the follicle. The most popular antibiotics in the treatment of acne are tetracycline, minocycline, and erythromycin. For milder cases, antibiotics can be used directly on the skin. For more advanced cases, they are taken orally.

Retin-A, a drug related to vitamin A, is an effective treatment for whiteheads and blackheads. It is often combined with benzoyl peroxide or antibiotics. Those with the most severe types of acne may be given a stronger vitamin-A-related drug called Accutane (isotretinoin). This drug has more serious side effects, including BIRTH DEFECTS, and requires strict medical supervision.

It's possible that some cases of acne can be controlled by regulating the androgen/estrogen hormone balance in those girls who have an increased activity of the enzyme that converts testosterone (a male hormone) into a more potent form that affects the oil glands. Since androgen has been implicated in the increased secretion of oil that starts a blemish, androgen blockers that reduce the size of oil glands may help girls whose acne is associated with other changes, such as excessive hair growth or balding. These drugs could be in the form of high-estrogen birth control pills.

Steroids are very effective for inflammatory or cystic acne when injected into a lesion; this can heal the cyst in about 24 hours.

acne, infant Acne is not unusual among newborns; it is triggered by hormones passed from the mother before birth. The hormones cause the glands in the skin to produce oil; if these glands become blocked and inflamed, whiteheads and pimples may develop on the newborn's face.

Newborn acne usually clears up on its own in three or four months. If it is troublesome or persistent, a pediatrician may prescribe a topical medication. Contrary to popular belief, infant acne is not associated with the development of acne in adolescence. Rarely, however, infantile acne becomes severe and persists for months or even a few years. This is usually associated with a family history of acne (usually in the father) and is often followed by severe acne in adolescence.

A doctor should evaluate the skin condition so as to rule out both SEBORRHEA dermatitis and MILIARIA.

acquired immunodeficiency syndrome See AIDS.

acyclovir (Zovirax) An antiviral drug introduced in 1982 that is used to treat viruses causing CHICKEN POX, SHINGLES, or HERPES simplex infection. It is officially approved for the acute management of chicken pox in children, for which it can slightly decrease the severity and duration of the infection. To be effective, therapy must be started within 24 hours of the onset of the rash. Its effect on the subsequent development of shingles is not known

When acyclovir is given in time, it decreases itching, the number of lesions, and the time until crusting. By the third day, all treated children, compared to 75 percent of untreated children, have no fever. Acyclovir does not work if given after the first 24 hours past the start of the rash.

Although acyclovir can decrease the duration and severity of varicella, it should not be given routinely to children who are otherwise healthy. Acyclovir is not indicated in youngsters under age two.

Currently, no data indicate that treating chicken pox with acyclovir hastens the return of children to school or parents to work; the rate of development of complications has not been diminished by active therapy.

Acyclovir has also been used to prevent the development of chicken pox in families in which one child has developed a rash before others; in one study, acyclovir given to exposed children seven to nine days after exposure for seven days protected 84 percent of children, who did not develop overt symptoms.

The American Academy of Pediatrics recommends against the routine use of acyclovir in cases of uncomplicated chicken pox in otherwise healthy children. The AAP does recommend acyclovir for susceptible teenagers who are not pregnant, or for those children over 12 months of age who are receiving long-term salicylate therapy because of the risk of Reye's syndrome, in those with chronic pulmonary or skin problems, and in those receiving aerosolized corticosteroids. However, the benefits of therapy in these groups has not been proven.

Side Effects

Adverse effects from acyclovir are uncommon. Taken by mouth, the drug may rarely cause stomach problems, headache, dizziness, or nausea and vomiting. The ointment may cause skin irritation or rash. Very rarely, acyclovir injections may lead to kidney damage.

ADD See ATTENTION DEFICIT HYPERACTIVITY DISORDER.

Adderall A stimulant medication prescribed for ATTENTION DEFICIT HYPERACTIVITY DISORDER (ADHD) that is a combination of dextramphetamine and amphetamine. Adderall can be used in children over the age of three.

The drug can improve attention span and decrease distractibility, and may decrease impulsivity, stubbornness, and aggression. The drug only needs to be taken once or twice a day; while the effects may be noted immediately, it may take up to six weeks to achieve its full benefit.

Adderall is usually prescribed as part of a treatment plan that includes educational and psychosocial treatment. It is sometimes prescribed in cases in which Ritalin or other stimulant medications have been ineffective. Because it has a fairly slow onset of action, there may be less chance of Adderall causing or worsening tics.

Adderall had earlier been approved and marketed by another company under a different name (Obetrol) as a weight control medication. The manufacturer was taken over by another company, which renamed the product Adderall in 1994. The drug was approved for the treatment of ADHD and reintroduced in 1996 as Adderall.

Side Effects

Most common side effects include appetite and weight loss, insomnia, and headache. Less frequently, a patient may experience dry mouth and nausea. Rare side effects include dizziness, irritability, stomach pain, increased heart rate, or hallucinations. As with most stimulants indicated for ADHD, there is a possibility of growth suppression and the potential for triggering motor tics and TOURETTE'S SYNDROME; in rare cases, worsening of psychosis has been reported.

As with all other stimulants used in treating ADHD, one of the more troublesome side effects is a decrease in brain growth. Although there is something of a rebound effect once the child is removed from the drug, the rebound generally does not bring the child back to the same level on the brain growth charts prior to drug treatment.

Drug Interactions

Adderall should not be taken with monoamine oxidase inhibitors (MAOI), because serious (even fatal) interactions can occur. At least 14 days must pass between taking MAOIs and Adderall. Acidifying agents such as guanethidine, reserpine, and fruit juices can interfere with the absorption of Adderall, whereas substances such as Diamox (acetazolamide) increase absorption. Tricyclic ANTIDEPRESSANTS such as Tofranil become more potent when taken with Adderall. Thorazine (chlorpromazine), lithium, and Haldol (haloperidol) can interfere with the effect of Adderall.

adenoid disorders Adenoids are small lumps of lymphatic tissue nestled above the tonsils that help protect against upper respiratory tract infections. Adenoid disorders—also known as adenoidism or adenoiditis—occur when the adenoids become swollen, making it hard to breathe or swallow.

Cause

Experts do not know why adenoidism is so common in toddlers and young children, although they suspect it may be due to frequent colds or allergies.

Symptoms

Typically, children with adenoid disorders speak with a nasal tone and breathe through their mouths. They may snore, have trouble swallowing, and periodically stop breathing while sleeping (a condition known as obstructive sleep APNEA). They also may have a raspy cough after awakening, bad breath, repeated ear infections or sore throats, persistent runny nose, labored and noisy breathing, snoring, or unusual sleep patterns.

Diagnosis

Adenoid disorders are hard to detect because of the location of the adenoids, which cannot be seen by looking into the mouth. A special viewing instrument is needed.

Treatment

In the past surgical removal of the adenoids (ADENOIDECTOMY) and tonsils in children was quite common. Today, before recommending surgery a doctor may first suggest waiting to see if a child outgrows the problem. Adenoids grow most quickly during the first five years of a child's life; after this, they begin to shrink until they disappear by adolescence.

If the adenoid swelling persists, however, the doctor may first recommend antibiotic treatment to eliminate possible bacterial infection. If the adenoid problem is caused by respiratory allergies, treatment may ease allergy symptoms and gradually reduce swelling.

If all other treatments fail and a child continues to suffer from an adenoid disorder, the doctor may recommend an adenoidectomy. The operation should be performed only after careful evaluation by an ear, nose, and throat specialist, or otolaryngologist. Most children should not have the operation until they reach school age. If a bacterial infection has occurred, surgery should be delayed until two to four weeks after it has cleared up.

According to the American Academy of Pediatrics, adenoid surgery is recommended if the swollen adenoids interfere with normal breathing or severely impair speech. Adenoid surgery should be considered if a child has had:

- seven severe episodes of STREP THROAT (or sore throat accompanied by high fever, swollen lymph nodes, and pus in the throat)
- five serious sore throats in each of two separate years, or three serious sore throats in each of three separate years
- swollen glands in the throat for six months or more despite antibiotic treatment
- recurrent EAR INFECTIONS that do not clear up even after treatment
- sleeping problems

adenoidectomy Surgical removal of the adenoids. In this procedure, after general anesthesia the otolaryngologist removes the adenoids using a small tool with a basket on the end. Pressure is applied to minimize bleeding but stitches are not necessary. The surgery usually takes less than 30 minutes.

Most of these procedures are done on an outpatient basis. ACETAMINOPHEN (Tylenol, Tempra, Panadol) can ease pain. During recovery, the doctor will recommend a soft, bland diet with no hot, spicy, or coarse foods for about a week. Most children completely recover in two to three weeks, although they should avoid strenuous exercise for about a month. See also ADENOID DISORDERS.

adenovirus A type of virus that causes upper respiratory infections producing symptoms resembling those of the common cold. Adenoviruses include 49 DNA-containing viruses identified by sequential letters and numbers that can cause infection in eyes, upper respiratory tract, and the gastrointestinal system.

Although characteristics of the adenoviruses vary, they are all transmitted either by direct contact, by fecal-oral transmission, or by contact with contaminated water. Respiratory infections caused by adenoviruses occur by contact with infectious material from another person or object; secretions from the respiratory tract may contain the virus. The virus also can survive for many hours on inanimate objects such as doorknobs, hard surfaces, and toys. Transmission of the digestive strain of the virus usually occurs by fecal-oral contact. This usually occurs from poor hand-washing or from eating or drinking contaminated food or water.

Some types of adenoviruses are capable of establishing persistent infections in tonsils, adenoids, and intestines without causing any symptoms; shedding can occur for months or years. After the initial illness fades away, the virus can persist in the tonsils, adenoids, and other lymph tissue. Adenoviruses do not become latent like the HERPES virus but instead reproduce constantly and slowly.

Epidemics of disease with fever and CONJUNCTIVITIS are associated with waterborne transmission of some adenovirus types, usually involving poorly chlorinated swimming pools and small lakes.

Symptoms
Respiratory infections may develop between two days and two weeks after exposure and are characterized by common cold symptoms, sore throat, fever, severe or nonproductive cough, swollen lymph nodes, and headache. Intestinal tract infections may appear from three to 10 days after exposure, usually among children under age four. They begin with an abrupt watery diarrhea, fever, and abdominal swelling and tenderness. These symptoms may last from one to two weeks.

Although outbreaks of adenovirus-associated respiratory disease have been more common in the late winter, spring, and early summer; these infections can occur throughout the year.

Treatment
Most infections are mild and do not need to be treated. Because there is no treatment specifically tailored to this virus, serious adenovirus illness can be managed only by treating symptoms and complications. Treatment for respiratory infection may include fluids, bronchodilator medications to open the airways, or supplemental oxygen through a mask, nasal prongs, or an oxygen tent. A child who becomes very sick with adenovirus may require mechanical ventilation or a respirator to assist with breathing for a period of time.

Treatment for intestinal infection may include fluids (water, formula, breast milk, and/or special electrolyte-containing fluids such as Pedialyte). Very young children should NOT be rehydrated with soda, juices, or sports drinks. Children may be given solid foods if they are able to tolerate them.

Complications

Children who develop PNEUMONIA from adenovirus may develop chronic lung disease. Very rarely, this strain of the virus has a 10 percent mortality rate. Children with weakened immune systems are at risk for developing a more severe infection from adenoviruses.

A severe complication of intestinal adenovirus is intussusception, an intestinal blockage that occurs when one part of the intestine slides over another section like a telescope. This is a medical emergency and most often occurs in infants under 1 year of age. The symptoms of intussusception may include bloody or "currant jelly" stool, vomiting, abdominal swelling, knees flexed to chest, loud cries of pain, weakness, and lethargy.

Prevention

Strict hand-washing is important to prevent the spread of adenoviruses to other infants, children, and adults. There are vaccines for adenovirus serotypes 4 and 7, but these are available only to prevent infection among military recruits. Strict infection control practices are effective at stopping outbreaks of adenovirus-associated disease in hospitals; adequately chlorinating pools can prevent swimming pool-associated outbreaks of adenovirus conjunctivitis.

ADHD See ATTENTION DEFICIT HYPERACTIVITY DISORDER.

adjustment disorder A maladaptive emotional or behavioral reaction to a stressful event or change in a child's life, such as a family move, divorce, loss of a pet, or birth of a sibling. The reaction must occur within three months of the stressful event to be considered an adjustment disorder. Because adjustment disorders are a reaction to stress, there is not a single direct cause between the stressful event and the reaction.

Children and adolescents vary in their temperament, past experiences, vulnerability, and coping skills. Their developmental stage and the capacity of their support system to meet their needs may contribute to their reaction to a particular stress.

Adjustment disorders are quite common in children and adolescents, but the characteristics of the disorder in those groups are different than they are in adults. Youthful symptoms of adjustment disorders are more behavioral—children are more likely to act out, while adults experience more depressive symptoms.

Symptoms

In all adjustment disorders, the reaction to the stress seems to be abnormally severe and significantly interferes with friends or school function. There are six subtypes of adjustment disorder based on symptoms:

adjustment disorder with depressed mood is characterized by depression, crying, and feelings of hopelessness.

adjustment disorder with anxiety may cause nervousness, worry, jitteriness, and fear of separation.

adjustment disorder with anxiety and depressed mood is a combination of symptoms from both of the above subtypes.

adjustment disorder with disturbance of conduct may be characterized by violating the rights of others, truancy, destruction of property, reckless driving, or fighting.

adjustment disorder with mixed disturbance of emotions and conduct involves a combination of all of the subtype symptoms (depressed mood, anxiety, and conduct).

adjustment disorder unspecified Reactions to stressful events that do not fit in one of the above subtypes is referred to as "unspecified" and may include behavior such as social withdrawal or reluctance to do homework or after-school chores.

Diagnosis

Because the symptoms of adjustment disorders may resemble other medical problems or psychiatric conditions, the child's physician should always be consulted for a correct diagnosis. A child psychiatrist or CHILD PSYCHOLOGIST usually makes the diagnosis after a comprehensive psychiatric evaluation and interview with the child and parents, including a detailed personal history describing development, life events, emotions, behaviors, and the identified stress. Early diagnosis and treatment can reduce the severity of symptoms, enhance the child's growth and development, and improve the quality of life.

Treatment

Individual psychotherapy uses cognitive-behavioral approaches to improve problem-solving skills, communication skills, impulse control, anger management skills, and stress management skills. Family therapy is often focused on making changes within the family system, such as improving communication skills and family interactions, as well as increasing family support among family members. Peer group therapy is often focused on developing and using social skills and interpersonal skills.

While medication has very little value in the treatment of adjustment disorders, it may be considered on a short-term basis if a specific symptom is severe and known to be responsive to medication.

adolescent immunization Experts recommend that all adolescents should have MEASLES, MUMPS, rubella (GERMAN) MEASLES, TETANUS, POLIO, and DIPHTHERIA immunizations. Teenagers with diabetes or chronic heart, lung, liver, or kidney disorders need protection against INFLUENZA and PNEUMONIA. CHICKEN POX vaccine is recommended for those not previously vaccinated who have no reliable history of the disease. HEPATITIS B vaccine is indicated for all adolescents up to age 18 who have not been vaccinated before. Hepatitis A vaccine is recommended for adolescents traveling to or working in countries where the disease is common, and for those living in communities with outbreaks of the disease. It is also recommended for adolescents who have chronic liver disease or clotting-factor disorders, use illegal injection drugs, or are male homosexuals.

Adolescents not previously vaccinated against measles, mumps, and rubella with two doses of MMR VACCINE require these. During childhood, teens should have received the DTaP vaccine against tetanus, diphtheria, and polio. Immunization against tetanus and diphtheria (Td vaccine) should be supplemented with a booster shot at age 11 or 12, and every 10 years thereafter. One dose of chicken pox vaccine is recommended for adolescents 11 or 12 years of age (or two doses for those 13 or older) if there is no proof of prior chicken pox disease or immunization.

The flu shot or nasal spray should be given each year to all adolescents—especially those at high risk for complications associated with influenza. High-risk teens should not be given the nasal spray version of the vaccine, however. Immunization against pneumococcal disease is recommended for adolescents with certain chronic diseases who are at increased risk for pneumonia or its complications; a booster dose is recommended 10 years after the initial dose for this group.

As with any medicine, there are very small risks that serious problems could occur after getting a vaccine. However, the potential risks associated with the diseases that these vaccines prevent are much greater than the potential risks associated with the vaccines themselves.

adoption Nearly 70,000 children are adopted in the United States each year, including 8,000 international children and 10,000 children with special emotional or physical needs.

Adoptions may be arranged independently or through an adoption agency. An independent adoption usually requires the participation of an adoption attorney or counselor, physician, or minister. Adoption laws vary significantly from state to state. Adopting between states or from a foreign country also is possible, but it is more complex. Many prospective Caucasian parents want to adopt healthy babies who come from a similar background, but in the United States there are very few healthy Caucasian infants available. Most Caucasian infants are placed through agencies and independent adoptions.

African-American, Hispanic, and mixed-race infants are available both through public and private adoption agencies. However, the adoption of Native American children of all ages by non-Indians is strictly limited by the Federal Indian Welfare Act (P.L.95-608).

Many children with special needs are available for adoption. These children may be older; they may have physical, emotional, or mental disabilities; or they may have brothers and sisters who should be adopted together. Usually children like these are being cared for by the state and are placed in foster care. Both public agencies and some private agencies place children with special needs.

Families can get help in adopting a child with special needs from national, regional, and state adoption exchanges. Adoption exchanges and agencies usually have photo listings and descriptions of available children, and many now provide information about waiting children on the Internet. In many cases, adoption subsidies are available to help parents pay for the legal, medical, and other costs that can occur when caring for a child with special needs.

International Adoption

Some parents may prefer to give a home to a child from another country. Most foreign-born children adopted in the United States come from Russia, China, Korea, India, and countries in Eastern Europe, Central America, and South America. More than 700 private U.S. agencies place children from foreign countries; a few countries allow families to work with attorneys rather than agencies.

However, it is not necessarily easier to look outside the borders of the United States for a child. There are strict immigration requirements for international adoptions, as well as substantial agency fees and transportation, legal, and medical costs.

Prospective parents should consider the emotional and social implications of adopting a child of a different nationality. Agencies seek families who will help a child learn about and appreciate his native culture because it is part of who he or she is.

Types of Agencies

An "agency adoption" is allowed in many states, and includes adoption through a local public agency or a licensed private agency. Many states also allow a couple to use an attorney or other intermediary; some states allow the use of adoption facilitators. Adoption laws vary from one state to the next. An adoption across state lines must comply with the laws in both states before the child can be adopted. The Interstate Compact for the Placement of Children governs how children can be placed across state lines in every state.

Agency adoptions offer the most assurance of monitoring and oversight since agencies are required to be licensed and follow certain procedures. A couple who chooses an independent adoption by an attorney at least is assured that the attorney must follow the standards of the Bar Association; some attorneys who specialize in adoption are members of the American Academy of Adoption Attorneys, a professional membership organization with standards of ethical practice. Adoptions by facilitators are the riskiest since they involve the least amount of supervision.

Open Adoption

Not so long ago, almost all U.S. adoptions were anonymous, but today many couples prefer open adoption. In an open adoption, there is an exchange of information and contact between the birth and adoptive parents. This is becoming more popular because keeping adoption a secret from an adopted child is generally not a good idea.

Costs

Fees and waiting times for infants vary tremendously, depending on the type of adoption involved. Public agency adoptions are often less expensive than private agency or independent adoptions, although private adoptions may take less time. Costs of adopting a healthy infant in the United States through a private agency range from $15,000 to $30,000. Foreign adoptions can be expensive as well; families pay between $10,000 and $20,000 in fees, and that may not include travel and living expenses while in the foreign country.

It is not expensive to adopt a child with special needs; often the agency has a sliding fee scale, and there may be little or no cost. After the adoption, the child may receive subsidies to cover medical and other expenses, although the family is still likely to incur costs for ongoing care.

Couples should obtain a written disclosure of all adoption fees and costs before going ahead with the adoption.

Who Can Adopt

Agencies recognize that many different kinds of people can be loving, effective parents. People considering adoption should be stable, sensitive, and be able to give a child love, understanding, and patience. An adoptive parent may be married or single, childless or already a parent. It is possible to adopt even if a person has been divorced, has had marital problems, received counseling, or has a disability—if the person can still care for a child. Agencies usually ask for proof of marriage, divorce, or death of a spouse, and applicants are generally asked to have a physical examination to document that their health permits them to care for a child.

The adoptive parent does not have to own a home or have a high income in order to provide permanence, stability, a lifetime commitment, and a chance to be part of a family. Children need one or more caring and committed individuals willing to meet their needs and raise them in a nurturing family environment.

More and more agencies and some foreign countries place children with single applicants, who have been proven to be as mature, independent, and supportive as couples. In fact, single adoptive parents are often the placement of choice for children who have trouble dealing with two parents due to a history of abuse or neglect.

For many infant adoptions in the United States, however, agency criteria for applicants are more restrictive. Often agencies will only consider couples married for at least one to three years, who are between ages 25 and 40, and who have good, stable jobs, although some agencies accept applicants who are older than 40.

Some agencies are more restrictive, requiring that the couple:

- have no other children
- are infertile
- have one at-home parent for at least six months after the adoption.

In some states a minor is allowed to adopt. A few states have special requirements for prospective adoptive parents: a certain age differential between the child and the adoptive parents; the adopting parent must live in the state for a certain period of time before being able to adopt; or the prospective adoptive parents and adoptee must live

together for a period of time prior to the adoption. In most states, adoption by "preferred" relatives or stepparents is simpler; waiting periods, home studies, and even the adoption hearing may be waived.

The Adoption and Safe Families Act of 1997 requires state agencies to speed up a child's move from foster care to adoption by establishing time frames for permanency planning and guidelines for when a child must be legally freed for adoption. The bill also removes geographic barriers to adoption by requiring that states not delay or deny a placement if an approved family is available outside the state. The 1995 Multi-Ethnic Placement Act bars any agency that receives federal funding and is involved in adoption from discriminating because of race when considering adoption opportunities for children.

Gay men and lesbians are adopting children both at home and abroad, as well as considering the adoption of younger children through private and international adoptions. The Family Pride Coalition and the ADOPTION RESOURCE EXCHANGE FOR SINGLE PARENTS (See Appendix I) can provide more information about single parent and nontraditional adoption.

The Process

When considering an option, a social worker will visit the couple's home to assess the potential adoptive parents physically, emotionally, and financially. This home study usually involves a series of meetings to provide more in-depth information about adoption and help prepare an applicant for parenting an adopted child. Social workers want to be sure that a person or couple can provide a safe and nurturing environment for a new child in their home.

The home study process varies from agency to agency. Some conduct individual and joint interviews with a husband and wife; others conduct group home studies with several families at one time. Most ask applicants to provide written information about themselves and their life experiences.

There is a waiting period for all adoptions. The time frame, like the cost, varies with the type of child being adopted. The wait is typically between two and seven years for a healthy infant. Children with special needs can often be adopted quickly, within a few months, if the prospective family has a completed home study.

Once an adoptive child is placed in the home, a legal application must be filed for an adoption with the court. After the child has been living in the home for some time, a social worker will visit the home again for a follow-up visit. After the adoption petition has been filed, a court hearing is held to review the case and grant the final adoption decree.

In order for a child to be adopted, the birth parents have to relinquish legal custody. With most agency adoptions, a child is already legally free for adoption before a placement occurs. While cases where parents change their minds (usually before an adoption is finalized) are highly publicized, they occur very rarely.

Adoption Resource Exchange for Single Parents, Inc. (ARESP)   A nonprofit organization founded in 1994 to help single people adopt special needs children. ARESP provides direct services to the Washington area but also serves single adults nationwide, and is a member of the North American Council on Adoptable Children, Adoption Exchange Association, Adoptive Families of America, and Families Adopting Children Everywhere.

The group advocates and promotes the adoption of older and special needs children in the foster care system while supporting the rights of single adoptive and foster parents. The organization assists in the process of adoption, the home study process, and the search for waiting children. It maintains listings and profiles of waiting children and gathers resources to be made available to prospective parents.

ARESP operates an Adoption Help Line, publishes a quarterly newsletter, offers seminars for prospective adoptive parents, conducts workshops at major adoption conferences, and helps prospective parents search for children. The organization believes that every child has a right to a loving and caring home, and any person willing to give a child love and support should be considered a prospective adoptive parent regardless of age, sex, race or ethnicity, creed, marital status, or sexual orientation. For contact information see Appendix I.

Advil   See IBUPROFEN.

Aerolate   See THEOPHYLLINE.

AIDS   A disease of the immune system caused by the human immunodeficiency virus (HIV) that has been a major cause of illness and death among children and teens worldwide. Nationally, AIDS has been the sixth leading cause of death in the United States among 15- to 24-year-olds since 1991; teens between 13 and 19 represent one of the fastest-growing HIV-positive groups. In recent years AIDS infection rates have been increasing rapidly among teens. Half of all new HIV infections in the United States occur in people under 25 years of age; thousands of teens in the United States become infected each year. According to the Centers for Disease Control (CDC), most new HIV cases in younger people are transmitted through unprotected sex; one-third of these cases are from sharing dirty, blood-contaminated needles.

In 2000 the CDC reported that more than 90 percent of current cases of AIDS in children, and almost all new HIV infections reported in young U.S. children, resulted from transmission of the HIV virus from the mother to her child during pregnancy, birth, or through breast-feeding. Between 6,000 and 7,000 children are born to HIV-infected mothers each year in the United States.

However, between 1992 and 1997 the number of infants who became HIV positive when born to an infected mother plummeted by 50 percent as a result of new antiretroviral medications now given to the mother before the baby is born. Because transmission often occurs during delivery, cesarean section may be indicated for some women. The virus also has been detected in breast milk, so infected mothers should not breast-feed.

Before 1985, a small group of children were infected with the virus by contaminated blood products. Since then, blood products have been screened for the virus and risk of infection from this route has been virtually eliminated.

In adolescents, HIV is most commonly spread by sexual contact with an infected partner. The virus enters the body through the lining of the vagina, vulva, penis, rectum, or mouth during sexual activity.

HIV is also spread by sharing needles, syringes, or drug use equipment with someone who is infected with the virus.

Cause

This disease results from infection with the human immunodeficiency virus (HIV), which infects and destroys a type of white blood cell involved in the body's immune response to invading germs. By destroying or impairing immune system cells, the virus progressively destroys the body's ability to fight infections and certain cancers.

Symptoms

Persistent or severe symptoms may not surface for 10 years or more after HIV infection first enters the body. This period of the infection varies from person to person, during this time the HIV is infecting and killing cells of the immune system. Its most obvious effect is a decline in the blood levels of CD4+ cells (also called T4 or "helper" cells)—the immune system's key infection fighters. The virus initially disables or destroys these cells without causing symptoms.

An HIV-infected child is usually diagnosed with AIDS when the immune system becomes severely damaged and other types of infections occur. As the immune system deteriorates, symptoms may include

- fatigue and lack of energy
- fevers and sweats
- enlarged lymph nodes for more than three months
- short-term memory loss
- pelvic inflammatory disease that does not respond to treatment
- persistent skin rashes or flaky skin
- persistent or frequent oral/vaginal yeast infections
- weight loss

Some children develop frequent and severe HERPES infections that cause mouth, genital, or anal sores, or SHINGLES.

Treatment

There are treatments to slow down the rate at which HIV weakens the immune system, but cur-

rently available antiretroviral drugs cannot cure HIV infection or AIDS, and all these drugs have severe side effects.

Some of the nucleoside reverse transcriptase (RT) inhibitors may deplete red or white blood cells, especially when taken in the later stages of the disease; some may also cause an inflammation of the pancreas and painful nerve damage. There have been reports of other severe reactions, including death, to some of the antiretroviral nucleoside drugs when used alone or in combination.

The most common side effects associated with protease inhibitors include nausea, diarrhea, and other gastrointestinal symptoms. In addition, protease inhibitors can interact with other drugs and cause serious side effects.

A major factor in reducing the number of deaths from AIDS in this country has been highly active antiretroviral therapy (HAART). HAART is a treatment regimen that combines reverse transcriptase inhibitors and protease inhibitors to treat AIDS patients.

While HAART is not a cure for AIDS, it has greatly improved the health of many children with AIDS, reducing the amount of virus circulating in the blood to nearly undetectable levels. However, researchers have shown that HAART cannot eradicate HIV entirely from the body.

A number of drugs are available to help treat opportunistic infections to which children with HIV are especially prone. These drugs include foscarnet and ganciclovir to treat cytomegalovirus eye infections, fluconazole to treat yeast and other fungal infections, and trimethoprim/sulfamethoxazole (TMP/SMX) or pentamidine to treat *Pneumocystis carinii* pneumonia (PCP).

Children can receive PCP preventive therapy when their T-cell counts drop to levels considered below normal for their age group, and they must take drugs for the rest of their lives to prevent an occurrence of the pneumonia.

air bags Since they were first placed in cars to serve as protective devices during accidents, 116 children have been killed by the force of deploying air bags, according to the National Highway Traffic Safety Administration. An air bag explodes out of the dashboard at rates of up to 200 miles per hour—faster than the blink of an eye—and can injure or kill a small child.

Because they were designed to protect adults, the force can be too strong for small children and can cause head and neck injuries in young riders. Still, the number of small children killed by air bags has fallen sharply in the past five years, suggesting that parents are getting the message that children are safest when riding in the backseat. There were only six child deaths caused by air bags in 2000, compared to 25 in 1996. In the same period, the number of cars with air bags rose from 22 million to more than 80 million.

The government began allowing switches to deactivate air bags in 1995 and recommends the passenger-side air bag be turned off if a child under age 13 is riding in the front seat. By September 1, 2003, all vehicles were required to have advanced air bags that deploy with less force or not at all when children are in the front seat.

Before riding in the front seat, a child should be

- at least 12 years of age
- at least 5 feet tall
- at least 110–120 pounds

Al-Anon/Alateen Al-Anon is a nonprofit organization that helps families and friends of alcoholics recover from the effects of living with the problem drinking of a relative or friend. Similarly, Alateen is a recovery program for young people, usually teenagers, whose lives have been affected by someone else's drinking. The groups are sponsored by Al-Anon members. Alateen helps young people share experience, strength, and hope with each other, discuss their problems, learn effective coping strategies, and help each other understand the principles of the Al-Anon program.

The program of recovery is adapted from Alcoholics Anonymous and is based upon the Twelve Steps, Twelve Traditions, and Twelve Concepts of Service. The only requirement for membership is that there be a problem of alcoholism in a relative or friend.

Al-Anon meetings are held in 115 countries; there are more than 24,000 Al-Anon and 2,300 Alateen groups worldwide.

See also Appendix I.

albinism A rare inherited condition present at birth in all races, that is characterized by the partial or total lack of the pigment melanin that gives color to skin, eyes, and hair. Children with albinism often have visual problems, are prone to skin inflammation, suffer severe sunburn, and tend to develop skin cancer.

The most common type of albinism affects hair, skin, and eyes; in the most severe form, hair and skin are snowy white throughout life. Less severely affected children may be born with white skin and hair that darkens slightly with age. Numerous freckles may develop on sun-exposed parts of the body. Whether mild or severe, the child's eyes cannot tolerate bright lights and often have abnormal flickering movements or nearsightedness. More rare types of albinism affect only skin, hair, or the eyes.

Less than 100,000 children in the United States and Europe are affected, although the prevalence is much higher in some parts of the world (about 20 per 100,000 in southern Nigeria, for instance).

The most serious complication of the disease is the lack of melanin, which protects the skin against the harmful radiation in sunlight. Because the skin cannot tan, it ages prematurely and is prone to skin cancers.

albuterol (Proventil, Ventolin) A drug used to open the airways in children with ASTHMA or chronic BRONCHITIS. It can be administered by mouth, injection, or inhalation. Side effects may include dizziness, tremor, nervousness, anxiety, and fast heart rate.

Alexander Graham Bell Association for the Deaf This private, nonprofit organization serves as an information center, publisher, and advocate of effective ways of teaching deaf and hard of hearing people improve their abilities to speak, speechread (lipread), use residual hearing, and process spoken and written language. It also works to empower children with hearing problems to function independently.

Although it began in 1890 as an active proponent of speech for deaf people, the organization has gradually expanded its interests to include research, family support, and financial assistance to help deaf students attend classes with hearing children. (For contact information, see Appendix I.)

allergic rhinitis   An inflammation of the mucous membrane lining the nose caused by an allergic reaction as inhaled allergens are trapped by the nasal filtration system. In allergic rhinitis, sneezing is a prominent feature and nasal symptoms may be accompanied by itchy watery eyes and intense itching of the nose and soft palate. The disease is triggered in susceptible children by allergic reactions to pollen, mold, dust mites, and other allergens.

Seasonal allergic rhinitis is called HAY FEVER or seasonal allergic rhinitis. In this condition, both the nose and the eyes are affected. Allergic rhinitis that occurs year-round is known as perennial allergic rhinitis. Seasonal pollen allergy may exacerbate symptoms of perennial rhinitis.

Allergic rhinitis is the most common chronic disease in children, affecting about one in five children by the age of two or three years; up to 30 percent are affected during adolescence. Boys are twice as likely to get allergic rhinitis than girls, but the prevalence of allergic rhinitis may vary greatly by region. A study in Tucson, Arizona, for example, found that 42 percent of children were diagnosed with allergic rhinitis by the age of six.

A family history of allergic rhinitis is the greatest known risk factor for the condition. Other risk factors include higher social class, male gender, breast-feeding for more than one month, being the first born, having a mother with asthma, and having a dog in the home.

Cause

Hay fever is triggered by windborne pollens such as grass and weeds as well as mold (fungal spores) in the summer and fall. Perennial allergic rhinitis is caused by house dust, feather pillows, cigarette smoke, animal dander, and upholstery.

Symptoms

Hay fever causes sneezing, profuse runny nose, and nasal obstruction or congestion. Nose and eyes may itch. Eyelids and the whites of the eyes may look red and swollen, and there may be headache or sinus pain, dark circles under the eyes, itchy throat, malaise, and fever. Perennial allergic rhinitis may cause dark circles under the eyes and chronic blocked nasal passages often extending to eustachian tube obstruction, particularly in children.

Children suffering from the disease may not sleep well or look well. An estimated one and a half million school days are lost each year due to allergic rhinitis, but even when children are at school, poorly treated allergic rhinitis can diminish their ability to learn, concentrate, and interact socially.

Diagnosis

Parents often are able to diagnose hay fever. While a common cold or upper respiratory infection can be confused with allergic rhinitis, parents should suspect rhinitis if the child has irritated eyes and no fever. Food allergies can also cause rhinitis symptoms in 70 percent of infants and young children, but with food allergies there are often other symptoms of skin or stomach irritation as well. A careful history usually reveals the seasonal nature of the complaint and the suspected role of seasonal allergens. Physical examination usually reveals puffy, reddened watery eyes, a red throat, and nostrils filled with clear watery mucus.

To determine what allergens an individual is allergic to, children may take a skin test in which they are exposed to various substances, such as pet dander, dust mites, or mold.

Treatment

Seasonal allergic rhinitis responds well to treatment. Ideally, avoiding the offending allergic substance is the first approach to managing any allergic disorder. However, it is usually impossible to avoid the offending pollen allergens that cause allergic rhinitis.

Steroid nasal sprays are the most effective type of drug treatment, but some doctors are still reluctant to use these medications because of potential side effects. The safety of steroid nasal sprays is a concern when treating children, since there is potential for some of these medications to enter the bloodstream, where they may affect bone metabolism and slow childhood growth. This potential adverse effect is of particular concern in children with both asthma and allergic rhinitis, who require long-term glucocorticoid therapy by both inhalation and nasal spray. Fluticasone (Flonase) is approved for children over age four. Mometasone (Nasonex) was recently shown to be safe and effective for children ages three and up.

Antihistamines are another treatment choice. The "second-generation" antihistamines can provide relief from symptoms while minimizing side effects, such as drowsiness or irritability. Children with chronic allergic rhinitis may need to take antihistamines every day. Otherwise, they should be taken before exposure to allergens. Cetirizine (Zyrtec) and loratadine (Claritin), both for ages two and up, are effective second-generation antihistamines for children, and fexofenadine (Allegra) is appropriate for children over age six. Claritin is now available without prescription. Clarinex is the same medication as Claritin but at half-strength; it is available by prescription only.

Decongestants, which unblock stuffy noses, may be prescribed as pills or sprays. They should be used with caution in young infants because of potential adverse reactions. Azelastine (Astelin) is a second-generation antihistamine available in a nasal spray for children over age six.

Allergen immunotherapy is a safe and effective treatment for long-term control of multi-seasonal, moderate-to-severe allergic rhinitis. Immunotherapy involves injections of allergens over a number of months until the body becomes accustomed to them. Because severe reactions are possible, immunotherapy is not recommended in very young children.

Complications

Left untreated, allergic rhinitis also can lead to other serious conditions, including ASTHMA, recurrent middle EAR INFECTIONS, sinusitis, sleep disorders, and chronic cough. Appropriate management of rhinitis is an important part of effectively managing these coexisting or complicating respiratory conditions.

allergies Overreactions of the immune system toward substances that are typically harmless to most people. In someone with an allergy, the body's immune system treats the substance (called an allergen) as an invader and reacts inappropriately—triggering the symptoms seen in allergies.

Everything from dust to cats to peanuts to cockroaches can cause allergies in children. Up to two million children have some type of allergy. It has been estimated that children miss more than two million school days per year because of allergies.

In the most common type of allergy, at the first exposure to an allergen, the immune system releases histamine and other chemicals to defend against the allergen "invader." It is the release of these chemicals that causes allergic reactions, as the body attempts to rid itself of the invading allergen.

Some of the most common allergies include those to food and to airborne allergens such as pollen, mold, dust mites, and animal fur or dander. Allergies can be seasonal, like pollen or certain molds, or year-round, like dust mites. Regional differences also occur since different allergens are more prevalent in different parts of the country or the world. For example, peanut allergy is unknown in Scandinavia, where peanuts are not eaten, but common in the United States, where the per capita consumption of peanuts is about eight pounds a year.

Children inherit allergic tendencies from their parents; if one parent has allergies, there is a one in four chance that a child will also have allergies. The risk increases if both parents have allergies. Allergies also tend to develop in response to multiple substances. If children are allergic to one substance, it is likely that they will be allergic to others.

Some children suffer from cross-reactions, so that a child who is allergic to birch pollen might have reactions when eating an apple because the apple contains protein similar to the pollen. Children who are allergic to latex are also more likely to be allergic to kiwi fruit or bananas.

The type and severity of allergy symptoms vary from child to child. Airborne allergens can cause ALLERGIC RHINITIS (sneezing, itchy nose or throat, nasal congestion, and coughing). These symptoms are often accompanied by "allergic conjunctivitis"—itchy, watery, red eyes, and dark circles around the reddened eyes. Allergic rhinitis occurs in about 15 percent to 20 percent of Americans and typically develops by age 10, reaching its peak in the early 20s. The symptoms of allergic rhinitis and conjunctivitis can be mild or severe and may occur only at certain times of the year or all year round. If symptoms occur with wheezing and shortness of breath, the allergy may have progressed to asthma, which can be a serious condition.

Food Allergies

Food allergies may cause only an itchy mouth and throat; other allergies trigger a rash or cramping, with nausea and vomiting or diarrhea, as the body attempts to flush out the irritant. Still other common allergic food symptoms include hives, and in more severe cases, shortness of breath. In severe reactions (such as in tree nut or peanut allergies), the child may develop a sudden, life-threatening reaction called anaphylactic shock. Severity of food allergies and when they develop depends on the quantity of the food eaten, the amount of exposure the child has had, and the child's sensitivity to the food. Common foods that may cause allergies include cow's milk, soy, egg, wheat, seafood, nuts, and peanuts. Severe symptoms or reactions to any allergen require immediate medical attention. Children with a severe allergy to foods must carry injectable epinephrine (Epipen), which can reverse anaphylactic shock. Fortunately, severe or life-threatening allergies occur only in a small group of children.

There is no cure for allergies, but it is possible to treat the symptoms. The easiest way is to eliminate exposure to allergens. If that is not possible, then medications may be given, such as ANTIHISTAMINES or a nasal spray steroid. In some cases, an allergist may recommend allergy shots to help desensitize a child. If a child is extremely sensitive to a particular food, or if the child has asthma in addition to the food allergy, his doctor will probably recommend that parents carry injectable epinephrine (Epipen) to counteract the allergic reaction in the event of an inadvertent exposure.

Food allergies are usually not lifelong, but reactions to nuts or seafood can last a lifetime. In these cases, avoiding the food is the only way to avoid symptoms while the sensitivity persists.

Airborne Allergens

Those who react to airborne allergens usually have allergic rhinitis and allergic conjunctivitis. Airborne allergens include dust mites, cockroach parts, pollens, and molds:

- *Dust mites* These microscopic creatures are one of the most common causes of allergies and are present year-round in most parts of the country, although they do not live at high altitudes. Dust mites live in bedding, upholstery, and carpets.
- *Cockroaches* The body parts and waste products of these insects are also a major household allergen, especially in inner cities. Asthma rates of inner city children are high, probably due to cockroach exposure in overcrowded buildings.
- *Pollen* Trees, weeds, and grasses release these tiny particles into the air to fertilize other plants. Most people know pollen allergy as hay fever or rose fever. Pollen allergies are seasonal, and the type of pollen a child is allergic to determines when he will be symptomatic. For example, in the mid-Atlantic states, tree pollination begins in February and March, grass from May through June, and ragweed from August through October. Pollen counts measure how much pollen is in the air. Pollen counts are usually higher in the morning and on warm, dry, breezy days; they are lowest when it is chilly and wet. Although they are not exact, the local weather report's pollen count can be helpful when planning outside activities.
- *Molds* These fungi thrive in warm, moist environments. As with pollen, mold spores are released into the air to reproduce. Outdoors, molds may be found in poor drainage areas, such as in piles of rotting leaves or compost piles; indoors they thrive in dark, poorly ventilated places, such as bathrooms and closets. Mold buildup may be found in damp basements or basements with water leaks. A musty odor suggests mold growth. Although molds can be seasonal, many thrive year-round, especially those indoors.

Animal Allergens

All warm-blooded, furry animals can cause allergic reactions, usually the result of proteins in their saliva, dander, and urine. When the animal licks itself, the saliva gets on the fur. As the saliva dries, protein particles become airborne and work their way into fabrics in the home. Cats often cause the most problems because their salivary protein is extremely small, and they tend to lick themselves as part of grooming more than other animals.

Allergy Skin Tests

An allergist can determine the cause of an allergy by using skin tests for the most common environmental and food allergens. In the test, a drop of a purified liquid form of the allergen is placed on the skin, or injected just under the skin. After about 15 minutes, if a reddened swelling appears at the injection site, the test is positive. Skin tests are less expensive and more accurate than blood tests for allergies, but blood tests may be required in children with skin conditions or those who are extremely sensitive to a particular allergen. Blood tests can also help determine if a child has outgrown a food allergy.

Alport's syndrome   A genetic disease that causes kidney inflammation in childhood, followed by a sensorineural hearing loss in young adulthood, and eye problems later in life. It is more common among boys than girls. There is no clear relationship between the extent of kidney disease and the onset of deafness. Alport syndrome affects about one in 5,000 Americans, striking boys more often and more severely than girls. There are several varieties of the syndrome, some occurring in childhood and others not causing symptoms until men reach their 20s or 30s. All varieties of the syndrome are characterized by kidney disease that usually progresses to chronic kidney failure and by uremia (the presence of excessive amounts of urea and other waste products in the blood).

Cause

Most cases of Alport's syndrome are caused by a defect in one or more genes located on the X chromosome. The syndrome is usually inherited from the mother, who is a normal carrier. However, in up to 20 percent of cases there is no family history of the disorder. In these cases, Alport's appears to be caused by a spontaneous genetic mutation.

Symptoms

Blood in the urine (hematuria) is a hallmark of Alport syndrome. Other symptoms that may appear in varying combinations include protein in the urine, hearing loss, eye problems, skin prob-

lems, platelet disorders, abnormal white blood cells, or smooth muscle tumors.

Not all patients with Alport syndrome have hearing problems. In general, those with normal hearing have less severe cases of Alport syndrome.

Diagnosis

The syndrome is diagnosed with a medical evaluation and family history, together with a kidney biopsy that can detect changes in the kidney. Urinalysis may reveal blood or protein in the urine. Blood tests can reveal a low platelet level. Tests for the Alport gene are also available and may be covered by health insurance. DNA tests can diagnose affected children even before birth, and genetic linkage tests tracing all family members at risk for Alport syndrome are also available.

Treatment

There is no specific treatment that can cure Alport syndrome. Instead, care is aimed at easing the problems related to kidney failure, such as the presence of too many waste products in the blood. To control kidney inflammation, patients should:

- restrict fluids
- control high blood pressure
- manage pulmonary edema
- control high blood levels of potassium

Rarely, patients with Alport syndrome may develop nephrotic syndrome, a group of symptoms including too much protein in the urine, low albumin levels, and swelling. To ease these symptoms, patients should drink less, eat a salt-free diet, use diuretics, and have albumin transfusions.

Treatment

Treatment for Alport syndrome is supportive. Eventually, dialysis and kidney transplant may be necessary; the disease is not known to recur after transplantation. Glucocorticoids and cytotoxic agents are not effective.

AMBER Alert Plan   A voluntary partnership between law-enforcement agencies and broadcasters to disseminate an urgent bulletin in the most serious child-abduction cases. Law enforcement and broadcasters use the Emergency Alert System (EAS; formerly called the Emergency Broadcast System) to air a description of the missing child and suspected abductor. This is the same concept used during severe weather emergencies. The goal of the AMBER Alert is to promptly involve communities to assist in the search for and safe return of abducted children.

The AMBER Plan was created in 1996 as a legacy to nine-year-old Amber Hagerman, who was kidnapped and brutally murdered while riding a bicycle in Arlington, Texas. Outraged residents contacted radio stations in the Dallas area to suggest they broadcast special alerts to help prevent similar incidents in the future. In response to the community's concern for the safety of local children, the Dallas/Fort Worth Association of Radio Managers teamed up with local law-enforcement agencies in northern Texas and developed this innovative early-warning system to help find abducted children.

How It Works

Once law enforcement has been notified about an abducted child, it must first determine if the case meets the criteria for triggering an alert. Local and state programs establish specific criteria; however, the National Center for Missing and Exploited Children suggests that before an alert is activated, law-enforcement officers should confirm a child has been abducted and believe that the circumstances surrounding the abduction indicate that the child is in danger of serious bodily harm or death.

There should also be enough descriptive information about the child, abductor, and/or suspect's car so that an immediate broadcast alert will help.

If these criteria are met, alert information must be put together for public distribution. This information can include descriptions and pictures of the missing child, the suspected abductor, a suspected vehicle, and any other information available to identify the child and suspect. The information is then transmitted to area radio and television stations and cable systems via the EAS, and it is immediately broadcast by participating stations to listeners. Radio stations interrupt programming to announce the Alert, and television stations and

cable systems run a "crawl" on the screen in addition to a picture of the child.

The AMBER Alert system is currently operated in 46 states and has been responsible for the recovery of 121 children as of January 2004. While most communities and states have AMBER Alert plans, many do not have comprehensive, statewide coverage or the ability to communicate state-to-state, a critical need when an abducted child is taken across state lines.

Although the AMBER Alert plan has been extremely successful since its initiation, it has not yet been implemented on a national level. National AMBER Alert Network legislation would help with state-to-state notification by establishing an AMBER Alert Coordinator within the Department of Justice to help states with their AMBER Alert plans. AMBER Alerts would continue to be issued by local and state law-enforcement agencies, and the coordinator would be responsible for facilitating regional coordination of AMBER Alerts, particularly with interstate travel situations. The coordinator also would help states, broadcasters, and police set up more AMBER Alert plans and set minimum voluntary standards to help states coordinate when necessary. In addition, the bill will provide for a matching grant program through the Department of Transportation for highway signage, education and training programs, and equipment to facilitate AMBER Alert systems.

The AMBER Alert message encourages the public to look for a missing child or suspect. In the event a citizen spots a child, adult, or car fitting an AMBER Alert description, the person should immediately call the phone number given in the AMBER Alert and report as much information as possible.

American Academy of Child and Adolescent Psychiatry (AACAP) The leading national professional medical association dedicated to treating and improving the quality of life for children, adolescents, and families affected by mental, behavioral, or developmental disorders. The nonprofit AACAP was established in 1953, with more than 6,500 child and adolescent psychiatrists and other interested physicians. Its members actively research, evaluate, diagnose, and treat psychiatric disorders.

The AACAP widely distributes information in a effort to promote an understanding of mental illnesses, advance prevention efforts, and assure proper treatment and access to services for children and adolescents.

The academy provides public information, acts as a government liaison, promotes education, and gives expert testimony on issues affecting children. The academy also offers continuing medical education through scientific meetings and institutes and works with managed care organizations to establish appropriate coverage for children and adolescents. The group promotes research and training opportunities and reviews training curricula for child and adolescent psychiatry training programs. (For contact information, see Appendix I.)

American Academy of Pediatrics (AAP) A nonprofit professional organization of pediatricians who dedicate their efforts and resources to the health, safety, and well-being of infants, children, adolescents, and young adults. The AAP has approximately 55,000 members in the United States, Canada, and Latin America, including pediatricians, pediatric medical subspecialists, and pediatric surgical specialists. More than 34,000 members are board-certified and called Fellows of the American Academy of Pediatrics (FAAP).

The AAP was founded in June 1930 by 35 pediatricians who met in Detroit in response to the need for an independent pediatric forum to address children's needs. When the AAP was established, the idea that children have special developmental and health needs was unusual. Preventive health practices now associated with child care, such as immunizations and regular health exams, were only just beginning to change the custom of treating children as "miniature adults."

The American Academy of Pediatrics works to attain the best physical, mental, and social health and well-being for all infants, children, adolescents, and young adults. The AAP currently has 51 sections with more than 29,000 members interested in specialized areas of pediatrics. This includes a section for resident physicians with more than 9,000 members. Sections present educational programs for both their members and the general membership of the AAP in order to highlight current research and practical knowledge in their respective subspecialties.

The AAP publishes a monthly scientific journal *Pediatrics,* a continuing education journal called *Pediatrics in Review,* and its membership newspaper *AAP News.* The AAP also produces patient education brochures and a series of child care books written by AAP members. The AAP executes original research in social, economic, and behavioral areas and promotes funding of research. It maintains a Washington, D.C., office to ensure that children's health needs are taken into consideration as legislation and public policy are developed. (For contact information, see Appendix I.)

American Association on Mental Retardation (AAMR) Since 1876, AAMR has been providing leadership, information, services, support, and advocacy in the field of mental retardation. The oldest and largest international interdisciplinary organization of professionals concerned about mental retardation and related disabilities, the association has more than 9,500 members in the United States and 55 other countries. AAMR promotes progressive policies, sound research, effective practices, and universal human rights for people with intellectual disabilities. (For contact information, see Appendix I.)

American Cleft Palate-Craniofacial Association (ACPA) An international nonprofit association of more than 2,500 health care professionals in more than 40 countries who are involved in treatment and/or research of birth defects of the face, including cleft lip, cleft palate, and other facial problems. The association is a multidisciplinary organization representing more than 30 disciplines.

ACPA holds a general scientific meeting every year to exchange information and ideas about how to improve the care and treatment of patients with clefts and craniofacial anomalies. The bi-monthly *Cleft Palate-Craniofacial Journal* is an international publication reporting on clinical and research activities in cleft lip/palate research, together with research in related laboratory sciences. While ACPA's focus is on professional education, its affiliated CLEFT PALATE FOUNDATION (CPF) provides information to affected individuals and their families and seeks to educate the public about facial differences. The quarterly ACPA/CPF newsletter reports on business affairs, meeting highlights, and member news. (For contact information, see Appendix I.)

American Diabetes Association The nation's leading nonprofit health organization providing diabetes research, information, and advocacy. The mission of the organization is to prevent and cure diabetes and to improve the lives of all people affected by diabetes. To fulfill this mission, the American Diabetes Association (ADA) funds research, publishes scientific findings, provides information and other services to people with diabetes, their families, health care professionals, and the public. The association is also actively involved in advocating for scientific research and for the rights of people with diabetes.

Founded in 1940, the American Diabetes Association conducts programs in all 50 states and the District of Columbia, reaching more than 800 communities. (For contact information, see Appendix I.)

American Juvenile Arthritis Organization (AJAO) A special council of the ARTHRITIS FOUNDATION that helps to serve the special needs of children, teens, and young adults with childhood rheumatic diseases and their families. Its members are parents, family members, doctors, nurses, occupational and physical therapists, social workers, young adults, and anyone with an interest in arthritis in young people. The AJAO serves as an advocate for and works to improve the quality of life for children with rheumatic diseases and their families by working toward better medical care, stimulating research, and providing education and support.

The organization tries to increase awareness of childhood arthritis, promotes access to care by pediatric rheumatologists, develops education and support programs, advocates the needs of those affected by childhood arthritis, and encourages research and funding toward prevention, control, and cure.

AJAO serves as a clearinghouse of information for the public on topics from medications and educational rights to social services and legislative issues. The group sponsors national and regional conferences and publishes educational materials ranging from free brochures to inexpensive self-help manuals. AJAO monitors and promotes legislation that affects children with arthritis, sponsors special events, and promotes public and legislative awareness of this serious medical condition. (For contact information, see Arthritis Foundation in Appendix I.)

American Lyme Disease Foundation (ALDF) A national organization dedicated to the prevention, diagnosis, treatment, and control of LYME DISEASE and other tick-borne infections. The foundation supports critical scientific research and plays a key role in providing reliable and scientifically accurate information about tick-borne diseases.

The ALDF hosts national, regional, and local conferences to educate medical and public health professionals. The foundation also provides key information about the importance of prevention and early intervention in avoiding complicated, expensive, and potentially debilitating long-term illness. The foundation offers information, community presentations, a physician referral service, and a Hispanic education service.

In 2001 the foundation awarded three research grants focusing on tick biocontrol methods, tick population surveillance and testing, and ecology of tick-borne disease agents. These grants ranged from $12,500 to $25,000 and were renewed annually (depending on initial progress and available funds) for a total of three years. (For contact information, see Appendix I.)

American SIDS Institute A national, nonprofit health care organization founded in 1983 that is dedicated to preventing SUDDEN INFANT DEATH SYNDROME (SIDS) and promoting infant health through an aggressive, comprehensive nationwide program. The institute promotes research about the cause of SIDS and methods of prevention, offers clinical services to help pediatricians in the medical management of high risk infants, provides information about prevention methods aimed at the public and medical community, and offers family support providing crisis phone counseling, grief literature, and referrals. (For contact information, see Appendix I.)

American Sleep Apnea Association (ASAA) A nonprofit organization founded in 1990 by persons with APNEA and concerned health care providers and researchers. The ASAA is dedicated to reducing injury, disability, and death from sleep apnea and enhancing the well-being of patients.

The ASAA promotes education and awareness, research, and the A.W.A.K.E. network of voluntary mutual support groups. As part of its endeavors to increase understanding of sleep apnea, the ASAA fulfills thousands of requests for information from the public each year and answers a multitude of questions about diagnosis and treatment options. The ASAA also works with other nonprofit organizations and societies for health care professionals to reach the undiagnosed. In addition, the ASAA serves as an advocate for people with sleep apnea and helps them live with this disorder.

The A.W.A.K.E. Network plays a crucial role in the ASAA's educational and advocacy efforts. "A.W.A.K.E." is an acronym for "Alert, Well, And Keeping Energetic," characteristics that are uncommon in persons with untreated apnea. Founded in 1988 as a support group for people affected by sleep apnea, the A.W.A.K.E. network is now composed of about 200 groups in nearly all states. A.W.A.K.E. meetings are held regularly and guest speakers are often invited to address the group. Topics may include advice on complying with treatment, legal issues affecting those with sleep apnea, weight loss, treatment options such as oral appliances, and new research findings. The ASAA also publishes the *WAKE-UP CALL* newsletter, a video, and a brochure that defines the disease, describes its symptoms, and explains the consequences of untreated apnea, together with a simple self-diagnostic test, the ASAA Snore Score. (For contact information, see Appendix I.)

American Speech-Language-Hearing Association (ASHA) The professional, scientific, and credentialing association for more than 99,000 speech-language pathologists, audiologists, and speech, language, and hearing scientists in the United States. The organization provides information and referrals to the public on speech, language, communication, and hearing disorders. (For contact information, see Appendix I.)

Americans with Disabilities Act (ADA) The legislation enacted in July 1990 that prohibits discrimination against individuals with disabilities. It guarantees equal opportunity for people with disabilities in jobs, public accommodations, transportation, and telecommunications, as well as other state services.

The Americans with Disabilities Act (ADA) represents a significant addition to the scope of protections defined by the Civil Rights Act of 1964, which was not intended to protect the rights of individuals with disabilities. It also augments other laws that address issues of disability and access to education and employment opportunities, such as the Individuals with Disabilities Education Act (IDEA) and the Rehabilitation Act (RA) of 1973.

While the ADA covers many areas of possible discrimination (including schools), it is used primarily to protect individuals with disabilities on the job. The IDEA and RA offer more specific protections and regulations in regard to schools and colleges.

On the job, employers are required to provide fair opportunities to individuals with disabilities if they are "otherwise qualified" for a position. For example, a person who is partly blind cannot perform the essential functions of an airline pilot. A person in a wheelchair, however, may be able to perform the essential functions of a bookkeeper and therefore should not be discriminated against based on physical limitations.

Employers and schools may also be required to provide accessibility to buildings for those who have physical disabilities. Employers with more than 15 employees also may be required to provide accommodations for employees with specific needs based on their disability, such as equipment or more frequent breaks. "Disability" is an important term from a legal perspective, as it distinguishes those with temporary limitations or less severe limitations from those for whom a physical or mental impairment limits major life activities.

For people with LEARNING DISABILITY, the ADA provides legislative support for accommodations within both educational and workplace settings. Unlike the federal legislation governing public education for children with learning disabilities, the ADA places a much greater burden of responsibility on the person seeking services or accommodations.

The ADA also clearly protects educational institutions and employers from being required to provide accommodations that place unreasonable burdens or that represent significant lowering of educational standards. At the same time, the ADA also provides broad protection for children with learning disabilities in a wide variety of contexts.

aminoglycosides A family of ANTIBIOTIC DRUGS used to treat infection caused by gram-negative bacteria that includes gentamicin, amikacin, kanamycin, neomycin, streptomycin, and tobramycin. These drugs have a narrow margin of safety and may be toxic to the nerve involved in balance and hearing; they also can damage the kidneys.

Amoxil See AMOXICILLIN.

amoxicillin (Amoxil, Moxilin, Wymox) A semisynthetic antibiotic that is effective against a broad spectrum of bacteria. Amoxicillin is used to treat infections of the ear, nose and throat, genitourinary tract, skin, and lower respiratory tract. It is also used to treat gonorrhea, although it is not considered to be the standard treatment.

Side Effects
As with other penicillins, some children may be allergic to this medication. Hypersensitivity reactions are more likely to occur in children who have previously demonstrated hypersensitivity to penicillins and in those with a history of allergy, ASTHMA, HAY FEVER, or hives. Nausea and vomiting also are common side effects.

ampicillin (Amcill, Omnipen, Polycillin, Principen) A penicillin-type semisynthetic antibiotic used to treat conditions caused by a broad spectrum of gram-negative and gram-positive organisms in the urinary, respiratory, and intestinal tracts. Some of these conditions include cystitis, BRONCHITIS, GONORRHEA, and ear and eye infections. It is inactivated by penicillinase and therefore cannot be used against bacteria that produce this enzyme.

Side Effects
Ampicillin may cause nausea and vomiting, fever, or diarrhea. Allergic reactions may include symptoms of rash, diarrhea, and (rarely) fever; swelling of the mouth and tongue; itching; or breathing problems.

anaphylaxis A severe, life-threatening allergic reaction that occurs rarely in those who have an extreme sensitivity to a particular substance or allergen. The reaction, which often includes an itchy red rash or hives, is most common after an insect sting or as a reaction to a drug such as PENICILLIN. It also may occur as an allergic reaction to certain foods, such as tree nuts or peanuts. As the allergen enters the blood, it triggers the release of massive amounts of histamine and other chemicals that affect the body by expanding blood vessels and lowering blood pressure.

Treatment
Anaphylaxis is a medical emergency. An injection of epinephrine (Epipen) can save the child's life, but it must be given as soon as possible. A person who experiences anaphylaxis after a drug or a sting should lie down with legs raised, to improve blood flow to the heart and brain.

anencephaly A NEURAL TUBE DEFECT in which the brain does not fully develop (or in some cases, is totally absent). This birth defect occurs in three out of 10,000 births and is almost always fatal.

Angelman syndrome A childhood disorder characterized by HYPERACTIVITY, seizures, laughter, and developmental delays. Initially presumed to be rare, it is now believed that thousands of children with Angelman syndrome (AS) have gone undiagnosed, or been misdiagnosed with CEREBRAL PALSY, AUTISM, or other childhood disorders.

In 1965 English physician Harry Angelman, M.D., first described three children with characteristics now known as Angelman syndrome, including stiff, jerky gait; lack of speech; excessive laughter; and seizures. Other cases were eventually published, but the condition was considered to be extremely rare and many physicians doubted its existence. The first reports from North America appeared in the early 1980s, and since then many new reports have appeared.

In the United States and Canada today, there are about 1,000 diagnosed individuals, but the condition has been reported throughout the world among divergent racial groups. In North America, however, most cases seem to occur in Caucasian children.

Angelman syndrome is usually not recognized at birth or in infancy, since the developmental problems are hard to spot at that time. Parents may first suspect the diagnosis after reading about AS or meeting a child with the condition. The most common age of diagnosis is between age three and seven, when the characteristic behaviors and features become evident.

Symptoms

Hyperactivity and a short attention span are probably the most typical behaviors, which affect boys and girls about equally. Infants and toddlers may be continually active, constantly keeping their hands or toys in their mouth, moving from object to object. In extreme cases, the constant movement can cause accidental bruises. Older children may grab, pinch, and bite. A child's attention span can be so short that it interferes with social interaction, since the child cannot pay attention to facial and other social cues.

Laughter is also quite common, which seems to be a reaction to physical or mental stimuli. Although AS children experience a variety of emotions, continual happiness is most common. Parents may first notice this laughter at the age of one to three months. Giggling, chortling, and constant smiling soon develop and appear to represent normal reflexive laughter, but cooing and babbling are delayed.

Other symptoms include

- developmental delay
- severe speech impairment with almost no use of words
- movement or balance disorder
- easily excitable personality, often with hand-flapping movements
- abnormally small head
- seizures

Treatment

Persistent and consistent behavior modification helps decrease or eliminate unwanted behavior. In milder cases, attention may be sufficient enough to learn sign language and other communication techniques. For these children, educational and developmental training programs are much easier to structure and are generally more effective. Most children do not receive drug therapy for hyperactivity although some may benefit from use of medications such as methylphenidate (RITALIN).

Angelman Syndrome Foundation This foundation provides information on diagnosis, treatment, and management of ANGELMAN SYNDROME, and offers support and advocacy through education, information exchange, and research. The group also offers local contacts and a newsletter. (For contact information, see Appendix I.)

angioedema An allergic reaction closely related to ANAPHYLAXIS characterized by hives (large, well-defined swellings) that appear suddenly in the skin and larynx. The swellings may last several hours (or days, if untreated).

Cause

The most common cause is a sudden response to certain foods (such as strawberries, peanuts, tree nuts, eggs, or seafood); less often it occurs in response to a medication (especially PENICILLIN), insect stings, snake bite, infection, emotional stress, exposure to animals, molds, pollen, or cold.

Symptoms

Angioedema may cause sudden breathing problems, difficulty swallowing, and obvious swelling of the lips, face, and neck. The swelling it produces in the throat may lead to suffocation by blocking the child's airway.

Treatment

Severe cases respond to injections of epinephrine, but use of a breathing tube or even tracheostomy may be necessary to prevent suffocation. In less severe cases, antihistamine drugs often ease symptoms.

animal bites See BITES, ANIMAL.

anorexia nervosa A serious, potentially life-threatening EATING DISORDER characterized by self-starvation, food preoccupation and rituals, compulsive exercising, and often in girls an absence of menstrual cycles. A child with anorexia nervosa is hungry but denies the hunger because of an irrational fear of becoming fat.

Anorexia affects one in every 100 to 200 adolescent girls and a much smaller number of boys. Approximately one percent of all adolescent American girls develop the problem, usually at puberty, which can be fatal if untreated. One in 10 cases ends in death from starvation, cardiac arrest, or suicide. The most common cause of death in a chronic anorexic is low potassium levels in the blood, which can cause an irregular heartbeat.

Anorexia is diagnosed when a girl is at least 15 percent below her normal body weight. Food and weight become obsessions, and for some, the compulsiveness shows up in strange eating rituals or the refusal to eat in front of others. Some girls with anorexia obsess about food, collecting recipes and preparing lavish gourmet feasts for family and friends while refusing any food themselves. They may adhere to strict exercise routines to keep off weight.

Cause

Certain personality characteristics seem to be associated with anorexia, including a fear of losing control, inflexible thinking, perfectionism, dissatisfaction with body image, and an overwhelming desire to be thin. Anorexia also has been linked to obsessive-compulsive tendencies, such as a preoccupation with food.

Symptoms

Anorexia nervosa is not a "fad" that the child will outgrow if left alone. Together with its associated syndrome, BULIMIA, these eating disorders are extremely widespread and dangerous problems. The chief symptoms are self-induced starvation and/or binge eating and purging. For many, this is a compulsive addiction, like alcoholism. Thousands of cases report ill health, psychological impairments, shame, guilt, withdrawal, and isolation.

Warning signs include:

- deliberate self-starvation with weight loss
- intense, persistent fear of gaining weight

- refusal to eat, except tiny portions
- continuous dieting
- excessive facial/body hair because of inadequate protein in the diet
- compulsive exercise
- abnormal weight loss
- sensitivity to cold
- absent or irregular menstruation
- hair loss

Because anorexia is basically self-starvation, the body is denied the essential nutrients it needs to function normally. As a result, it is forced to slow down all of its processes to conserve energy. This "slowing down" can have serious medical consequences, including an abnormally slow heart rate and low blood pressure. The risk for heart failure rises as heart rate and blood pressure levels sink lower and lower. Thyroid function slows, menstrual periods stop, and even breathing slows down. Nails and hair become brittle, the skin dries and yellows. Girls may become very thirsty and urinate often, as dehydration contributes to constipation and reduced body fat leads to lowered body temperature.

Children with anorexia also can develop osteoporosis, muscle loss and weakness, severe dehydration leading to kidney failure, fainting, fatigue, and overall weakness, hair loss, and growth of a downy layer of hair called lanugo all over the body, including the face. As the girl's weight plummets, vital organs such as the brain and heart can be damaged.

Treatment

Fortunately, the above symptoms can be reversed once normal weight is reestablished. The first step in treating anorexia is to get the girl to put on weight; the greater the weight loss, the more likely she will need hospitalization.

Increasing awareness of the dangers of anorexia, backed by medical studies and extensive media coverage, has led many girls to seek help. Nevertheless, many girls with anorexia refuse to admit that there is a problem and reject treatment.

Friends, relatives, teachers, therapists, dietitians, peer support groups, and physicians all play an important role in helping a child with anorexia stick with a treatment program. Encouragement, caring, and persistence, as well as information about eating disorders and their dangers, may be needed to convince the child to get help, stick with treatment, or try again.

Outpatient programs have become common, including day programs requiring patients to stay eight hours a day, five days a week. Anorexic patients are given a carefully prescribed diet, starting with small meals and gradually increasing the caloric intake. A patient is given a goal weight range, and as she approaches her ideal weight, more independence in her eating habits is allowed. However, if she falls below the set range, greater supervision may be reinstated.

As she gains weight, she will usually begin individual and group therapy. Counseling typically involves education about body weight regulation and the effects of starvation, clarification of dietary misconceptions, and work on the issues of self-control and self-esteem. Length of treatment varies among different programs and ranges from short-term therapy of just 10 sessions to long-term psychotherapy lasting two or three years or more. Some researchers employ family therapy with a team approach. Others recommend two to three years of psychotherapy aimed at improving problems of low self-esteem, guilt, anxiety, depression, and helplessness. Family therapy (which may take about six months) focuses on changing the patterns of family interaction. Hypnosis is used by some therapists but may be resisted by many children with anorexia who fear the loss of self control. Some success is claimed by those teaching self-hypnosis and biofeedback techniques during three to six months of hospitalization.

Even after the eating disorder has been controlled, follow-up counseling for the child as well as her family may be recommended. While many girls can recover, relapse is common and may occur months or years after treatment has ended. Girls with anorexia tend to do better if they are younger when they become sick, or if they have more self-esteem or do not deny their condition as much.

anthrax   A potentially fatal bacterial infection that can cause either a skin or respiratory infection. In the past the bacteria affected primarily livestock, but in 2001 infection with anthrax spores was used as a potential terrorist weapon. During the autumn of 2001 numerous pieces of mail tainted with anthrax spores sickened and killed Americans on the east coast; one infant became infected with skin anthrax after visiting a New York City office contaminated by anthrax spores.

Cause

Anthrax is caused by the bacterium *Bacillus anthracis,* which produces spores that can remain dormant for years. When reactivated, anyone can contract the disease who breathes in the spores or who comes in contact with the spores on the skin.

Symptoms

The most common symptom of skin anthrax is a raised, itchy area at the site of entry, progressing to a large blister and then a black scab with swelling of surrounding tissue. Respiratory anthrax, which is a much more serious infection, begins with flu-like symptoms and can kill within days if untreated.

Diagnosis

Anthrax is diagnosed by isolating *B. anthracis* from the blood, skin lesions, or respiratory secretions, or by measuring specific antibodies in the blood.

Treatment

Prompt treatment with antibiotics such as ciprofloxin or penicillin can cure anthrax, although the death rate for inhaled anthrax is high even with treatment. Less is known about the prognosis in children.

Prevention

While the government does not provide anthrax vaccinations for civilians, it did offer vaccination for postal workers considered to be at high risk for infection due to the terrorist use of anthrax-contaminated mail.

Because anthrax is considered to be a risk of biological warfare, the Department of Defense systematically vaccinates all U.S. military personnel. The anthrax vaccine is reported to be 93 percent effective in protecting against anthrax and is given in three subcutaneous injections two weeks apart followed by three more injections given at six, 12, and 18 months. Annual booster injections of the vaccine are recommended thereafter.

About 30 percent of recipients experience mild local reactions and slight tenderness and redness at the injection site. Severe local reactions are infrequent and consist of extensive swelling of the forearm in addition to the local reaction. Systemic reactions occur in fewer than 0.2 percent of recipients.

antibacterial drugs A group of drugs used to treat infections caused by bacteria. These drugs share the same actions of antibiotic drugs, but (unlike the antibiotics) have always been produced synthetically. The largest group of antibacterial agents are the sulfonamides.

Antibacterial ointments contain combinations of the "nonabsorbable" antibiotics (bacitracin, neomycin, polymyxin B, and gramicidin). While these may help for mild skin wounds, more extensive bacterial skin infections require systemic antibiotics.

Bacitracin is effective against organisms including *Streptococcus, Staphylococcus,* and *Pneumococcus.* Neomycin is effective against most gram-negative organisms; it is about 50 times more active against *Staphylococcus* than bacitracin, but bacitracin is 20 times more active against *Streptococcus.* However, neomycin causes more allergic contact sensitivity than any other topical antibiotic.

Gentamicin is also effective against *Staphylococcus aureus* and group-A or group-B hemolytic streptococci. While it may be used topically, it is no better than other drugs mentioned above, and it may produce an allergic reaction.

antibiotic drugs A group of drugs used to treat infections caused by bacteria. Originally prepared from molds and fungi, antibiotic drugs are now made synthetically. Antibiotics help fight infection when the body has been invaded by harmful bacteria or when the bacteria present in the body begin to multiply uncontrollably. More than one kind of antibiotic may be prescribed to increase the efficiency of treatment and to reduce the risk of antibiotic resistance.

Some bacteria develop resistance to a once-useful antibiotic. Resistance is most likely to develop if a person fails to take an antibiotic as directed, during long-term treatment, or if the drugs are overprescribed by physicians. Some drugs, known as broad-spectrum antibiotics, are effective against a wide range of bacteria, while others are useful only in treating specific types.

Bacteria and other microorganisms that have developed resistance to antimicrobial drugs include:

- methicillin/oxacillin-resistant *Staphylococcus aureus*
- vancomycin-resistant enterococci
- extended-spectrum beta-lactamases (which are resistant to cephalosporins and monobactams)
- penicillin-resistant *Streptococcus pneumoniae*
- penicillin-resistant *Hemophilus influenzae*

Among the newest antibiotics in development are self-assembling antibiotics—small rings of amino acids that can assemble themselves into tubes that punch holes in bacteria. Other research is focusing on tiny viruses that target and infect bacteria, which could someday be the source of a new class of antibiotics. Some of these viruses, which are known as bacteriophages, produce a protein that wreaks havoc with a bacterium's ability to construct its cell wall. The viruses infect a bacterium, replicate and fill the bacterial cell with new copies of the virus, and then break through the bacterium's cell wall, causing it to burst.

Side Effects

Because these agents may kill "normal" bacteria naturally present in the body, fungi may grow in their place, causing oral, intestinal, or vaginal candidiasis (thrush). Some patients sometimes experience a severe allergic response, causing facial swelling, itching, or breathing problems.

Types

Some of the most well-known antibiotics include the penicillins (amoxicillin, penicillin V, and oxacillin), the aminoglycosides (gentamicin and streptomycin), the cephalosporins (cefaclor and cephalexin), the tetracyclines (doxycycline and oxytetracycline), erythromycin, and neomycin.

anticonvulsant drugs Medications that have been used for many years to treat seizure disorders.

More recently these medications have also been used to treat mood and psychiatric disorders, including acute manic, impulse control disorders, and aggressive behavior.

Anticonvulsants include carbamazepine (Tegretol), phenobarbital, phenytoin (Dilantin), primidone (Mysoline), valproic acid (Depakene), sodium valproate (Depakene syrup), valproic acid (Depakene), divalproex sodium valproic acid and sodium valproate (Depakote), gabapentin (Neurontin), and lamotrigine (Lamictal).

Side Effects

Common side effects include sleepiness, dizziness, tremor, and minor stomach symptoms such as decrease or increase in appetite, nausea, vomiting, and diarrhea. Taking an anticonvulsant with meals can lessen the side effects. Valproate may may induce weight gain and hair loss. Rarely, but most seriously, life-threatening side effects may occur, including a decrease in blood cell production (carbamazepine, valproate) causing unusual bruising or bleeding, or infections with fever and sore throat and severe skin rash (carbamazepine, lamotrigine), and liver damage, unusual tiredness, weakness, and abdominal pain.

Several of these medications (carbamazepine, valproate) require periodic blood tests to determine the level of the drug in the blood and to monitor its effects, if any, on the liver and blood cells.

antidepressants Medications that alleviate the symptoms of DEPRESSION. There are many different types of antidepressant drugs that are very effective in treating depression in children, especially when combined with psychotherapy. Up to one and a half million children and adolescents suffer from depression in the United States, and the number of prescriptions for popular drugs such as Prozac is rising each year.

Antidepressants appear to work by correcting a chemical imbalance or dysfunction in the brains of depressed patients. An antidepressant boosts the level of brain chemicals called neurotransmitters that are important in alleviating depression—especially serotonin, dopamine, and norepinephrine.

Each of the major classes of antidepressants— selective serotonin reuptake inhibitors (SSRIs), structurally unrelated antidepressants, cyclics, and monoamine oxidase inhibitors—affects different groups of neurotransmitters in a different way. The SSRIs and the structurally unrelated drugs are the newest class of antidepressants and include Prozac, Zoloft, Celexa, Luvox, and Paxil. The SSRIs primarily affect serotonin and have been found to be effective in treating depression and anxiety without as many side effects as some older antidepressants.

Approval of a medication by the Federal Drug Administration (FDA) means that adequate data have been provided by the drug manufacturer to show safety and efficacy for a particular therapy in a particular population. Based on the data, a label indication for the drug is established that includes proper dosage, potential side effects, and approved age.

Although in some cases there is extensive clinical experience in using medications for children or adolescents, in many cases there is not. Everyone agrees that more studies in children are needed to better understand appropriate dosages, how a drug works in children, and what effects the drugs may have on learning and development. Despite the effectiveness of antidepressants in children, some experts are worried that not enough studies have been done investigating the safety of these drugs in very young children. In particular, there is some concern about a possible increase in suicide attempts in some children taking some antidepressants.

As a result, federal regulators are taking the first steps in requiring drug companies to test popular antidepressant drugs for their long-term effects on children. Short-term studies of Prozac and Paxil have indicated that they are safe and effective in children, but more studies need to be done with other drugs as well.

Many medications have not been officially approved by the FDA for use in children, but they can still legally be prescribed for children as an "off label" use. In the past medications were not studied in children because of ethical concerns about involving children in clinical trials. However, this meant that there was a lack of knowledge about the best treatments for children. In clinical settings where children are suffering from mental or

behavioral disorders, medications are being prescribed at earlier and earlier ages. The FDA has
been urging that products be appropriately studied
in children and has offered incentives to drug manufacturers to carry out such testing.

Following is a list of antidepressants and the
FDA-approved age at which they can be safely
prescribed.

Brand Name	Generic Name	Approved Age
Anafranil	clomipramine	10 and older (for OCD*)
BuSpar	buspirone	18 and older
Effexor	venlafaxine	18 and older
Luvox (SSRI)	fluvoxamine	8 and older (for OCD)
Paxil (SSRI)	paroxetine	18 and older
Prozac (SSRI)	fluoxetine	18 and older
Sinequan	doxepin	12 and older
Tofranil	imipramine	6 and older (for bed-wetting)
Wellbutrin	bupropion	18 and older
Zoloft (SSRI)	sertraline	6 and older (for OCD)

*obsessive-compulsive disorder

antidiarrheal drugs Medications that treat diarrhea. The drug loperamide (Imodium A-D) slows
the passage of stools through the intestines. Adsor-
bents such as attapulgite (Kaopectate) pull diarrhea-causing substances from the digestive tract.
Bismuth subsalicylate (Pepto-Bismol) decreases
the secretion of fluid into the intestine and inhibits
the activity of bacteria. It not only controls diarrhea but also relieves the cramps that often accompany diarrhea.

Patients should not use antidiarrheal drugs for
more than two days unless told to do so by a doctor.

Bismuth subsalicylate may cause the tongue or
the stool to temporarily darken harmlessly. Children with flu or CHICKEN POX should not be given
bismuth subsalicylate because it can lead to REYE'S
SYNDROME, a life-threatening condition that affects
the liver and central nervous system. Children may
have unpredictable reactions to other antidiarrheal
drugs; loperamide should not be given to children
under six, and attapulgite should not be given to

children under three years, unless directed by a
physician.

Children with a history of liver disease or who
have been taking antibiotics should check with a
doctor before taking the antidiarrheal drug loperamide. Loperamide should not be used by people
whose diarrhea is caused by certain infections,
such as salmonella or shigella.

Side Effects

The most common side effects of attapulgite are
constipation, bloating, and fullness. Bismuth subsalicylate may cause ringing in the ears, but that
side effect is rare. Possible side effects from loperamide include skin rash, constipation, drowsiness, dizziness, tiredness, dry mouth, nausea,
vomiting, and swelling, pain, and discomfort in the
abdomen. Some of these symptoms are the same as
those that occur with diarrhea, so it may be difficult to tell if the medicine is causing the problems.
Children may be more sensitive than adults to certain side effects of loperamide, such as drowsiness
and dizziness. Other rare side effects may occur
with any antidiarrheal medicine.

antifungal/antiyeast agents A group of drugs
prescribed to treat infections caused by either fungi
or yeasts (and sometimes both in one product) that
can be administered directly to the skin or taken
orally or by injection. They are commonly used to
treat different types of TINEA, including ATHLETE'S
FOOT, JOCK ITCH, and scalp ringworm. They are also
used to treat THRUSH and rare fungal infections
such as cryptococcus.

Side Effects

Agents applied to the skin, scalp, mouth, or vagina
may sometimes increase irritation, and antifungal
agents given by mouth or injection may cause more
serious side effects, damaging the kidney or liver.

Types

Antifungal agents are available as creams, injections, tablets, lozenges, suspensions, and vaginal
suppositories. The most common antifungals
include amphotericin B, cyclopirox, clotrimazole,
econozole, griseofulvin (by mouth only), itraconazole (by mouth and IV only), fluconazole (by
mouth and IV only), ketoconazole, miconazole,

and tolnaftate. While amphotericin B is the standard drug for treating fungal infections, it is usually given in the hospital because of the danger of side effects. On the other hand, itraconazole and fluconazole are the two most recently approved drugs to enter the antifungal arsenal. These two cause fewer side effects and can be taken orally on an outpatient basis.

Nonprescription creams such as Monistat 7 and Gyne-Lotrimin may be helpful in remedying candidal vaginal yeast infections, but fatal candidal infections affecting the brain, kidney, or other organs may occur in immuno-compromised patients in the hospital.

Antiyeast agents such as Nystatin do not kill most fungi, but most antifungals kill yeasts as well—except for griseofulvin. Drugs that are used for both systemic fungal and yeast infections include fluconazole, ketoconazole, amphotericin B, and itraconazole.

Most yeast infections are superficial. Systemic, life-threatening yeast infections do NOT occur in normal individuals.

antihelminthics A group of drugs used to treat worm infestations. Because the body's immune system does not fight worms well, persistent infestations are not uncommon. The antihelminthic drugs eliminate the worms from the body, preventing the complications that occur in untreated individuals.

Different types of antihelminthic drugs are used to treat infestation by different types of worms; they include niclosamide, niridazole, piperazine, praziquantel, and thiabendazole.

The drugs work by either killing or paralyzing the worms so that they cannot grip onto the intestinal walls. They are then moved out of the body in the feces. To speed up this process, laxatives may be used at the same time. In other tissues, antihelminthics kill worms by boosting their vulnerability to the immune system; once these worms have died, they may need to be surgically removed along with any cysts that they have caused.

Side Effects

Potential adverse effects include nausea and vomiting, stomach pain, headache, dizziness, and rash.

antihistamines A family of drugs used to treat allergic conditions, such as itching and hives. The drugs work by blocking the action of histamine, a chemical that is released during an allergic reaction. Examples of antihistamines include diphenhydramine, promethazine, terfenadine, and chlorpheniramine.

Without treatment, histamine dilates small blood vessels, causing redness and swelling; antihistamines block this effect, while preventing the irritation of nerve fibers that would otherwise cause itching. Antihistamines are the most effective treatment for hives.

Side Effects

Some antihistamines cause drowsiness and dizziness, but new versions (such as Claritin and Clarinex) do not reach the brain and thus do not cause these side effects. Other possible side effects common to most antihistamines include appetite loss, nausea, dry mouth, blurry vision, and urination problems.

anti-inflammatory drugs A family of drugs used to help decrease inflammation and pain without affecting the cause of the inflammation. This class of drugs includes ANTIHISTAMINES, NONSTEROIDAL ANTI-INFLAMMATORY DRUGS (NSAIDs) such as IBUPROFEN (Motrin, Advil), and corticosteroids.

antimalarial drugs Medications that can prevent MALARIA; they should be taken by anyone traveling to another part of the world where malaria is endemic. Travelers to malaria-risk areas in South America, Africa, the Indian subcontinent, Asia, and the South Pacific should take one of the following drugs: mefloquine (Lariam), doxycycline, or Malarone.

Antimalarials, which should be obtained before leaving the United States, should be taken exactly on schedule without missing doses. Because overdosage of antimalarials can be fatal, these drugs should be kept in childproof containers out of the reach of children.

Mefloquine

The first dose of Mefloquine should be taken one week before arrival in the malaria-risk area. It should then be taken once a week, on the same day of the week, while in the malaria-risk area, and then once a week for four weeks after leaving the malaria-risk area.

Mefloquine rarely causes any side effects. The most commonly reported minor side effects include nausea, dizziness, difficulty sleeping, and vivid dreams. Mefloquine has very rarely been reported to cause serious side effects, such as seizures, hallucinations, and severe anxiety. Minor side effects usually do not require stopping the drug. Travelers who have serious side effects should see a health care provider.

Travelers should not take mefloquine if they have seizure disorders such as epilepsy, a history of severe mental illness or other psychiatric disorders, or have been diagnosed or treated for an irregular heartbeat.

Travelers to the borders of Thailand with Burma (Myanmar) and Cambodia, the western provinces of Cambodia, and in the eastern states of Burma (Myanmar) should be aware that mefloquine resistance has been reported in these areas and either doxycycline or Malarone would be the recommended antimalarial drug.

Doxycycline

Doxycycline should not be given to children under the age of eight, because it may permanently stain the teeth. The first dose of doxycycline should be taken one or two days before arrival in the malaria-risk area. It should then be taken once a day, at the same time each day, while in the malaria-risk area, and then once a day for four weeks after leaving the malaria-risk area.

Taking doxycycline may cause travelers to sunburn faster than normal. The drug should be taken on a full stomach to lessen nausea; travelers should not lie down for one hour after taking the drug to prevent the drug from backing up into the esophagus.

Malarone

This new antimalarial drug is a combination of two drugs (atovaquone and proguanil) and is an effective alternative for travelers who cannot or choose not to take mefloquine or doxycycline. Infants weighing less than 24 pounds should not be given Malarone.

The first dose of Malarone should be taken one to two days before travel to the malaria-risk area. It should then be taken once a day while in the malaria-risk area, and once a day for seven days after leaving the malaria-risk area. Each dose should be taken at the same time each day with food or milk.

Although side effects are rare, abdominal pain, nausea, vomiting, and headache can occur. Malarone should not be taken by patients with severe kidney problems.

Chloroquine (Aralen)

Travelers to malaria-risk areas in Mexico, Haiti, the Dominican Republic, and certain countries in Central America, the Middle East, and Eastern Europe should take chloroquine or hydroxychloroquine sulfate as their antimalarial drug. The first dose of chloroquine should be taken one week before arrival in the malaria-risk area. It should then be taken once a week, on the same day of the week, while in the malaria-risk area, and once a week for four weeks after leaving the malaria-risk area.

Chloroquine should be taken on a full stomach to minimize nausea. Although side effects are rare, nausea and vomiting, headache, dizziness, blurred vision, and itching can occur. Chloroquine may worsen the symptoms of PSORIASIS.

Hydroxychloroquine Sulfate (Plaquenil)

Travelers to malaria-risk areas in Mexico, Haiti, the Dominican Republic, and certain countries in Central America, the Middle East, and Eastern Europe should take hydroxychloroquine sulfate or chloroquine as their antimalarial drug.

The first dose of hydroxychloroquine sulfate should be taken one week before arrival in the malaria-risk area. It should then be taken once a week, on the same day of the week, while in the malaria-risk area, and once a week for four weeks after leaving the malaria-risk area.

Hydroxychloroquine sulfate should be taken on a full stomach, for example, after dinner, to minimize nausea. While hydroxychloroquine sulfate may be better tolerated than chloroquine, rare side effects may include nausea and vomiting, headache, dizziness, blurred vision, and itching. Hydroxychloroquine sulfate may worsen the symptoms of psoriasis.

antimicrobial drugs Drugs that destroy or inhibit the growth of microorganisms.

antipsychotic drugs Medications used to treat psychosis. Standard antipsychotic drugs appear to be effective for children and adolescents with SCHIZOPHRENIA. Clozapine is helpful for at least half of those who do not respond to typical drugs. In a few cases psychotic symptoms seem to disappear entirely. Unfortunately, children may be more susceptible than adults to the toxic effects of clozapine; about one-third of them have to stop taking it because of the side effects. Newer antipsychotic drugs that may be safer and just as effective are now being tested.

antipyretic drugs A type of medication designed to lower fever by reducing the body temperature. Most popular types of antipyretics include ACETAMINOPHEN, ASPIRIN, and other NONSTEROIDAL ANTI-INFLAMMATORY DRUGS (NSAIDS), such as IBUPROFEN.

antiseptic A germicide used for human skin or tissue (not inanimate objects) that inhibits the growth and reproduction of microorganisms. It will weaken microbes but does not usually kill them. Health-care antiseptics in soaps or other products help prevent the spread of infection in medical facilities. Antiseptics include alcohol (ethanol or isopropanol), iodine (iodophor), povidone-iodine (Betadine), hydrogen peroxide, chlorhexidine, or hexachlorophene (Phisohex).

Over-the-counter antiseptics applied to the skin can help prevent infection in minor cuts, scrapes, or BURNS. Antiseptics can be kept in the first aid kit to pour on an animal bite, after cleaning it with soap and water, or to apply to a dirty cut after washing it out with soap and water. Normal cuts and scratches do not require antiseptics.

However, if an injury is extensive, it should be treated by a doctor. Antiseptics should not be used for cuts that are deep, that keep bleeding, or that require stitches. In addition, antiseptics should not be used for scrapes with imbedded particles that cannot be flushed away, large wounds, or serious burns. Over-the-counter antiseptics should not be used for more than one week on an injury; if the

wound does not heal or worsens, the child should be taken for medical care.

Experts advise against using hydrogen peroxide as an antiseptic, since it does not kill bacteria and interferes with capillary blood flow and wound healing. Other experts note that ethyl alcohol is not a good wound antiseptic because it irritates already-damaged tissue and causes a scab to form that may protect bacteria.

The U.S. Food and Drug Administration (FDA) advisory review panel has found some antiseptics that are not generally recognized as safe and effective. These products include mercury, cloflucarban, fluorosalan, and tribromsalan.

antiserum A preparation containing antibodies that combine with specific foreign proteins (antigens)—usually components of microorganisms such as viruses or bacteria. Antiserum is usually used (together with immunization) as an emergency treatment when someone has been exposed to a dangerous infection but has not previously been immunized against it.

Antiserum is prepared from the blood of animals or humans who have already been immunized against the organism.

The antiserum helps to provide some immediate protection against the microorganisms, while full immunity develops. However, these measures are not as effective in preventing disease as is immunization before exposure.

antitoxin An antibody produced by the body to fight off a toxin formed by invading bacteria or a biological poison such as BOTULISM. Antitoxins are also produced commercially to contain an antibody that can combine and neutralize the effect of a specific toxin released into the blood by bacteria (such as those that cause TETANUS or DIPHTHERIA). Antivenin is a type of antitoxin specifically made to combat snakebite poison. Antivenins are specific for each poisonous snake.

Antitoxins are prepared by injecting animals (usually horses) with specific toxins that provoke the animal's immune system into producing antibodies that neutralize the toxin. Then extracts are taken of the animal's blood to be used as antitoxins.

When used in treatment, antitoxins are usually injected into the muscle of the patient. Occasionally, the antitoxin may cause an allergic reaction or (even more rarely) anaphylactic shock.

antitussive drugs A type of medication used to suppress coughing, possibly by reducing the activity of the child's cough center in the brain or by depressing breathing. These drugs include both narcotics and nonnarcotics that act on the central and peripheral nervous systems to suppress the cough reflex. Because the cough reflex is important in clearing secretions from the upper respiratory tract, antitussives should not be used with a cough that produces mucus.

Codeine and hydrocodone are strong narcotic antitussives. Dextromethorphan is equally effective but does not carry the danger of inducing dependence as the narcotics do.

Antitussives are given by mouth (usually in a syrup with an expectorant and some alcohol). The medications also may be given as a capsule combined with an antihistamine and a mild painkiller.

antiviral drugs A group of drugs used to treat viral infections that include ACYCLOVIR, famcyclovir, VALACYCLOVIR, and AZT (zidouvine, prescribed for the treatment of AIDS). Until the development of these drugs, no effective way to treat viruses existed.

To this point no drugs have been developed that eradicate viruses and cure the illnesses they cause. This is because viruses live only within cells; a drug capable of killing a virus would also kill its host cell. New antiviral agents interfere with viral replication or otherwise disrupt chemical processes of viral metabolism; some prevent viruses from penetrating cells. They are effective treatments for a variety of infections.

Relatively newly developed antivirals including acyclovir and famcyclovir are especially effective in treating HERPES family (HSV) infections. Antiviral drugs reduce the severity of the herpes symptoms and may shorten the course of the infection, but the drugs cannot eliminate the virus completely. Recently scientists have been testing several varieties of a vaccine that appears to lessen the severity of herpes attacks. The vaccine is a combination of alum and a genetically engineered protein, glycoprotein D (gD2) that sits on the outer surface of the herpesvirus and is targeted by the body's immune cells.

AZT, a drug used in the treatment of AIDS, works by interrupting the replication cycle of the HIV virus and has demonstrated effectiveness in delaying the progression of HIV infection.

Side Effects

Most antiviral drugs have few side effects, although the creams and ointments may irritate skin. Oral antiviral drugs can cause nausea and dizziness. Acyclovir, if not given with significant fluids, can crystalize in the kidneys, causing kidney damage.

anxiety A feeling of apprehension, fear, or worry not connected to a specific threat. Many experts believe that anxiety is a learned response to stress. For example, a child who has been stung by a bee will run away crying on the next appearance of a flying buzzing insect. Should the avoidance continue to be reinforced, the anxiety will continue and may develop into a PHOBIA.

Cognitive psychologists believe that anxiety is the result of inappropriate thoughts. For someone who has an irrational fear of snakes, a picture of a snake can cause anxiety even though it is not possible to be hurt by a two-dimensional picture.

Children with LEARNING DISABILITIES may often have accompanying problems with anxiety, especially in connection to school work. Reading aloud, taking timed tests, or trying to start a writing assignment all may trigger anxiety and cause even further problems with the required task. Someone experiencing a high level of anxiety may "freeze up" and find it impossible to perform at all, or may show signs of restlessness and agitation, leading to erratic and inconsistent performance.

There is also a significant link between attention deficits and anxiety. To some degree, it can be hard to tell the difference between the two. An inability to focus and sustain attention may often lead to anxiety, and anxiety itself can make it very difficult for a child to pay attention to a task. In some cases, attention deficit disorders coexist with anxiety disorders.

It is also possible for someone with an anxiety disorder to be misdiagnosed with attention deficit hyperactivity disorder (ADHD). In evaluating ADHD, a differential diagnosis for anxiety may be important. It is equally important that those who work with individuals with ADHD take into account the possibility that anxiety may underlie some expressions of learning, communication, and social difficulties. (See also ANXIETY DISORDERS.)

anxiety disorders   Mental health disorders characterized by persistent worry. Anxiety disorders are the most common type of mental health disorder in children, affecting as many as 10 percent of young people. Studies suggest that children or adolescents are more likely to have an anxiety disorder if their parents have the same condition.

All children experience ANXIETY occasionally; for example, from about eight months of age through the preschool years, healthy youngsters may show intense anxiety when separated from their parents. Young children may have short-lived fears of the dark, storms, animals, or strangers.

Anxiety becomes a problem when it interrupts a child's normal activities, such as separating from parents, attending school, and making friends. Parents should consider seeking the evaluation and advice of a child and adolescent psychiatrist.

Symptoms

Anxious children are often overly tense. Some may seek a lot of reassurance, and their worries may interfere with activities. Because anxious children may also be quiet, compliant, and eager to please, their problems may be overlooked. Parents should be alert to the signs of severe anxiety so they can intervene early to prevent complications.

There are several types of anxiety disorders that affect children, including generalized anxiety disorder, SEPARATION ANXIETY DISORDER, SOCIAL PHOBIA, OBSESSIVE-COMPULSIVE DISORDER, and POST-TRAUMATIC STRESS DISORDER.

Generalized Anxiety Disorder

Children with generalized anxiety disorder have recurring fears and worries that they find difficult to control. They worry unnecessarily about almost everything—school, sports, being on time, even

natural disasters. They may be restless, irritable, tense, or easily tired, and they may have trouble concentrating or sleeping. Children with generalized anxiety disorder usually are very eager to please others and may be "perfectionists," dissatisfied with their own less-than-perfect performance.

Separation Anxiety Disorder

Children with separation anxiety disorder have intense anxiety about being away from home or caregivers to the point where social or school functioning is affected. Such children have a great need to stay at home or close to their parents. When they are apart, these children may worry excessively about their parents, and when they are together, the children may cling to parents, refuse to go to school, or be afraid to go to sleep. Repeated nightmares about separation and physical symptoms such as stomachaches and headaches are also common.

Social Phobia

Social phobia usually emerges in the mid-teens and typically does not affect young children. Children and adolescents with this disorder have a constant fear of social or performance situations, like speaking in class or eating in public. They are always afraid of being embarrassed in these situations. This fear is often accompanied by physical symptoms, such as sweating, blushing, heart palpitations, shortness of breath, or muscle tenseness.

Young people with this disorder typically respond to these feelings by avoiding the frightening situation, such as staying home from school or not going to parties.

Young people with social phobia are often overly sensitive to criticism, have trouble being assertive, and have low self-esteem. Social phobia may be limited to certain situations so that the adolescent may experience a sense of dread in relation to dating or recreational events but may be confident in school and work situations.

Obsessive-Compulsive Disorder

Children with obsessive-compulsive disorder have frequent and uncontrollable thoughts ("obsessions") and/or perform routines or rituals ("compulsions"), usually to get rid of the thoughts. This disorder often involves repeating behaviors to avoid some imagined consequence, so that a child might constantly wash hands because of a fear of germs. Other common compulsions include: counting, repeating words silently, and rechecking completed tasks. The obsessions and/or compulsions may take up a lot of time and cause a child much anxiety. Typically, this disorder begins in adolescence.

Post-Traumatic Stress Disorder

Children who experience a physical or emotional trauma, such as witnessing a shooting, surviving physical or sexual abuse, or being in a car accident, may develop post-traumatic stress disorder (PTSD). Children are more easily traumatized than adults: An event that may not be traumatic to an adult might be to a child, such as a turbulent plane ride. As a result of the trauma, a child may "reexperience" the event through nightmares, constant thoughts about what happened, or by reenacting the event while playing. A child with PTSD will experience symptoms of general anxiety, including trouble sleeping and eating or being irritable. Many children may exhibit other physical symptoms as well, such as being easily startled.

Treatment

Anxiety disorders are treatable, especially with early diagnosis. Effective treatment for anxiety disorders may include some form of psychotherapy, behavioral therapy, or medications. Children who exhibit persistent symptoms of an anxiety disorder should be referred to and evaluated by a mental health professional who specializes in treating children. The evaluation may include psychological testing and consultation with other specialists. A comprehensive treatment plan should be developed with the family, and whenever possible, the child should be involved in making treatment decisions.

Apgar score   A test devised in 1952 by the late pediatrician Virginia Apgar to quickly assess the clinical status of a newborn infant. Newborns are rated at one minute, five minutes, and 10 minutes after delivery on five qualities:

- Appearance (color)
- Pulse (heartbeat)
- Grimace (reflex)
- Activity (muscle tone)
- Respiration (breathing).

A score is determined by awarding zero, one, or two points in each category. The higher the score, the better the baby's condition—scores of seven and over indicate the baby is in good condition.

Although the APGAR test is medically useful, it does have its limits. While the score should improve from one test to the next, in most cases long-term behavior of the baby should not be predicted based upon the APGAR score. While the score is a good quick way to assess a newborn's health, parents should not put too much emphasis on the score as a predictor of the baby's future intellect or performance.

aplasia cutis   The absence of small areas of skin that may occur any time from before birth to early childhood. These localized birth defects are usually found on the back of the scalp, although they may occur anywhere on the body. At birth, the affected area may be covered by a tough, smooth membrane or it may be raw and crusted.

Symptoms

On the scalp, the areas tend to be hairless with sharp margins that heal slowly, eventually to be replaced by a flat scar. Occasionally there may be an infection, hemorrhage, or an underlying defect in the bone that will heal on its own during the baby's first two years of life.

Cause

The defect may be inherited, but it usually appears spontaneously. It is sometimes seen with syndromes such as the chromosome disorder trisomy 13.

Treatment

There is no known treatment other than to cut out the hairless area or, better still, to transplant normal skin and hair follicles.

apnea   Brief pauses in the breathing pattern during sleep. Usually these brief breathing pauses are normal, but it can become a problem when breathing stops for more than 20 seconds. The word *apnea* comes from the Greek word meaning "without wind." There are three types of apnea: obstructive, central, and mixed. In addition apnea of prematurity can be either obstructive, central, or mixed. Apnea of infancy is a type of persistent apnea of unknown origin.

Obstructive Apnea

An obstruction of the airway (such as enlarged tonsils and adenoids) may affect up to three percent of otherwise healthy preschoolers. This is a common type of apnea in children, especially in those who are obese.

Symptoms Snoring is the most common symptom; other signs include color changes, labored breathing or gasping for air during sleep or sleeping in unusual positions. Because obstructive sleep apnea may disturb sleep patterns, these children may wake up sleepy and continue to complain of fatigue and attention problems throughout the day that may affect school performance. One recent study suggests that some children diagnosed with attention deficit hyperactivity disorder (ADHD) actually have attention problems in school because of disrupted sleep patterns caused by obstructive sleep apnea.

Treatment Obstructive apnea can be cured by keeping the child's throat open to improve airflow. This may be done by surgically removing the tonsils and adenoids, or by providing continuous positive airway pressure (CPAP). CPAP is provided by having the child wear a nose mask while sleeping.

Central Apnea

This type of apnea occurs when the part of the brain that controls breathing does not properly start or maintain the breathing process. It is the least common form of apnea, although it is fairly common in very premature infants with an immature respiratory center in the brain. Often there is a neurological cause. A few short central apneas are normal, particularly after a deep breath.

Mixed Apnea

As its name implies, this is a combination of central and obstructive apnea commonly observed in infants or young children who have abnormal control of breathing. Mixed apnea may occur when a child is awake or asleep.

Apnea of Prematurity (AOP)

Premature infants may have an immature brain or respiratory system and may not be able to regulate breathing normally. Apnea of prematurity (AOP) can be obstructive, central, or mixed.

Treatment The condition can be improved by keeping the infant's head and neck straight, giving drugs such as aminophylline, caffeine, or doxapram to stimulate the respiratory system, and providing CPAP to keep the airway open with the help of forced air through a nose mask.

Apnea of Infancy (AOI)

Persistent apnea of unknown origin is called apnea of infancy, and occurs in children younger than age one who were born after a full-term pregnancy. Infants with this condition can be observed at home with a special monitor prescribed by a sleep specialist that records chest movements and heart rate, relaying readings to a hospital apnea program for future examination. The apnea usually goes away on its own; if it does not cause any problems (such as low blood oxygen), it may be considered part of the child's normal breathing pattern.

Apparent Life-Threatening Events

In addition to the above types of apnea, the cessation of breathing also can occur in connection with Apparent Life-Threatening Events (ALTEs). An ALTE itself is not a sleep disorder but an event that is a combination of apnea, change in color, change in muscle tone, choking, or gagging. Most ALTEs can be frightening to see, but they usually are uncomplicated and do not recur. However, some ALTEs (especially in young infants) are associated with medical conditions such as gastroesophageal reflux (GERD), infections, or neurological disorders. These medical conditions require treatment, so all children who experience an ALTE should be seen by a doctor immediately.

appendicitis Infection of the appendix, a small piece of tissue that connects to the beginning of the large intestine, usually at the lower right side of the abdomen. Appendicitis is the most common reason for a child to need emergency abdominal surgery. Young people between the ages of 11 and 20 are most often affected, and most cases of appendicitis occur in the winter between October and May. A family history of appendicitis may increase a child's risk for the illness, especially in boys. Having CYSTIC FIBROSIS also increases a child's risk for appendicitis.

Cause

The inside of the appendix usually opens into the large intestine. When the inside of the appendix is blocked by a piece of stool or something that a child swallowed, the appendix becomes swollen and easily infected by bacteria. If the infected appendix is not removed, an abscess may form and eventually burst or perforate. This may happen as soon as 48 to 72 hours after symptoms begin.

Symptoms

In older children, the classic symptoms of appendicitis are abdominal pain, fever, and vomiting. Abdominal pain usually begins in the center of the abdomen near the navel; often the pain then moves down and to the right, roughly where the appendix is located in the lower right part of the abdomen. After the abdominal pain begins, children with appendicitis usually develop a slight fever, lose their appetite, and may vomit. The fact that abdominal pain begins before nausea and vomiting instead of after is one clue to suspect appendicitis rather than an intestinal infection.

Other symptoms that may be seen in older children with appendicitis include diarrhea (small stools with mucus), urinating often or having an uncomfortably strong urge to urinate, constipation, and sometimes breathing problems.

In children younger than age two, the most common symptoms are vomiting and a bloated or swollen abdomen. There may be abdominal pain, but children may be too young to describe this pain. Because appendicitis is rare in infants, and their symptoms are not "classic," the diagnosis of appendicitis is often delayed.

Diagnosis

Correctly diagnosing appendicitis can be difficult, since symptoms may mimic many other more common conditions, such as gastrointestinal infections. Even the most experienced physicians and surgeons are not able to diagnose appendicitis 100 percent of the time. Children between ages five and nine with appendicitis are often misdiagnosed

with either gastroenteritis or a respiratory infection, which are much more common illnesses in this age group.

A diagnosis of appendicitis is made based on a physical examination, together with tests of blood and urine. To help support or eliminate the diagnosis, a doctor may also order X rays of the abdomen and chest. No laboratory test is specifically designed to identify appendicitis. Instead, surgeons are beginning to rely on CT scans of the appendix to confirm appendicitis when the diagnosis is not clear. Ultrasound tests are even more accurate in correctly diagnosing appendicitis.

Complications

If appendicitis is not treated, the infected appendix may break open and spread the infection to the rest of the abdomen. If perforation does occur, the child's abdominal pain may spread out to involve the whole abdomen, and fever may spike. Once symptoms of appendicitis begin, it takes as little as 24 hours for an infected appendix to perforate. Perforation with appendicitis is more common with younger children. It is a life-threatening complication.

Treatment

Appendicitis is a medical emergency that must be treated surgically; it cannot be treated at home. A child with a suspected case of appendicitis should see a doctor immediately. Since the doctor will need to examine the child's abdomen for signs of pain and tenderness, no pain medication should be given without a doctor's permission. If there is a suspicion of appendicitis, no food or liquids should be given as possible preparation for surgery.

The decision whether to operate or not is most often based on history and physical exam. Surgeons have the option of removing a child's appendix either through the traditional abdominal incision, or by using a small surgical device called a laparoscope to create a smaller opening in the abdomen. However, if the appendix has perforated, surgery becomes more complex and the risk of complications increases.

If the appendix is removed surgically before it perforates, complications are rare. After the surgery the child usually must remain in the hospital between one and three days. Even if the appendix has not perforated, the doctor may prescribe antibiotics to decrease the risk for wound infection after surgery.

However, if the infected appendix perforates, a longer hospital stay is needed.

Prevention

There is no way to prevent appendicitis. Although appendicitis is rare in countries where people eat a high-fiber diet, experts have not yet proven that a high-fiber diet definitely prevents appendicitis.

arboviral infections   Infections caused by any of a number of viruses transmitted by arthropods such as mosquitoes and ticks, such as WEST NILE VIRUS, ENCEPHALITIS, eastern equine encephalomyelitis, St. Louis encephalitis, and California encephalitis. The term *arboviral* is short for arthropod-borne. These types of infections usually occur during warm weather months when mosquitoes are active.

Children are especially susceptible to getting an arboviral infection. Most of these type of infections are spread by infected mosquitoes, but only a few types of mosquitoes are capable of transmitting disease—and only a few of these actually carry a virus. Infection with one arbovirus can provide immunity to that specific virus and may also protect against other related viruses.

Symptoms

Symptoms of the different types of arboviruses are usually similar, although they differ in severity. Most infections do not cause any symptoms at all; mild cases may involve a slight fever or headache. Severe infections quickly cause a severe headache, high fever, disorientation, coma, tremor, convulsions, paralysis, or death. Symptoms usually occur between five and 15 days after exposure.

Treatment

Because there are no specific treatments for these kinds of viral infections, treatment is typically aimed at relieving symptoms.

Prevention

The arboviral diseases can be prevented by using insect repellents when outdoors in mosquito-infested areas, using screening, and community control programs.

arthritis   A group of more than 100 different diseases that is considered to be one category of rheumatic diseases. Rheumatic diseases may cause pain, stiffness, and swelling in the joints and other supporting body structures, such as muscles, tendons, ligaments, and bones. However, rheumatic diseases also can affect other areas of the body, including internal organs. When the immune system does not function properly, it leaves the body susceptible to an array of diseases, including juvenile rheumatoid arthritis.

Arthritis and rheumatic disease can affect anyone, at any age, or of any race. There are nearly 300,000 children in America with some form of arthritis or rheumatic disease. Juvenile rheumatoid arthritis affects children between two and 16 years of age more frequently. Septic arthritis is diagnosed in 6.5 percent of all pediatric arthritis cases and occurs at a slightly higher rate in boys.

The impact of arthritis on school, social life, family relationships, dating, sports, and almost every other aspect of an active, growing child's life raises special concerns. New coping skills for living with the everyday challenges of arthritis must be learned.

Symptoms

Pain and stiffness over a joint is the primary symptom. Many children experience a period of stiffness when they get up each day. This morning stiffness can be one of the best measures of disease activity; the longer the stiffness lasts, the more active the disease. Taking a hot bath or shower, sleeping in a sleeping bag or water bed, doing range-of-motion exercises, or using a hot or cold pack can help relieve pain. Although most children do better with warmth, there are a few who respond to cold.

Cause

The cause of most types of arthritis remains unknown and, in many cases, varies depending on the type of disease present. However, researchers believe that some or all of the following may play a role in the development or aggravation of one or more types of rheumatic diseases:

- genetics and family history (i.e., inherited cartilage weakness)
- trauma

- infection
- brain disturbances
- metabolic disturbances
- excessive wear and tear and stress on a joint(s)
- environmental triggers
- hormones

Treatment

Exercise Getting plenty of exercise is a very important part of treatment for juvenile arthritis. For children with arthritis, exercise helps to keep joints mobile, keep muscles strong, regain lost motion or strength in a joint or muscle, make everyday activities like walking or dressing easier, and improve general fitness and endurance. While medications reduce pain and inflammation, only therapeutic exercise can restore lost motion in a joint. These exercises can make it easier for children to walk and perform other activities of daily living such as walking, eating, and writing. Range-of-motion exercises keep joints flexible and are especially important for children who have lost motion in a joint, or whose joints have become fixed in a bent position. Strengthening exercises build muscles.

Strong muscles and joint protection are the keys to participating in sports. Although contact sports are never recommended, even aggressive sports such as soccer and basketball may not be off limits. Special exercises and protective equipment can further reduce the risk of injury and help children with arthritis play sports.

Splints Splints can help keep joints in the correct position and relieve pain. If a joint is becoming deformed, a splint may help stretch that joint gradually back to its normal position. Commonly used splints include knee extension splints, wrist extension splints, and ring splints for the fingers. An occupational or physical therapist usually makes the splint, which can be adjusted as the child grows. Arm and hand splints are made from plastic; leg splints are sometimes made of cast material.

Medication Prescribing and administering medication for children with arthritis can be completely different from prescribing medication to adults with arthritis. Children will most likely require different dosages of medication, and they may have different or additional side effects to the same drug.

Surgery An operation is rarely used to treat juvenile arthritis in the early course of the disease, but it can be used to ease pain, release joint malformation, or replace a damaged joint. The latter procedure is used primarily with older children who have stopped growing and whose joints have been badly damaged by arthritis. This operation, which is usually used to replace the hip, knee, or jaw joints, can reduce pain and improve function.

Instead of replacement, soft tissue release may sometimes help to improve the position of a joint. In this operation, the surgeon cuts and repairs the tight tissues that caused the initial contracture, allowing the joint to return to a normal position. (See also ARTHRITIS, JUVENILE PSORIATIC; ARTHRITIS, JUVENILE RHEUMATOID.)

Arthritis Foundation The only national non-profit organization that supports the more than 100 types of ARTHRITIS and related conditions with advocacy, programs, services, and research. The foundation also supports a special council devoted to juvenile arthritis, called the AMERICAN JUVENILE ARTHRITIS ORGANIZATION.

Since 1948 the foundation has spent more than $244 million to support some 2,000 scientists and physicians in arthritis research. Organized as the Arthritis and Rheumatism Foundation, the organization's name was changed in 1964 to the Arthritis Foundation.

Arthritis Foundation efforts center on the three-fold mission of the organization: research, prevention, and quality of life. The Arthritis Foundation currently provides nearly $20 million in grants to nearly 300 researchers to help find a cure, prevention, or better treatment for arthritis. The Arthritis Foundation's sponsorship of research for more than 50 years has resulted in major treatment advances for most arthritis diseases.

The foundation offers videotapes, brochures, and booklets about arthritis and publishes a national, bimonthly consumer magazine, *Arthritis Today*. In addition, the Arthritis Foundation provides community-based services nationwide, including self-help courses, water- and land-based exercise classes, support and home study groups, and continuing education courses and publications for health professionals. (See also ARTHRITIS, JUVENILE PSORIATIC; ARTHRITIS, JUVENILE RHEUMATOID; Appendix I.)

arthritis, juvenile psoriatic A type of ARTHRITIS linked to PSORIASIS. While the chronic rash of psoriasis is a common skin condition, only about 12 to 14 percent of people with psoriasis will develop related arthritis.

Causes

Genetic and environmental factors play a strong role in the development of psoriatic arthritis. A family history of psoriasis is linked to many children with juvenile psoriatic arthritis, as well as a family history of other forms of spondyloarthropathy, but there is little relationship between the severity of a rash and the risk of getting juvenile psoriatic arthritis.

Symptoms

Symptoms include pitting or thickening and yellowing of the fingernails and toenails, a small round scaly patch on the scalp, belly button, or buttocks; joint problems in large joints such as the hip, either on just one side or in the same joints on both sides of the body; swelling of fingers or toes.

Because eye inflammation occurs in between 10 and 20 percent of cases, children with juvenile psoriatic arthritis should be examined by an ophthalmologist annually to check for eye problems.

Diagnosis

Juvenile psoriatic arthritis can be tricky to diagnose. In some children with the condition, symptoms of arthritis appear before the rash. In these cases, diagnosis can be so difficult that it may take up to 10 years to be certain of a definite diagnosis.

Complications

While many children have no long-term consequences of juvenile psoriatic arthritis, there are a number of possible complications, including eye problems; decreased range of joint motion; shortening or lengthening of a limb, finger, or toe; damaged cartilage; or enlargement of a joint. (See also ARTHRITIS, JUVENILE RHEUMATOID; ARTHRITIS FOUNDATION.)

arthritis, juvenile rheumatoid The most common type of juvenile ARTHRITIS, which is an inflammation of the joints characterized by swelling, heat, and pain. Arthritis can be short-term or chronic, and in rare cases it can last a lifetime. Juvenile arthritis is the term used for all the types of arthritis that affect more than 285,000 children in the United States. Juvenile rheumatoid arthritis (JRA) affects about 75,000 American children.

Cause

Doctors do not know what causes rheumatoid arthritis (also called idiopathic arthritis) in children, but research suggests that it is an autoimmune disease. In autoimmune diseases, white blood cells lose the ability to tell the difference between the body's own healthy cells and tissues and harmful bacteria and viruses. The immune system, which is supposed to protect the body from invasion, instead releases chemicals that can damage healthy tissues and cause inflammation and pain.

Symptoms

JRA usually appears between the ages of six months and 16 years. The first signs are often joint pain or swelling and reddened or warm joints. Rashes may suddenly appear and disappear, developing in one area and then another. High fevers that tend to spike in the evenings and suddenly disappear are characteristic of systemic JRA.

There are several types of JRA; which type a child has is determined by the pattern of symptoms that occurs within the first six months. About half the time children eventually outgrow the disease, but it is hard to predict who will continue to suffer with symptoms. Often the more joints that are affected, the more severe the disease and the less likely that the symptoms will eventually go away.

The three major types of JRA are polyarticular arthritis, pauciarticular JRA, and systemic JRA.

polyarticular arthritis primarily affects girls, causing swelling or pain in five or more joints. The small joints of the hands are affected as well as the weight-bearing joints such as the knees, hips, ankles, feet, and neck. There may be a low-grade fever as well as bumps on the body in areas subjected to pressure from sitting or leaning.

pauciarticular JRA affects fewer than four joints; the knee and wrist joints are most often involved. Symptoms include pain, stiffness, or swelling of affected joints. In this subtype of JRA, an inflammation of the iris of the eye may occur with or without active symptoms. This eye inflammation, called iridocyclitis or iritis or uveitis, can be detected by an ophthalmologist.

systemic JRA affects the entire body, with high fevers that rise at night and then suddenly drop to normal. During the onset of fever, the child may feel very ill, appear pale, or develop an intermittent rash. The spleen and lymph nodes may become enlarged. Eventually many of the body's joints are affected by swelling, pain, and stiffness.

Diagnosis

To effectively manage and minimize the effects of arthritis, an early and accurate diagnosis is essential. Many viral infections can cause a brief bout of arthritis that then disappears. If the arthritis has not cleared within six weeks, a rheumatologist or other specialist should be consulted.

Diagnosis begins with a detailed medical history and a thorough physical examination. X rays or blood tests may be used to exclude other conditions that can mimic JRA. Tests may include:

- a complete blood count to evaluate all the basic cellular components of blood, including red blood cells, white blood cells, and platelets. Abnormalities in the numbers and appearances of these cells can be useful in the diagnosis of many medical conditions.

- a blood culture to detect bacteria that cause infections in the bloodstream. A blood culture may help rule out infections.

- bone marrow examination reveals the condition of blood where it is being formed to rule out conditions such as leukemia.

- erythrocyte sedimentation rate checks how rapidly red blood cells settle to the bottom of a test tube. This rate often increases in people when inflammation is occurring in the body.

- rheumatoid factor, an antibody produced in the blood of children with some forms of JRA. Rheumatoid factor is much more common in adults.

- antinuclear factor (ANA), a blood test to detect autoimmunity that can predict which children are likely to have eye disease with JRA

- X rays and bone scans can detect changes in bone and joints to evaluate the causes of unexplained bone and joint pain.

Treatment

JRA is treated with a combination of medication, physical therapy, and exercise. Sometimes a child may need surgery or corticosteroid shots into the joint. The goals of treatment are to relieve pain and inflammation, slow down or prevent the destruction of joints, and restore use and function of affected joints.

NONSTEROIDAL ANTI-INFLAMMATORY DRUGS (NSAIDs) may be prescribed for inflammation and pain. Although swelling and pain may temporarily improve, it is important to continue medication until a doctor decides that the disease is fully controlled. If NSAIDs do not control inflammation of the joints, other medications such as methotrexate may be prescribed.

New biological agents are available to treat some forms of chronic arthritis in children. Etanercept, Enbrel, and Remicads are approved for use in children with polyarticular JRA, while infliximab is currently being tested for use in some types of childhood arthritis.

A physical therapy program is essential in managing any type of arthritis, including activities and exercises suited to a child's specific condition. Range-of-motion exercises can restore flexibility in stiff, sore joints, and other exercises will build strength and endurance. It is very important for children with arthritis to maintain a regular exercise program so that muscles are kept strong and healthy to help support and protect joints. Regular exercise also helps to maintain range of motion of joints and prevent cycles of pain and depression. Safe activities include walking, swimming, and bicycling (especially on stationary bikes). However, some sports (especially impact sports) can be hazardous to a child whose arthritis has weakened joints and bones.

A child with arthritis should also be sure to eat a balanced diet that includes plenty of calcium to promote bone health. (See also ARTHRITIS, JUVENILE PSORIATIC.)

Asian flu   See INFLUENZA.

Asperger syndrome (Asperger's disorder)   A condition characterized by sustained problems with social interactions and social relatedness, and the development of restricted, repetitive patterns of interests, activities, and behaviors. The disorder is named after Hans Asperger, a Viennese pediatrician who first documented this cluster of characteristics in the 1940s.

One type of AUTISM SPECTRUM DISORDER, Asperger's is a milder form of AUTISM but without the delays in cognitive or language development. In 1994 Asperger's was first classified as a pervasive developmental disorder, a designation that also includes autistic disorder.

Many children with pervasive developmental disorders such as Asperger's disorder also meet the diagnostic criteria for ATTENTION DEFICIT HYPERACTIVITY DISORDER (ADHD). However, ADHD should not be diagnosed when there is Asperger's, since all the ADHD symptoms can be attributed to the other condition. Clinicians who overlook other symptoms of Asperger's tend to diagnose these children as having ADHD.

Like many learning disorders, Asperger's is believed to be more common in boys, although more research needs to be done to understand its genetic origins. According to the National Institutes of Health, Asperger's disorder occurs in one out of every 500 Americans—more often than multiple sclerosis, DOWN SYNDROME, or CYSTIC FIBROSIS. It is estimated that more than 400,000 families are affected by this condition.

Symptoms

Often there are no obvious delays in language or cognitive development or in age-appropriate self-help skills. While these individuals possess attention deficits, problems with organization, and an uneven profile of skills, they usually have average and sometimes gifted intelligence.

Individuals with Asperger's syndrome may have problems with social situations and in developing peer relationships. They may have noticeable difficulty with nonverbal communication, impaired use of social gestures, facial expressions, and eye contact. There may be certain repetitive behaviors or rituals. Though grammatical, speech is peculiar due to abnormal inflection and repetition. Clumsiness (and a lack of motor planning) is prominent both in speech and physical movements. Individuals with this disorder usually have a limited area of interest that usually excludes more age-appropriate, common interests. Some examples of these single-minded obsessions may include cars, trains, Russian literature, doorknobs, hinges, astronomy, or history.

Asperger's vs. Autism

Clumsiness and single-minded interests are more common in Asperger's, and verbal IQ is usually higher than performance IQ. In autism, the reverse is usually true. The outcome is usually more positive for Asperger's than for autism.

Cause

Biological factors are of crucial importance in the etiology of autism, and frontal lobe abnormalities have been found. Associated medical conditions such as FRAGILE X SYNDROME, tuberous sclerosis, neurofibromatosis, and hypothyroidism (sluggish thyroid) are less common in Asperger's disorder than in classical autism. Therefore, scientists suspect there may be fewer major physical brain problems associated with Asperger's than with autism.

Treatment

While there is no cure, early intervention has been proven to be effective. The need for academic and social supports increase through the school years, and by adolescence many children develop symptoms of depression and anxiety. It is important to continue supports into adulthood to ensure that affected adults can lead productive lives.

Symptoms can be managed using social skills training and individual psychotherapy to help the individual to process the feelings aroused by being socially handicapped. Other treatments may include parent education and training, behavioral modification, educational interventions, and medication. For treating hyperactivity, inattention, and impulsivity, stimulants such as methylphenidate, dextroamphetamine, metamphetamine, pemoline, clonidine, desipramine and nortriptyline may be used. For irritability and aggression, mood stabilizers (valproate, carbamazepine, lithium), beta blockers (nadolol, propranolol), and neuroleptics (risperidone, haloperidol) are effective. To treat preoccupations, rituals, and compulsions doctors may prescribe antidepressants such as fluvoxamine, fluoxetine, or clomipramine. To treat anxiety doctors may prescribe antidepressants (sertraline, fluoxetine, imipramine, clomipramine, or nortriptyline).

Asperger Syndrome Coalition of the United States A national nonprofit support and advocacy organization for ASPERGER SYNDROME and related disorders that is committed to providing the most up-to-date and comprehensive information on the condition. (For contact information, see Appendix I.)

aspergillosis A rare infection with the fungus *Aspergillus fumigatus* (found in old buildings or decaying plants) that can attack the mucous membranes of the nose or urethra, the lungs, liver, or kidneys. It is an occasionally fatal opportunistic infection among children with impaired immune systems, especially if the infection has spread throughout the body. The fungus is found everywhere in soil and proliferates rapidly. Inhalation of *A. fumigatus* and *A. flatus* is common but infection is rare.

Treatment
Topical fungicides can be used on the skin; amphotericin B is used to treat systemic aspergillosis, especially if it has spread to the lungs.

aspirin A widely used drug that relieves pain, inflammation, and fever. Children and teenagers should never take aspirin, or products containing aspirin or other salicylates, if they have chicken pox or flu symptoms or are recovering from these or other viral illnesses. Aspirin use in children sick with a virus has been associated with REYE'S SYNDROME, a rare but serious condition that can cause death. The incidence of Reye's syndrome has dropped dramatically since children stopped taking aspirin regularly.

The U.S. Food and Drug Administration has proposed adding a more descriptive warning label on aspirin and other products containing salicy-lates to describe symptoms of Reye's syndrome in more detail than it does now.

To reduce fever safely in children, parents should use ACETAMINOPHEN (Tylenol) or IBUPROFEN (Motrin, Advil).

Association for the Education and Rehabilitation of the Blind and Visually Impaired The only international membership organization dedicated to providing support to professionals who work in education and rehabilitation of blind and visually impaired children. The group was formed in 1984 as the result of a consolidation between the American Association of Workers for the Blind and the Association for Education of the Visually Handicapped. It is a private nonprofit association that coordinates biennial international conferences, assists in membership promotion and development, provides information and referrals about blindness, and works closely in planning activities and providing services to its divisions, chapters, and regions. (For contact information, see Appendix I.)

Association of Birth Defect Children, Inc. This nonprofit group provides information and support to families of children with BIRTH DEFECTS caused by their mothers' exposure to environmental agents such as drugs, chemicals, or radiation. The association sponsors a National Birth Defects Registry, which contains demographic data and medical histories from member families in the United States and Canada and matches families of children with similar disabilities. The association provides information about drug use during pregnancy and the care and rehabilitation of children with birth defects. Families of children with genetic birth defects are also eligible for membership. (For contact information, see Appendix I.)

asthma A chronic inflammatory disease characterized by airways that have become sensitive to substances that trigger an allergic reaction: First, the lining of the airways become swollen and inflamed, the muscles that surround the airways tighten, and mucus production increases. All of these factors cause the airways to narrow, making it hard for the child to breathe air out of the lungs.

Asthma affects more than 4.8 million children in the United States, making it the most common serious and chronic disease among children; it is the third most common cause of childhood hospitalizations under the age of 15. Alarmingly, asthma cases and asthma deaths have been increasing. From 1979 to 1996, asthma deaths have risen 120 percent from 2,598 to 5,667. Hospitalizations for asthma have increased 256 percent from 1979 to 1996, to 474,100 people annually.

Although any child may develop asthma, it most commonly occurs in children by the age of five, a child with a family history of asthma, children with other allergies, or children exposed to secondhand tobacco smoke. Asthma is 26 percent more common in African-American children than in Caucasian children, and African-American children with asthma generally experience more severe disability from asthma and have more frequent hospitalizations.

Cause

The exact cause of asthma is not known, but experts believe it may be inherited; however, asthma also involves many other environmental, infectious, and chemical factors. Each child has different triggers that cause the asthma to worsen. Some children have exercise-induced asthma, which is triggered during or shortly after exercise.

The changes that occur in asthma are believed to happen in two phases: An immediate response to the trigger leads to swelling and narrowing of the airways, making it hard for the child to breathe. A later response, which can happen four to eight hours after the initial exposure to the allergen, leads to further inflammation of the airways and obstruction of airflow.

Symptoms

Each child may experience symptoms differently. It is important to remember that some children do not exhibit the characteristic wheeze of asthma—they may only cough. The cough may be either constant or intermittent, there may be wheezing (a whistling sound that may be heard while your child is breathing), or a child may have trouble breathing or experience shortness of breath while playing or exercising. Some children may complain that their chests hurt or feel tight. Other symptoms include fatigue, night-time cough, and noisy breathing.

Because the symptoms of asthma may resemble other problems or medical conditions, a physician or respiratory specialist should make the diagnosis.

Diagnosis

To diagnose asthma and distinguish it from other lung disorders, physicians rely on a combination of medical history, physical examination, and laboratory tests, which may include

- spirometry—the evaluation of lung function—one of the simplest, most common pulmonary function tests
- peak flow monitor—a device that measures the amount of air a child can blow out of the lungs. This is very important in evaluating how well or how poorly the disease is being controlled.
- chest X ray (to rule out PNEUMONIA)
- blood tests to analyze the amount of carbon dioxide and oxygen in the blood (less common unless child is hospitalized)
- allergy tests
- pulse oximetry to analyze the oxygen content of the blood

Asthma and Allergy Foundation of America A patient organization dedicated to improving the quality of life for children with ASTHMA and ALLERGIES through education, advocacy, and research. The Asthma and Allergy Foundation of America (AAFA) a not-for-profit organization founded in 1953, provides practical information, community-based services, support, and referrals through a national network of chapters and educational support groups. AAFA also sponsors research toward better treatments and a cure for asthma and allergic diseases. (For contact information, see Appendix I.)

athlete's foot A common fungal condition causing the skin between the toes (usually the fourth and fifth toes) to itch, peel, and crack with diffuse scaling and redness of the soles and sides of the foot. Associated with wearing shoes and sweating, the condition is rare in young children and in places of the world where people do not wear shoes. It is primarily found in adolescent and older men, especially boys who wear sneakers without socks. A person with athlete's foot is infectious for as long as the lesions exist.

Itchy skin on the foot is probably not athlete's foot if it occurs on the top of the toes. If the foot is red, swollen, sore, blistered, and oozing, it is more likely some form of contact dermatitis although inflammatory fungal infections can sometimes look like this.

Causes

The fungi that are responsible for athlete's foot are called dermatophytes; they live only on dead body tissue (hair, the outer layer of skin, and nails). The two dermatophytes responsible for athlete's foot are *Trichophyton rubrum* and *T. mentagrophytes.* The condition occurs both by direct and indirect contact; it can be passed in locker rooms, showers, or shared towels or shoes.

Symptoms

Symptoms may include scaling and cracking of the skin between the toes and the sides of the feet; the skin may itch and peel. There may be small water blisters between the toes; it can spread to the instep or the hands. There is usually an odor present.

Diagnosis

Scrapings from the affected area will be examined under a microscope for certain fungal characteristics.

Treatment

The condition may clear up without any attention, but it usually requires treatment. An untreated fungal infection can lead to bacteria-inviting cracks in the skin. The affected area should be kept dry, clad in dry cotton socks or sandals, or kept uncovered. A number of nonprescription fungicide sprays will cure athlete's foot, including: clotrimazole (Lotrimin), ketoconazole (Nizoral), miconazolenitrate (Monistatderm), sulconazole (Exelderm), or tolnaftate (Tenactin). Before applying, the feet should be bathed well with soap and water, and then well dried (especially between the toes). The sprays should be applied to all sides of the feet twice a day for up to four weeks. After the spray has been applied, the feet should be covered in clean, white cotton socks. For cases that do not respond to the sprays, a physician may prescribe an oral medicine (griseofulvin) or Ketoconazole.

When the acute phase of the infection passes, the dead skin should be removed with a bristle brush in order to destroy the living fungi. All bits of the skin should be washed away.

Prevention

Good hygiene is the best way to prevent athlete's foot. Disinfecting the floors of showers and locker rooms can help control the spread of infection.

Once an infection has cleared up, the patient should continue using antifungal cream now and then—especially during warm weather. Plastic or too-tight shoes and any type of footwear treated to keep out water should be avoided. Natural materials (cotton and leather) and sandals are the best choices, while wool and rubber can make a fungal problem worse by trapping moisture.

Shoes should be aired out regularly in the sun and wiped inside with a disinfectant-treated cloth to remove fungi-carrying dead skin. The insides of shoes should then be dusted with antifungal powder or spray (Desenex). Those individuals who perspire heavily should change socks three or four times daily. Only natural white cotton socks should be worn, and they should be rinsed thoroughly during washing.

Feet should be air dried after bathing and then powdered. It is important to wear sandals or flip-flops in public bathing areas.

attention deficit hyperactivity disorder (ADHD) A condition that may occur in both children and adults who consistently display inattention, HYPERACTIVITY, and impulsivity. People who are inattentive may have trouble keeping their minds focused and may get bored with a task after just a few minutes. Those who are hyperactive seem to feel restless and are constantly in motion, finding it hard to sit still. People who are impulsive have a problem with curbing their immediate reactions and tend to act before they think. Other symptoms may include problems in school, with friends, and with behavior.

ADHD and LEARNING DISABILITY frequently occur together, but they are not the same. Learning disabilities include difficulty with receiving, organizing, processing, understanding, remembering, and offering information. ADHD involves difficulty with paying attention to information. Between 10 percent and 20 percent of all school-age children have learning disabilities. Of those with learning disabilities, between 4 percent and 12 percent of all school-age children will also have ADHD, making it the most common childhood neurobehavioral disorder.

Although ADHD is a common childhood behavioral disorder, it can be difficult to diagnose and even harder to understand. Once viewed as a disorder of childhood primarily involving hyperactivity and the inability to pay attention, ADHD is now seen as a lifelong condition that may not include physical restlessness or hyperactive behavior at all. It may also be the source of unusual talents or giftedness in specific areas.

In recent years there has been growing interest in ADHD as well as concerns about possible over-diagnosis. In surveys among pediatricians and family physicians across the country, wide variations were found in diagnostic criteria and treatment methods for ADHD. Indeed, the definition and treatments of ADHD continues to evolve; since the early 1990s there has been an extraordinary surge in the level of focus on ADHD and in the incidence of diagnosis among children and adults. It is likely that the present level of understanding of the disorder, as well as current methods of diagnosis and treatment, will continue to develop rapidly in the coming years.

Once thought to be a disorder primarily affecting young hyperactive boys, ADHD is both more complicated and more pervasive. In particular, experts now know that children do not typically "outgrow" the condition, nor does it affect only boys. The present gender ratio ranges from three to one to seven to one boys to girls, but this is hampered by inconsistent standards for diagnosis and insufficient research samples.

Cause

ADHD is presumed to be a brain condition that affects between three percent and seven percent of the population. Since the early 1990s scientists have worked to pinpoint the differences found in brain scans between the normal brain and the ADHD brain. Recently, scientists have been able to localize the brain areas involved in ADHD, finding that areas in the frontal lobe and basal ganglia are reduced by about 10 percent in size and activity in children with ADHD.

Studies in the past few years have shown that boys with ADHD tend to have brains that are more symmetrical. Three structures in the brains of boys with ADHD were smaller than in non-ADHD boys of the same age: prefrontal cortex, caudate nucleus, and the globus pallidus. The prefrontal cortex is thought to be the brain's "command center"; the other two parts translate the commands into action.

There is also evidence that not only are some of the structures slightly varied, but the brain may use these areas differently. Watching brain scans, researchers discovered that boys with ADHD have an abnormal increase of activity in the frontal lobe and certain areas below it. These areas work in part to control voluntary action. This meant that the ADHD boys were working harder to control their impulses than non-ADHD boys. Once given Ritalin, this abnormal activity quieted down. This effect was not seen in the non-ADHD boys. This means that Ritalin may act differently on ADHD brains compared to "normal" brains.

Although a brain scan (called functional magnetic resonance imaging or fMRI), is expensive and may not be covered by insurance, it may provide a more accurate way to diagnose ADHD. As scientists explore more of the brain, ADHD may be thought of more as a disorder than a behavioral problem.

Dopamine pathways in the brain, which link the basal ganglia and frontal cortex, also appear to play a major role in ADHD. The National Institute of Mental Health has released the results of a major clinical trial focusing on ADHD that found that medication that boosts the level of dopamine in the brain is the most successful type of treatment.

Experts believe that at least some cases of ADHD may be inherited, and that it may involve both brain structures in the frontal lobe related to attention, impulse control, and executive functions, as well as neurotransmitters and subtle imbalances in brain chemistry. Other children may experience abnormal fetal development that affects the areas of the brain controlling attention and movement.

Diagnosis

ADHD is primarily diagnosed through a combination of individual and family history, individual behavioral assessments, and information about behavior from parents, teachers, rating scales, and others. Some tests also contain factors for inattention, distractibility, and memory that can be affected by ADHD and may contribute to a diagnosis.

In addition, certain medical conditions such as hypothyroidism, juvenile diabetes, and seizure disorders must be ruled out as causes for the child's inability to pay attention. Increasingly, psychologists and physicians are reluctant to make the diagnosis alone, favoring a joint diagnosis after they have gathered all necessary medical, psychological, and behavioral information.

Formerly called attention deficit disorder, with or without hyperactivity, this disorder was recently renamed attention deficit hyperactivity disorder (ADHD) and includes three subtypes:

- *Inattentive subtype* (formerly known as attention deficit disorder, or ADD) with signs that include being easily distracted, an inability to pay attention to details, not following directions, losing or forgetting things like toys, notebooks, or homework
- *Hyperactive-impulsive subtype* (formerly known as attention deficit hyperactivity disorder, or ADHD) includes fidgeting, squirming, blurting out answers before hearing the full question, difficulty waiting, running or jumping out of a seat when quiet behavior is expected
- *Combined subtype* (the most common of the subtypes) includes those signs from both of the subtypes above and can be seen with or without hyperactivity.

To be considered for a diagnosis of ADHD, a child must display these behaviors before age seven and the behaviors must last for at least six months, and they must be considered "maladaptive." For a diagnosis, the behavior must also negatively affect at least two areas of a child's life, such as school, home, or friendships.

ADHD is diagnosed using the criteria in the *Diagnostic and Statistical Manual of Mental Disorders, Fourth Edition (DSM-IV)*. Diagnostic criteria include:

Inattention

- often fails to give close attention to details or makes careless mistakes in schoolwork, work, or other activities

- often has difficulty sustaining attention in tasks or play activities
- often does not seem to listen when spoken to directly
- often does not follow through on instructions and fails to finish schoolwork, chores, or duties in the workplace (not due to oppositional behavior or failure to understand instructions)
- often has difficulty organizing tasks and activities
- often avoids, dislikes, or is reluctant to engage in tasks that require sustained mental effort (such as schoolwork or homework)
- often loses things necessary for tasks or activities (such as toys, school assignments, pencils, books, or tools)
- is often easily distracted by extraneous stimuli
- is often forgetful in daily activities

Hyperactivity-Impulsivity

- often fidgets with hands or feet or squirms in seat very tight
- often leaves seat in classroom or in other situations in which remaining seated is expected
- often runs about or climbs excessively in situations in which it is inappropriate (in adolescents or adults, may be limited to subjective feelings of restlessness)
- often has trouble playing or engaging in leisure activities quietly
- is often on the go
- talks excessively
- often blurts out answers before questions have been completed
- often has difficulty awaiting turn
- often interrupts or intrudes on others

The American Academy of Pediatrics recently developed new guidelines for the diagnosis of ADHD with input from a panel of medical, mental health, and educational experts. The new guidelines, designed for primary care physicians diagnosing ADHD in children aged six to 12 years, include the following recommendations:

- ADHD evaluations should be performed by the primary care clinician for children who show signs of school difficulties, academic under-achievement, troublesome relationships with teachers, family members, and peers, and other behavioral problems.

• Questions to parents, either directly or through a pre-visit questionnaire, regarding school and behavioral issues may help alert physicians to possible ADHD.

• In diagnosing ADHD, physicians should use DSM-IV criteria, which require that symptoms be present in two or more of a child's settings, and that the symptoms interfere with the child's academic or social functioning for at least six months.

• The assessment of ADHD should include information obtained directly from parents or care-givers, as well as a classroom teacher or other school professional, regarding the core symptoms of ADHD in various settings, the age of onset, duration of symptoms, and degree of functional impairment.

• Evaluation of a child with ADHD should also include assessment for coexisting conditions: learning and language problems, aggression, disruptive behavior, depression, or anxiety.

• Because as many as one-third of children diagnosed with ADHD also have a coexisting condition, other diagnostic tests (sometimes considered positive indicators for ADHD) have been reviewed and considered not effective. These tests include lead screening, tests for generalized resistance to thyroid hormone, and brain image studies.

Of course, all children sometimes have trouble paying attention, following directions, or being quiet, but for children with ADHD, these behaviors occur more frequently and are more disturbing.

Symptoms

Although the primary symptoms associated with ADHD are inattention, distractibility, and hyperactivity, some current researchers now recognize ADHD as a condition that primarily affects impulse controls that delay response to external or internal stimuli. The inability of impulse controls to delay response has a significant effect on memory and executive functions that involve holding verbal or visual information in mind in order to process it, reflecting on previous experience and learning to change behavior based on it, and reconstituting prior emotional states as a means to self-understanding and development.

Symptoms of ADHD may include failing to sustain attention while playing or performing tasks, difficulty completing tasks, difficulty with organization and planning, difficulty with impulsive behavior, such as blurting out answers, acting inappropriately, and/or fidgeting and restlessness. There may also be an inability to self-monitor or self-regulate behavior, and an impaired sense of the passage of time. Individuals with ADHD frequently have difficulty getting started, lose focus, and do not finish projects. Short- and long-term planning abilities may be greatly diminished, and disorganization can result from an inability to mindfully plan, act, and complete even the most basic tasks, such as cleaning a room. Individuals with ADHD often display risk-taking or conflict-seeking behaviors and may exhibit poor judgment in social or interpersonal contexts.

At the same time, individuals with ADHD may also display paradoxical behaviors, such as the ability to focus intensively on a task over a period of time, very strong intellectual, verbal, and problem-solving skills, and extraordinary creativity. Characteristically, both types of behavior may occur within a single place, such as a class or work environment. Because the performance of individuals with ADHD can be strong, especially when they are very interested, subsequent failure to perform at the same level is often perceived as a lack of self-discipline or effort. Adults who are diagnosed late in life often report severe and lifelong problems in school, job, or with personal relationships. They may feel misunderstood and are frequently misdiagnosed, given the range of varying symptoms that can develop as a result of an attention disorder or a coexisting condition.

ADHD and Other Disorders

ADHD can coexist with a number of psychological conditions, including conduct disorders, mood disorders (such as depression), anxiety disorders, and impulse control disorders (such as eating disorders and alcohol abuse). Some children may be depressed as a result of having ADHD, whereas others may have a mood disorder that exists independently of ADHD. Nearly half of all children with ADHD also have oppositional defiant disorder characterized by stubbornness, outbursts of temper, and defiance.

Many children with ADHD also have a specific learning disability, which means that they might have trouble mastering language or other skills, such as math, reading, or handwriting. Although ADHD is not categorized as a learning disability, its interference with concentration and attention can make it even more difficult for a child to perform well in school. The issue of coexisting conditions makes diagnosis, treatment, and understanding of ADHD particularly complex.

Treatment

There is no cure for ADHD, but a combined program of medication and behavioral therapy can help and is often prescribed to treat ADHD. With the advice and cooperation of a child's pediatrician, teachers, counselors, and family members, the child can have a normal life in spite of this disorder.

For most children and adults with ADHD, medication is an important part of treatment that is not used to "control" behavior but to ease the symptoms of ADHD and to help the child cope. Stimulants appear to work by altering the levels of transmitters in the brain by which the different nerve cells communicate.

Between 70 and 80 percent of children with ADHD respond positively to these medications, with improvements in attention span, impulsivity, and behavior, especially in structured environments. Some children also demonstrate improvements in frustration tolerance, compliance, and even handwriting. Relationships with parents, peers, and teachers may also improve.

This medication may also be effective in adults who have ADHD. The reaction to these medications can be similar to that experienced by children with ADHD—a decrease in impulsivity and an increase in attention. Many ADHD adults treated with medication report that they are able to bring more control and organization to their lives. Other medications, such as antidepressants, can be help-

ful when depression, phobic, panic, anxiety and/or obsessive-compulsive disorders are present.

The newest drug used to treat ADHD is STRATTERA (atomoxetine), the first nonstimulant medication approved for the treatment of ADHD in children, adolescents, and adults. Strattera is a selective norepinephrine reuptake inhibitor, a class of drugs that works differently from the other ADHD medications available. It works by selectively blocking the reuptake of norepinephrine, a chemical neurotransmitter, by certain nerve cells in the brain. This action increases the availability of norepinephrine, which experts believe is essential in regulating impulse control, organization, and attention. The precise mechanism by which Strattera works on ADHD is not known.

Because Strattera does not appear to have a potential for abuse, it is not classified as a controlled substance, although it is a prescription drug. Strattera is an oral capsule and can be taken once or twice a day to provide full-day relief from ADHD symptoms. While parents may notice improvements in ADHD symptoms after the first week of use, it may take up to a month to see the full therapeutic benefit of the medication.

The drugs usually include regular, fairly small doses of stimulants such as RITALIN (methylphenidate), Dexedrine or Dextrostat (DEXTROAMPHETAMINE), ADDERALL (single entity amphetamine), or CYLERT (pemoline). While these drugs can be addictive in teenagers and adults, they do not seem to be addictive in children. Nine out of 10 children improve on one of these stimulants, so if one does not work, others are tried. It may seem strange to give stimulants to children with hyperactivity and attention deficit problems, but instead of making the child act out more, these drugs reduce the hyperactivity and increase the attention span. The drugs also help children with ADHD control their behavior. A child using these drugs actually becomes quieter and more attentive.

Sometimes, however, none of these medications work. In this case, some children may respond well to antihistamines usually prescribed for allergies, or antidepressants like Elavil, Prozac, Tofranil, or Norpramin. Clonidine, a drug normally used to treat high blood pressure, may ease some symptoms of ADHD. With any of these medications, adjusting the dosage for each child is vital for treating the symptoms of ADHD.

Stimulant drugs do cause side effects. Most doctors feel the potential side effects should be carefully weighed against the benefits before prescribing drugs to children with ADHD. While taking these medications, some children may lose weight, have stomachaches or have less appetite, and temporarily grow more slowly. Others may have trouble falling asleep and become irritable. Some doctors worry that stimulants may worsen the symptoms of TOURETTE'S SYNDROME, although recent research suggests this is not true. Many doctors believe if they carefully monitor a child's height, weight, and overall development, the benefits of medication far outweigh the potential side effects. Side effects that do occur can often be handled by reducing the dosage.

Unfortunately, the long-term effects of taking these drugs is not known. Cylert may cause more serious side effects and is therefore not considered to be a first-line medication for ADHD. Otherwise, side effects are usually dose related.

Still, the use of stimulants for children with ADHD—especially Ritalin—is not without controversy. Critics worry that Ritalin and other stimulant drugs are prescribed unnecessarily for too many children, since many things—including anxiety, depression, allergies, seizures, or problems at home or school—can make children seem overactive, impulsive, or inattentive. They argue that many children who do not have ADHD are drugged anyway as a way to control disruptive behaviors.

Critics also worry that so many of the nation's children are given these drugs without any real understanding of the future side effects. Although Ritalin is one of the most commonly prescribed drugs for children, there are concerns about its long-term effects.

There are no studies on children who have taken Ritalin for more than 14 months. Ritalin affects the brain in a way very similar to cocaine, one of the most addictive substances known. Critics worry that children who take Ritalin may be more likely to use illegal drugs in the future, or that they might be more likely to smoke as adults. These concerns are fueled by research showing that rats who were exposed to stimulants were more likely to choose cocaine, suggesting that early exposure to some drugs may make a person more likely to abuse drugs in the future. However, the data on whether there is a link between Ritalin and later substance abuse are controversial. Some studies show that Ritalin makes people more prone to addiction to certain substances, but other researchers insist that ADHD children are not more likely to use drugs of any type later in life.

Many experts believe that the best way to manage the symptoms of ADHD is to combine drug treatment with behavioral methods. Medication can help to control some of the behavior problems that may have led to family turmoil, but more often there are other aspects of a child's problem that medication will not affect.

Even though ADHD primarily affects a person's behavior, the simple fact of having ADHD can trigger serious emotional problems as well. Some of these children have very few experiences that build their sense of worth and competence. If they are hyperactive, they are often punished for being disruptive. If they are too disorganized and unfocused to complete tasks, they may be branded "lazy." If they are impulsive, shove classmates, and interrupt, they may lose friends. If they are unlucky enough to have a related conduct disorder, they may get in trouble at school or with the police.

The daily frustrations that are a part of having ADHD can make people feel abnormal or stupid. In many cases, the cycle of frustration and anger has persisted for so long that it may take years to alleviate.

For this reason, parents and children may need special help to develop techniques to manage the behavior patterns that have become ingrained. In such cases, mental health professionals can help the child and family develop new attitudes and ways of relating to each other.

Behavior treatments include coaching, a process of individual support that focuses on understanding maladaptive patterns of behavior, identifying goals and strategies for change, and providing consistent reinforcement and feedback. For younger children, such an approach may involve behavioral rating scales, consistent feedback, and reinforcement for positive behavioral change. For adults, the approach may focus on identifying and describing goals and strategies. In either case, focusing on the role of individual responsibility and choice is a vital component, as is developing a consistent pattern of feedback and reinforcement.

In individual counseling, the therapist helps children or adults with ADHD learn to feel better about themselves. The therapist can also help people with ADHD identify and build on their strengths, cope with daily problems, and control their attention and aggression.

In group counseling, people learn that they are not alone in their frustration and that others want to help. Sometimes only the child with ADHD needs counseling, but often the entire family can benefit from support. If the child is young, parents can learn techniques for coping with and improving their child's behavior.

Several intervention approaches are available and different therapists tend to prefer one approach or another. Knowing something about the various types of interventions makes it easier for families to choose the best therapist for their own situation.

In psychotherapy, patients talk with the therapist about their thoughts and feelings, explore problem behaviors, and learn different ways to handle their emotions. If someone who has ADHD wants to gain control of symptoms more directly, more direct kinds of intervention are available.

Cognitive-behavioral therapy helps people directly change their behavior instead of only concentrating on understanding their feelings and actions. The therapist may help an individual learn to think through tasks and organize work, or encourage new behavior by giving praise each time the person acts in the desired way. A cognitive-behavioral therapist can use these techniques to help an ADHD child learn to control his fighting, or an impulsive teenager to think before speaking.

Social skills training can help children learn new behaviors by watching the therapist model appropriate behavior like waiting for a turn, sharing toys, or responding to a bully.

Support groups can also be helpful, linking people who have common concerns. Many adults with ADHD and parents of children with ADHD find it useful to join a local or national support group.

Many groups deal with issues of children's disorders. Members of support groups share frustrations and successes and provide referrals.

Because ADHD affects all aspects of a child's home and school life, experts recommend parent education and support groups to help family members learn how to help the child cope with frustrations, organize environments, and develop problem-solving skills. Special parenting skills are often needed because children with ADHD may not respond as well to typical parenting practices—especially punishment. Instead, children with ADHD should learn how to reinforce their positive behaviors themselves and also learn how to solve problems. Children who take medications and practice these behavior techniques do better than those who rely on medication alone.

Parental Training

Parenting skills training, offered by therapists or in special classes, gives parents tools and techniques for managing their child's behavior. One such technique is the use of "time-out" when the child becomes too unruly or out of control. During time-outs, the child is removed from the agitating situation and sits alone quietly for a short time to calm down. Parents may also be taught to give the child quality time each day, in which they share a relaxed activity. During this time together, the parent looks for opportunities to point out what the child is doing right and to praise strengths and abilities. An effective way to modify a child's behavior is through a system of rewards and penalties. The parents or teacher identify a few desirable behaviors that they want to encourage in the child, such as asking for a toy politely. The child is told exactly what is expected in order to earn a small reward, which is awarded when he performs the desired behavior. The goal is to help children learn to control their own behavior and to choose the more desired behavior. The technique works well with all children, although children with ADHD may need more frequent rewards.

Parents also may learn to structure situations in ways that will allow their child to succeed. If a child is easily overstimulated, parents may try allowing only one or two playmates at a time. If the child has trouble completing tasks, parents may help the child divide a large task into small steps, then praise the child as each step is completed.

Stress management methods such as meditation, relaxation techniques, and exercise can increase the parents' tolerance for frustration, enabling them to respond more calmly to their child's behavior.

Other behavioral treatments that may be helpful in treating children with ADHD include play therapy and special physical exercise. Play therapy may help a child who has fears and anxieties, but these are not the key problems among most ADHD children. Special physical exercises usually try to boost coordination and increase a child's ability to handle activities that can be overstimulating. Most ADHD children do have problems in these areas, but this is not the cause of ADHD. While these exercises may help, they seem to work mostly because they get parents to pay more attention to the child, which boosts self-esteem.

In addition to more traditional treatments, there are a range of controversial therapies that may sound reasonable. Some come with glowing reports, and a few are outright quackery. Some are developed by reputable doctors or specialists but when tested scientifically, the results cannot be proven.

One of the most widely used controversial treatments is a special diet based on the unproven idea that certain foods cause ADHD. These diets look at specific groups of foods, such as additives, sugar, and foods to which children are commonly allergic, such as corn, nuts, chocolate, shellfish, or wheat. While there is scientific evidence that these diets do not work, many parents strongly believe they help. Some of these diets are healthy and will not hurt, but most experts agree that no special diet alone can solve the problems of ADHD and should not be used as the only treatment for a child's behavior.

Other types of treatment that have not been scientifically shown to be effective in treating the majority of children or adults with ADHD include:

- biofeedback
- allergy treatments
- drug treatments for inner ear problems
- megadoses of vitamins
- chiropractic treatments
- yeast infection treatment
- eye training or special colored glasses

ADHD occurs in children with all levels of intelligence, yet even bright or gifted children with ADHD may experience school failure. Despite their natural ability, problems with inattentiveness, impulsivity, and hyperactivity often lead to poor grades, retention, suspension, and expulsion. Without proper diagnosis, accommodations, and intervention, children with ADHD are more likely to experience negative consequences.

Children suspected of having ADHD must be evaluated at the school's expense and, if found to be eligible, provided services under either of two federal laws, the Individuals with Disabilities Education Act, Part B [IDEA] and Section 504 of the Rehabilitation Act of 1973. These two laws guarantee children with ADHD a free and appropriate public education. Both laws also require that children with disabilities be educated to the maximum extent appropriate with children who do not have disabilities. Because there are different criteria for eligibility, different services available, different procedures for implementing the laws, and different procedural safeguards, it is important for parents, educators, clinicians, and advocates to be well aware of the variations between these laws and to be fully informed about their respective advantages and disadvantages.

The most substantial difference between these two laws is that eligibility for IDEA mandates that a child have a disability requiring special education services, while eligibility for Section 504 may occur when the child needs special accommodations or related services. Because of this distinction, children covered under Section 504 include those who typically either have less severe disabilities than those covered under IDEA or have disabilities that do not neatly fit within the categories of eligibility under IDEA. Most students classified as ADHD are served under the Rehabilitation Act.

Some of the services that could be provided to eligible children include modified instructions, assignments, and testing; help from a classroom aide or a special education teacher; assistive technology; behavior management; and the development of a behavioral intervention plan.

Adjustments may be necessary for a child with ADHD in the classroom, such as having the child sit in front of the room so as to help him pay better attention. The teacher can try to limit open spaces in the classroom, which may encourage hyperactive behaviors. Teachers should provide clear instructions and have the child write down homework assignments in a notebook. Both parent and teacher should keep oral instructions brief and provide written instructions for tasks that involve many steps.

Formal feedback and reward programs (such as a star chart) can be used to reinforce positive behaviors and progress even if it falls a little short of the goal. The child should work hard on organization, establishing daily checklists.

Parents and teachers also can help the child with ADHD:

- *Control impulses* Urge him to slow down when answering questions and to check his homework before turning it in.
- *Foster self-esteem* The child should be encouraged and not be asked to perform a task in public that is too difficult.
- *Design a specific behavior program* that focuses on a few unacceptable behaviors with clear and consistent consequences. These consequences should not be publicly humiliating (hand signals can warn a child that his behavior is inappropriate).
- *Encourage active learning* by having the child underline important passages in his school books as he reads and to take notes in class.

Even when suspended or expelled, children covered by IDEA are still entitled to education services that meet the standards of a free appropriate education. Parents can request an impartial due process hearing when they disagree with a school's decision.

Under a separate provision, a child can remain in the then-current educational placement until all administrative proceedings are concluded, unless the child has brought a weapon or drugs to school or is proven to be substantially likely to harm himself or others.

If a child's behavior interferes with learning, IDEA requires that a functional behavior analysis be conducted and a positive behavior plan be developed. IDEA prohibits schools from suspending such a child for more than 10 days or expelling students whose behavior results from their disability, unless drugs or weapons are involved or the child is a danger to himself or others.

Attention Deficit Information Network, Inc. A nonprofit volunteer organization offering information to families of children and adults with ADD, and professionals, through a network of Attention Deficit Information Network (AD-IN) chapters. AD-IN was founded in 1988 by several parent support group leaders. Today it acts as a community resource for information on training programs and speakers for those who work with individuals with ADD.

The organization also presents conferences and workshops for parents and professionals on current issues, research, and treatments for ADD and makes an annual, postsecondary scholarship award. (For contact information see Appendix I.)

Augmentin An antibiotic that combines AMOXI-CILLIN and clavulanate potassium to treat infections of the lower respiratory tract, middle ear, sinus, skin, and urinary tract caused by certain specific bacteria. Augmentin ES-600 is a stronger, oral-suspension form of the drug that is prescribed for certain stubborn ear infections if previous treatment has failed to clear up the infections in children two and under, or those attending day care.

A doctor should be consulted before giving Augmentin to any child who is allergic to either PENI-CILLIN or cephalosporin antibiotics in any form. Children who are allergic to penicillin or cephalosporin may also be allergic to Augmentin, and if a reaction occurs it could be extremely severe.

Side Effects

While Augmentin and other penicillin-like medicines are generally safe, anyone with liver, kidney, or blood disorders is at increased risk when using this drug. More common side effects may include diarrhea/loose stools, nausea, skin rashes, and hives.

autism This complex developmental disorder of brain function causes impaired social interaction, problems with verbal and nonverbal communication, and unusual or severely limited activities and interests. Symptoms of autism usually appear during the first three years of childhood and continue throughout life. Although there is no cure, appropriate early educational intervention may improve social development and reduce undesirable behaviors.

The result of a neurological communication disorder that affects the functioning of the brain, autism and its associated behaviors have been estimated to occur in an estimated 10 to 20 of every 10,000 people, depending on the diagnostic criteria used. Most estimates that include people with similar disorders are two to three times greater. The condition is four times more common in boys than girls and is not related to race, ethnic origin, family income, lifestyle, or education.

Autism significantly impairs a child's ability to communicate and socialize with others. While severity and symptoms vary according to age, the disorder is significant and sustained. The mildest forms of autism resemble a personality disorder associated with a perceived learning disability. The most severe cases are marked by extremely repetitive, unusual, self-injurious, and aggressive behavior that may persist and prove very difficult to change, posing a tremendous challenge to those who must live with, treat, and teach these individuals.

Children with autistic disorder demonstrate little interest in friends or social interactions, often failing to develop verbal and nonverbal communication skills. Typically, these children function at a low intellectual level; most experience mild to severe mental retardation. About half of people with autism score below 50 on IQ tests, 20 percent score between 50 and 70, and 30 percent score higher than 70. However, estimating IQ in young children with autism is often difficult because problems with language and behavior can interfere with testing.

However, this is by no means true for all individuals with autistic disorder; the condition may be accompanied by average or strong abilities in an isolated area such as reading or computation. A small percentage of people with autism are savants, with limited but extraordinary skills in areas like music, mathematics, drawing, or visualization.

During the course of childhood and adolescence, children with this condition usually make some developmental gains. Those who show improvement in language and intellectual ability have the best overall outlook. Although some individuals with autism are able to live with some measure of partial independence in adulthood, very few are able to live entirely on their own.

Cause

Autism impacts the normal development of the brain in the areas of social interaction and communication skills. Although a single specific cause of autism is not known, current research links autism to biological or neurological differences in the brain.

Studies of people with autism have found abnormalities in several regions of the brain, including the cerebellum, amygdala, hippocampus, septum, and mamillary bodies. Neurons in these regions appear smaller than normal and have stunted nerve fibers, which may interfere with nerve signaling. These abnormalities suggest that autism results from disruption of normal brain development early in fetal development. Other studies suggest that people with autism have abnormalities of serotonin or other neurotransmitters in the brain. However, these findings are preliminary and require further study.

In a few cases, disorders such as FRAGILE X SYNDROME, tuberous sclerosis, untreated PHENYLKETONURIA (PKU), and congenital GERMAN MEASLES cause autistic behavior. Other disorders, including TOURETTE'S SYNDROME, LEARNING DISABILITY, and attention deficit disorder often occur with autism but do not cause it. While people with SCHIZOPHRENIA may show some autistic-like behavior, their symptoms usually do not appear until the late teens or early adulthood. Most people with schizophrenia also have hallucinations and delusions, which do not occur in autism.

In many families there appears to be a pattern of autism or related disabilities—which suggests that there is a genetic basis to the disorder. Although at this time no gene has been directly linked to autism, researchers have identified a number of genes that may play a role in the disorder. Scientists think that the genetic basis is complex and probably involves several combinations of genes.

Scientists estimate that in families with one autistic child, the risk of having a second child with the disorder is about one in 20, which is greater than the risk for the general population. In some cases, parents and other relatives of an autistic person show mild social, communicative, or repetitive behaviors that allow them to function normally but appear to be linked to autism. Evidence also suggests that some emotional disorders occur more frequently than average in families of people with autism.

Autism is NOT a mental illness or a behavior problem, and it is not caused by bad parenting. No known psychological factors in the development of the child have been shown to cause autism.

Symptoms

Characteristics of autism can appear in a wide variety of combinations from mild to severe, but the primary feature of autism is impaired social interaction. Although autism is defined by a certain set of behaviors, children and adults can exhibit any combination of behaviors in any degree of severity. Two children with the same diagnosis can act very differently from one another and have varying skills.

Children and adults with autism typically have problems in verbal and nonverbal communication, social interactions, and leisure or play activities.

- *Communication* Language develops slowly or not at all; uses words without attaching the usual meaning; communicates with gestures instead of words; short attention span

- *Social interaction*   Spends time alone rather than with others; shows little interest in making friends; less responsive to social cues such as eye contact or smiles

- *Sensory impairment* May have overly sensitive sight, hearing, touch, smell, and taste

- *Play* Lack of spontaneous or imaginative play; does not imitate others or initiate pretend games

- *Behavior* May be overactive or very passive; throw tantrums for no apparent reason; show an obsessive interest in a single item, idea, activity, or person; lack common sense, show aggression, often has difficulty with changes in routine.

The disorder makes it hard for children to communicate with others and relate to the outside world. There may be repeated body movements (hand flapping, rocking), unusual responses to people or attachments to objects, and resistance to changes in routines. In some cases, there may be aggressive or self-injurious behavior. Autism may affect a child's range of responses and make it more difficult to control how their bodies and minds react. Sometimes visual, motor, or processing problems make it hard for these children to maintain eye contact, and some use peripheral vision rather than looking directly at others. Sometimes touching or being close to others may be painful to a person with autism. Because they cannot make sense of the world in a normal way, people with autism may experience anxiety, fear, and confusion.

In addition, people with autism may have other disorders that affect brain function, such as EPILEPSY, MENTAL RETARDATION, DOWN SYNDROME or genetic disorders such as FRAGILE X SYNDROME or TOURETTE'S SYNDROME.

Symptoms in many children with autism improve with treatment or age. Some people with autism eventually lead normal or near-normal lives. The teen years may worsen behavior problems in some children with autism, who may become depressed or increasingly unmanageable. Parents should be ready to adjust treatment for their child's changing needs.

Diagnosis

Autism is classified as one of the pervasive developmental disorders. Because it varies widely in its severity and symptoms, autism may go unrecognized, especially in mildly affected individuals or in those with multiple handicaps.

Because there are no medical tests for autism, an accurate diagnosis must be based on observing the person's communication, behavior, and developmental levels. However, because many of the behaviors associated with autism are similar to other disorders, various medical tests may be ordered to rule out or identify other possible causes of symptoms.

Because the characteristics of the disorder vary, a child should be evaluated by a team including a neurologist, psychologist, developmental pediatrician, speech/language therapist, occupational therapist, or other professionals experienced in autism. Problems in recognizing autism often lead to a lack of services to meet the complex needs of these individuals.

It is important to include history from parents and caregivers in coming to an accurate diagnosis. Some people with autism may seem to have developmental disabilities, a behavior disorder, problems with hearing, or eccentric behavior. It is important to distinguish autism from other conditions, since early identification is required for an effective treatment program.

Specific diagnostic categories have changed over the years as research progresses and as new editions of the DSM (Diagnostic and Statistical Manual) have been issued. Some frequently used criteria include:

- Absence or impairment of imaginative and social play
- Impaired ability to make friends with peers
- Impaired ability to initiate or sustain a conversation with others
- Stereotyped, repetitive, or unusual use of language
- Restricted patterns of interests that are abnormal in intensity or focus
- Apparently inflexible adherence to specific routines or rituals
- Preoccupation with parts of objects

Children with some symptoms of autism, but not enough to be diagnosed with the classical form of the disorder, are often diagnosed with PERVASIVE DEVELOPMENTAL DISORDER—not otherwise specified (PDD—NOS). People with autistic behavior but well-developed language skills are often diagnosed with ASPERGER SYNDROME. Children who appear normal in their first several years but then lose skills and begin showing autistic behavior may be diagnosed with childhood disintegrative disorder (CDD). Girls with RETT SYNDROME, a sex-linked genetic disorder characterized by inadequate brain growth, seizures, and other neurological problems, also may show autistic behavior.

PDD—NOS, Asperger's disorder, CDD, and Rett syndrome are referred to as "autism spectrum disorders."

Since hearing problems can be confused with autism, children with delayed speech development should always have their hearing checked, although children may have hearing problems in addition to autism.

Treatment

While there is no "cure" for the brain abnormalities that cause autism, patients can learn coping mechanisms and strategies to ease various symptoms. With appropriate treatment, many problem behaviors can be changed so that the child may appear to no longer have autism. However, most patients continue to show some faint symptoms to some degree throughout their entire lives. The best-studied therapies include educational/behavioral and medical interventions. Although these treatments do not cure autism, they often bring about substantial improvement.

Early intervention is crucial, and can provide dramatic improvements for young children with autism. While various preschool models may differ, all emphasize early, appropriate, and intensive educational interventions for young children. Other common factors may be

- Some degree of inclusion, mostly behaviorally based interventions
- Programs that build on the interests of the child
- Extensive use of visuals to accompany instruction
- Structured activities
- Parent and staff training
- Transition planning
- Follow-up

Studies show that individuals with autism respond well to a highly structured, specialized education program tailored to individual needs. A well-designed treatment approach may include work on communication and social skills, sensory integration therapy, and applied behavior analysis by autism experts.

More severely ill children may require a structured, intensive education and behavior program with a one-on-one teacher to student ratio. However, many other children with autism may do well in a normal education environment with appropriate support.

Because of the nature of autism, no single approach can ease symptoms in all cases. Educational/behavioral interventions emphasize highly structured and often intensive skill-oriented training tailored to the individual child. Therapists work with children to help them develop social and language skills. Because children learn most effectively and rapidly when very young, this type of therapy should begin as early as possible. Recent evidence suggests that early intervention has a good chance of favorably influencing brain development.

In addition, doctors may prescribe a variety of drugs to reduce self-injurious behavior or other troublesome symptoms of autism, as well as associated conditions such as epilepsy and attention disorders. Most of these drugs affect levels of serotonin, dopamine, or other signaling chemicals in the brain.

Many other interventions are available, but few, if any, scientific studies support their use. These therapies include applied auditory integration training, special diets, discrete trial teaching, music therapy, physical therapy, speech/language therapy, and vision therapy. Some of these treatments are controversial and may or may not reduce a specific person's symptoms. Parents should use caution before subscribing to any particular treatment. Counseling for the families of people with autism also may assist them in coping with the disorder.

In addition to an academic program, children with autism should be trained in functional living skills at the earliest possible age. Learning to cross a street, to buy something in a store, or ask for help are critical skills and may be hard even for those with average intelligence. Training is aimed at boosting a person's independence and providing opportunity for personal choice and freedom.

Prognosis

Contrary to popular belief, many children and adults with autism can make eye contact and can show affection and demonstrate a variety of other emotions in varying degrees. Like other children, they respond to their environment in both positive and negative ways. With appropriate treatment, some behaviors associated with autism may lessen over time. Although communication and social problems will continue in some form throughout life, difficulties in other areas may improve with age, education, or stress level. Many individuals with autism enjoy their lives and contribute to their community in a meaningful way, as they learn to compensate for and cope with their disability.

Some adults with autism live and work independently in the community, can drive a car, earn a college degree, and even get married. Some may only need some support for daily pressure, while others require a great deal of support from family and professionals.

Adults with autism may live in a variety of residential settings ranging from an independent home or apartment to group homes, supervised apartment settings, with other family members, or in more structured residential care.

More and more support groups for adults with autism are appearing, and many patients are forming their own networks to share information, support each other, and speak for themselves. Individuals with autism (such as animal scientist Temple Grandin, Ph.D.) are providing valuable insight into the challenges of this disability by publishing articles and books and appearing on TV to discuss their lives and experiences.

Autism Society of America   A nonprofit organization that seeks to promote lifelong access and opportunities for persons within the AUTISM spectrum and their families, to be fully included, participating members of their communities through advocacy, public awareness, education, and research related to autism.

Founded in 1965 by a small group of parents, the society has been the leading source of information and referral on autism and the largest collective voice representing the autism community for more than 33 years. Today more than 24,000 members are connected through a volunteer network of more than 240 chapters in 50 states. (For contact information, see Appendix I.)

Autism Society of America Foundation (ASAF)
A fund-raising organization founded in 1996 by the AUTISM SOCIETY OF AMERICA, the largest and

oldest organization representing people with AUTISM. The ASAF was established to raise and allocate funds for research to address the many unanswered questions about autism.

The ASAF has implemented action on several autism research priorities, such as developing up-to-date statistics; developing a national registry of individuals and families with autism who are willing to participate in research studies; and implementing a system to identify potential donors of autism brain tissue for research purposes and facilitating the donation process. In addition, the foundation contributes money for applied and biomedical research in the causes of and treatment approaches to autism. (For contact information, see Appendix I.)

Aveeno bath   A range of moisturizers, cleansers, and bath additives that are formulated from oatmeal, which has been used for centuries for its natural, soothing anti-itching action. All Aveeno products are specially formulated for dry and sensitive skin, and they are particularly effective in helping to relieve the itch associated with many skin conditions such as CHICKEN POX, HIVES, RASHES, PSORIASIS, POISON IVY, and so on. Aveeno products are safe for children and babies.

babesiosis (babesiasis) A rare, sometimes fatal disease caused by a tick-borne virus similar to both LYME DISEASE and human granulocytic ehrlichiosis (HGE). Also known as Nantucket fever, it is most often seen in the elderly and those with impaired immune systems. Severe cases have been diagnosed in those who have had their spleen removed.

Most cases of babesiosis have been reported in summer and fall in the northeastern United States, especially Nantucket, Massachusetts; Shelter Island, New York; and nearby islands. However, cases have recently been identified in the upper Midwest, the Pacific Coast states, and Europe. A related species has caused a babesiosis-like illness in Washington and California.

The protozoa causing babesiosis was first identified by Roman bacteriologist Victor Babes, for whom the organism and the disease was named.

Cause

Babesiosis is caused by protozoa similar to those that cause MALARIA (the species *Babesia microti*); it is passed via the bite of ticks of the species *Ixodes dammini*. The tick is carried by meadow voles, mice, and deer. The disease can also be transmitted via contaminated blood transfusions.

Symptoms

Babesiosis typically causes mild illness in otherwise healthy people, but it can be overwhelming to those with impaired immune systems. Within one to 12 months after infection, symptoms appear, including fever, fatigue, and hemolytic anemia lasting from several days to several months. A person may also have the disease with no symptoms at all. It is not known if a past infection renders a patient immune.

Diagnosis

Molecular tests are being developed, but currently the disease is diagnosed by microscopic examination of blood smears.

Treatment

Standardized treatments have not been developed; however, a combination of ANTIMALARIAL DRUGS such as quinine and an antibiotic (clindamycin) are usually the drugs of choice.

Prevention

The spread of babesiosis can be curtailed with the control of rodents around houses and the use of tick repellents.

bacillary dysentery See SHIGELLOSIS.

backpacks The popularity of carrying books in a backpack is almost universal in American schools, but overloading the packs can be harmful. Some studies have shown that as many as half of all teenagers suffer from back pain, which may be caused by the improper use of backpacks. While many factors may cause back pain, such as increased level of competition in sports, poor posture while sitting, and long periods of inactivity, far too many children are also carrying backpacks that exceed 15 percent of the child's body weight. Therefore, a 60-pound child should carry no more than nine pounds of books on the back.

Backpacks can be a helpful tool if they are used properly, since they can help children stay organized while toting their books and papers from home to school and back again. Compared to shoulder bags or purses, backpacks are better because the strongest muscles in the body, the back and the abdominal muscles, support the weight of the pack. Because the weight is evenly distributed across the child's body, shoulder and neck injuries are less common than if the child carried a briefcase.

When a backpack is too heavy, the child arches the back or leans the head and body forward to compensate for the weight of the bag. This stresses the muscles in the neck and back, increasing the risk of injury. Using only one strap, as many youngsters do, affects the spine's natural shock absorption abilities.

Most doctors and physical therapists recommend that children carry no more than 10 percent to 15 percent of their body weight in their packs.

Girls and younger children may be especially at risk for backpack-related injuries because they are smaller and may carry loads that are heavier in proportion to their body weight.

A backpack is too heavy if the child has to struggle to get a backpack on or off, has back pain, has to lean forward to carry a pack, or has numbness or weakness in arms or legs.

The safest backpack has two wide, padded straps that go over the shoulders, a padded waist or chest belt to distribute weight more evenly across the body, multiple compartments to distribute the weight of the load, and is not wider than the child's body. Backpacks with a metal frame are a good choice, but many lockers will not accommodate a pack that large. No matter how well designed the backpack, children need to keep the backpack loads reasonable.

Newest backpacks have wheels and allow students to roll, rather than carry, books and other materials.

A child should be encouraged to visit a locker or desk often throughout the day instead of carrying the entire day's worth of books in a backpack. Children should not carry unnecessary items such as laptops, CD players, and video games. If a child does have to carry something heavy in the pack, it should be placed closer to the back of the pack, next to the body.

As with any heavy weight, a child should bend at the knees and grab the pack with both hands when lifting it to his shoulders. Another way to prevent back injury is to strengthen the stabilizing muscles in the lower back and abdomen. Weight training and yoga can help strengthen the core muscles.

bacteremia The presence of bacteria in the bloodstream, which is a common occurrence a few hours after minor surgery. It may also occur with such infections as TONSILLITIS. If a child's immune system has been weakened, either by illness or by major surgery, the presence of bacteria in the blood may lead to SEPTICEMIA and shock. In those with abnormal heart valves because of rheumatic fever or a congenital defect, the bacteria may cause endocarditis. Bacteremia usually resolves without treatment.

In children under the age of 24 months, bacteremia accounts for about 10 percent of all cases of fever over 101.3°F. If a child this age runs a fever without localized signs, a blood test is usually taken.

bacteria Neither plants nor animals, bacteria are microbes whose nuclei are not enclosed in thin tissue like plants or animals. Some bacteria feed on other organisms, some make their own food (as plants do), and some bacteria do both. Some need air to survive and others exist without air (anaerobic). Some move by themselves, and others cannot move at all. Bacteria also come in a variety of shapes, colors, sizes, and ways of living. Some of the more serious types of bacterial infections include GONORRHEA, MENINGITIS, WHOOPING COUGH, PNEUMONIA, and TUBERCULOSIS. Bacteria are of incredible importance because of their extreme flexibility, capacity for rapid growth and reproduction, and their ancient age—the oldest known fossils are those of bacteria-like organisms that lived nearly three-and-a-half billion years ago.

It is important to remember that not all bacteria are harmful; most are helpful, such as those that break down dead plant and animal matter in the soil. Some (like the actinomycetes) produce antibiotics such as streptomycin and nocardicin. Plants cannot grow without nitrogen, and bacteria help nitrogen to form in the soil. Bacteria are also used to make cheese out of milk, and leather out of animal hide. Grazing animals use bacteria in their stomachs to digest grass.

Bacteria can be found in the air, the water, food, and everyday objects. Since few of these are harmful, humans are seldom bothered by them.

When harmful bacteria do enter the body, the immune system most of the time can kill the invading microbes.

Unfortunately, bacteria are beginning to become resistant to many of the antibiotics doctors use to treat the infections. A 1996 World Health Organization report found that drug-resistant strains of microbes causing MALARIA, TUBERCULOSIS, PNEUMONIA, CHOLERA, and diarrhea are on the rise. Strong new types of microbes in the United States cause up to 60 percent of hospital-acquired infections, the report adds.

The problem occurs when antibiotics are prescribed when they are not needed, or when patients do not take the full course of medication, allowing a few microbes to survive.

bacterial endocarditis An infection of the lining of the heart that may occur in any infant or child, whether or not there is any heart disease present. Bacterial endocarditis does not occur very often, but when it does, it can cause serious heart damage, so it is important to prevent this infection if possible.

Cause
Bacterial endocarditis is caused by bacteria that enter the blood, lodging inside the heart where they multiply and cause infection. A normal heart has a smooth lining that is hard for bacteria to attach to, but children with congenital heart disease may have a roughened area on the heart lining caused by pressure from an abnormal opening or a leaky valve. Even after surgery, roughened areas may remain as a result of scar tissue formation or patches used to redirect blood flow. These rough areas make perfect places for bacteria to build up and multiply.

Bacteria that cause this problem may get into the blood during dental procedures, tonsillectomy, or ADENOIDECTOMY, examination of the respiratory passageways with a rigid bronchoscope, or during certain types of surgery on the respiratory passageways, the gastrointestinal tract, or the urinary tract.

Any infant or child who has congenital heart disease that has not yet been repaired can develop bacterial endocarditis. Some children who have already had a heart defect repaired may also need to take precautions against bacterial endocarditis

for the rest of their lives, while others may no longer need to observe these precautions. Heart problems that put children at risk for developing bacterial endocarditis include mitral valve prolapse, having artificial heart valves, a previous history of endocarditis, complex cyanotic congenital heart disease due to insufficient oxygen in the blood, and surgically constructed systemic pulmonary shunts. Other heart problems linked to endocarditis may include acquired valve dysfunction, such as is due to rheumatic heart disease or collagen vascular disease, or an enlarged heart muscle that causes impeded blood flow.

Diagnosis
In addition to a complete medical history and physical examination of the child, diagnostic procedures may include echocardiogram, a complete blood count (CBC), and a blood culture to assess the specific type of bacteria in the bloodstream, if any.

Prevention
Helping children maintain excellent oral hygiene is an important step in preventing bacterial endocarditis. Regular visits to the dentist for professional cleaning and checkups are essential. Proper oral hygiene is crucial, including regular brushing and flossing.

One dose of an antibiotic is often given prior to any procedure that would put a child at risk with a follow-up dose six hours after the procedure. In most cases, the antibiotics can be given by mouth.

Treatment
Specific treatment is based on the child's age, overall health, and medical history; the extent and cause of the infection; the child's tolerance for procedures or treatments; and how the child's doctor expects the infection to progress. In most cases, the infection is treated with strong antibiotics given through an IV over the course of several weeks. However, heart damage may still occur before the infection can be controlled.

bacterial pneumonia See PNEUMONIA.

bed-wetting Known medically as nocturnal enuresis, this is the inability of a child to control urinating at night. Some children do not attain nighttime control for several years after they have been completely potty trained during the day. In fact, bed-wetting is not considered abnormal until after age five, and even then the situation eventually improves on its own.

Bed-wetting occurs in 15 to 20 percent of all five-year-old children, for an estimated 5 to 6 million children. About 15 percent of these problems will fade away on their own in each subsequent year, so that only 1 to 2 percent of adolescents by age 15 still wet at night. Moreover, 20 percent of children with this problem have some element of daytime wetting.

Cause

Bed-wetting is not a behavioral problem, nor is it related to how a child sleeps. Instead, bed-wetting is caused by a developmental delay in the normal process of achieving control at night. Normally, a hormone called vasopressin is released that prompts the kidneys to slow down production of urine during sleep. Many children who have a problem with staying dry at night do not secrete enough of this hormone. Researchers also have discovered some genetic links that suggest heredity may play a role.

Diagnosis

Any child over age five who is still wetting the bed should be examined by a pediatric urologist to ensure that there are no other underlying problems that may be causing the problem, such as bladder instability or posterior urethral valves. Because between 18 and 39 percent of children have symptoms of bladder instability, a careful history of the child's complete urinating and bowel habits will be important.

Other studies may include an X ray that examines the urinary tract, called a voiding cystourethrogram (VCUG), a renal bladder ultrasound, or a urodynamics study to assess how the bladder and urethral sphincter function in accordance with the brain and spinal cord during the stages of bladder filling and emptying.

Treatment

Because there are several theories about what causes bed-wetting, there are a variety of treatments based on the premise of each of these theo-ries. There is not one proven theory or treatment that is successful all the time. Often a combination of treatments are needed to control the problem. On the other hand, bed-wetting will eventually stop on its own without specific treatment. Bed-wetting is not harmful to a child in any way other than its impact on self-esteem. A child who is embarrassed to attend camp or a sleepover may benefit from treatment that includes restricting fluids after 6 P.M., conditioning therapy using a bed-wetting alarm, drug therapy to replace vasopressin, or psychotherapy.

Benadryl   See ANTIHISTAMINES.

benzoyl peroxide   An antibacterial agent that is considered to be the most effective nonprescription ACNE treatment, suppressing the bacterium *Propionibacterium acnes* associated with acne. This extremely effective topical antibacterial agent draws peroxide into the pore where it releases oxygen, killing the bacteria that can aggravate acne. Benzoyl also suppresses fatty acid cells that irritate pores and helps to unplug blocked pores. It is most effective for teenagers with inflammatory acne; by inhibiting bacteria, it decreases the inflammation in the skin.

Benzoyl peroxide is usually sold in strengths ranging between 5 percent and 10 percent, but dermatologists usually advise patients to start with a 5 percent product. The lower concentration is just as effective and is less likely to cause irritation.

Most over-the-counter products contain benzoyl peroxide in a lotion base; the prescription items contain the chemical in a gel base. A fairly new prescription preparation combining 3 percent erythromycin with a 5 percent benzoyl peroxide in a gel base may be more effective than either component by itself.

Side Effects

Its safety for children under age 12 has not been established. Because benzoyl peroxide is a bleach, it will discolor most fabrics and hair. Most patients experience some burning, itching, or peeling, but benzoyl peroxide can produce a stronger reaction in some people with very sensitive or very fair skin. It is normal to experience a warm or stinging feeling, with some dryness or peeling, but if the skin turns very red, or there is pain, a lot of scaling, and swelling, an adverse reaction has occurred and the product should not be used.

The stronger the product, the greater the chance of a reaction. Benzoyl peroxide should never be applied near the eyes, where it can cause swelling or irritation. Hands should be thoroughly washed after using the product, and eyes should never be rubbed with contaminated fingers.

Some studies have reported that benzoyl peroxide is carcinogenic, although this conclusion is controversial and inconclusive.

bike safety Each year, nearly one million children are treated for bicycle-related injuries in U.S. hospitals, and almost half of all bicyclist deaths occur to children age 16 or younger. One in seven children suffers head injuries in bicycle-related accidents. Each state has its own bike regulations, which usually govern equipment, safety features, and rules of the road.

In order to ride safely, it is important to ride a bike that is the right size. The bike, which should have a bell or horn, should not be too big or complicated, and the child should be able to place the balls of the feet on the ground when sitting on the seat.

Rules of the Road

Bike riders should stop before riding into traffic from a driveway, sidewalk, parking lot, or other street. They should ride on the far right of the road, with traffic, and be visible to cars by wearing brightly colored clothes, especially at night. Bikes should not be ridden in the dark, or during bad weather. Children who do ride at night should be sure to have a headlight, a flashing taillight, and reflectors.

Helmet Standards

It is imperative that every child wear a safety helmet when riding a bike. Seventeen states and more than 55 localities in the United States have mandatory helmet laws, as do parts of Canada. As long as they are fitted securely and buckled during a crash, a helmet can prevent up to 88 percent of cyclists' brain injuries.

When buying a helmet, consumers should check for safety approval, since helmet standards test for things that cannot be judged in a store, like impact performance and strap strength. The U.S. Consumer Product Safety Commission's bike helmet standard is law for every helmet made after March 1999. A bike helmet may carry approvals by the American National Standards Institute (ANSI), the American Society for Testing and Materials (ASTM), or the U.S. Consumer Product Safety Commission (CPSC).

The helmet should fit the child's head so that when the straps are snug, the helmet does not move. The front edge of the helmet should be two finger widths above the eyebrows. Front and back straps of the helmet should form a V just below the ear, and front straps should be vertical and the rear straps should be flat. The chin strap should be snug when the child opens the mouth (one finger should fit between the chin and chin strap when the mouth is closed).

For younger children, it is possible to find many types of helmets designed for ages one to five. However, there are no tiny helmets on the market for children under age one because nobody recommends taking a very young infant on a bicycle.

A helmet should be replaced after a bike accident, if it is more than 20 years old, if the outside is just foam or cloth instead of plastic, if it lacks a CPSC, ASTM, or Snell sticker, or if it cannot be made to fit correctly.

Some helmets are "multisport," which can be used for in-line skating, skateboarding, bicycling, or other wheel sports. Helmets that specifically are called "bicycle helmets" are designed only for that sport. Helmets come in many sizes and varieties. They also are equipped with sponge pads that adjust to fit the head.

bilirubin A substance produced when red blood cells are broken down. Usually the bilirubin is taken up by the liver and then excreted. However, the liver of newborn babies is immature and cannot do a good job of getting rid of bilirubin, so it remains in the blood, making the skin appear yellow. These babies are then diagnosed with JAUNDICE, which is very common among newborns.

Occasionally the bilirubin level is so high it can be dangerous to the brain, especially if the mother's and baby's blood types are different. In addition to the A and B antigens possibly present on a baby's red cells, there is another class of protein called the Rh antigen. If a mother has Rh-negative blood (which means she does not have the Rh antigen on her blood cells), but she carries a fetus whose blood type is Rh-positive, cells from the baby can migrate across the placental barrier and stimulate the production of a maternal antibody that can cross back into the baby's system and trigger the destruction of the baby's red blood cells. This is termed hemolytic anemia. The resultant flood of bilirubin from the breakdown of these red cells overwhelms the baby's ability to cleanse the bloodstream of bilirubin.

Usually, the abnormal antibody poses little threat to the first Rh-positive baby born to an Rh-negative mother. However, subsequent Rh-positive babies are at risk. Fortunately, this problem is now very rare due to an immunization given to Rh-negative mothers after delivery of an Rh-positive baby. This shot (RhoGam) blocks the formation of high levels of the abnormal anti-Rh antibody and protects subsequent pregnancies with a high degree of efficiency. The degree of jaundice can be measured by a simple blood test. If treatment is necessary, allowing the newborn to sleep under fluorescent lights or under a special "light blanket" usually resolves the problem.

binge eating disorder An EATING DISORDER that resembles BULIMIA but without the vomiting (purging). Girls with binge eating disorder feel that they lose control of themselves when eating, gorging themselves with huge amounts of food until they are uncomfortably full. Usually, they have more problem losing weight and keeping it off than do girls with ANOREXIA or bulimia. In fact, most girls with the disorder are obese and have a history of weight fluctuations. About 3 percent of all teenage girls develop binge eating disorder.

Girls with this condition are usually overweight, so they are prone to the serious medical problems associated with obesity. They also tend to have high rates of other psychiatric illnesses, especially DEPRESSION.

bioterrorism and children Children are at particular risk when exposed to biological weapons, and the time available for treatment is much shorter than for adults. Although the effects of bioterrorism weapons such as ANTHRAX and SMALLPOX are the same for children as for adults, children are particularly susceptible to these agents because of their size and stage of development.

The severity of the effect depends on the stage of life. Very young children are most likely to suffer severe effects because they have a faster breathing rate, a higher skin-to-mass ratio, more permeable skin, and less fluid reserve.

Although public health authorities are not recommending large-scale smallpox vaccination for children, the vaccine is available if needed. Treatment guidelines also are in place for possible anthrax exposure, in which antibiotics would be administered in appropriate doses for children to prevent disease.

bipolar disorder Popularly known as "manic depression," this condition is characterized by manic episodes alternating with DEPRESSION. Mood swings are often dramatic and unpredictable. Almost one-third of six- to 12-year-old children diagnosed with major depression will develop bipolar disorders within a few years.

Because the manic periods (with impulsive behavior and bursts of energy) can be similar to symptoms of ATTENTION DEFICIT HYPERACTIVITY DISORDER, a good diagnosis is important for any child experiencing repeated episodes of mania or depression. The feelings of depression, inadequacy, fatigue, and sadness are also similar to emotions experienced by children with other disorders.

While everyone experiences normal mood changes during everyday life, bipolar disorder is a medical condition in which people have mood swings totally unrelated to things going on in their lives. These swings affect thoughts, feelings, physical health, behavior, and functioning.

Bipolar disorder, which affects about 1 percent of the adult population of the United States, is in the same family of illnesses (called "affective disorders") as clinical depression. Unlike depression, which affects more girls than boys, bipolar disorder seems to affect boys and girls equally.

For a clinical definition of bipolar disorder, symptoms must include one or more manic episodes accompanied by one or more major depressive episodes, which usually occur in cycles.

Cause

Bipolar disorder usually begins in adolescence or early adulthood, although it can sometimes start in early childhood. There is no single, proven cause of bipolar disorder, but research strongly suggests that it is often an inherited problem related to a lack of stability in the transmission of nerve impulses in the brain. This biochemical problem makes people with bipolar disorder more vulnerable to emotional and physical stresses. This means that if a person experiences stress, substance use, lack of sleep, or too much stimulation, the normal brain mechanisms for restoring calm functioning do not always work properly.

Bipolar disorder tends to run in families, and a number of genes have been linked to the condition, suggesting the presence of several different biochemical problems. If one parent has bipolar disorder and the other does not, there is a one in seven chance that the couple's child will develop the condition. The chance may be greater if one spouse has several relatives with bipolar disorder or depression.

Symptoms

A child with bipolar disorder may experience any or all of four different kinds of episodes—mania, mild mania (hypomania), depression, or a combination ("mixed episode").

Mania (manic episode): This episode often begins with a pleasant sense of high energy, creativity, and social confidence, which becomes more intense until it develops into a full-blown manic episode. Children with mania typically lack insight and deny that anything is wrong, angrily blaming anyone who suggests otherwise. A manic episode is characterized by feeling unusually euphoric or irritable for at least a week, plus at least four (and often almost all) of the following symptoms:

- Needing little sleep yet having great amounts of energy
- Talking fast
- Having racing thoughts
- Being easily distracted

- Having an inflated feeling of power, greatness, or importance
- Doing reckless things without concern about possible negative consequences, such as spending too much money or (for teenagers) engaging in inappropriate sexual activity
- Psychotic symptoms may occur in very severe cases, such as hallucinations or delusions

Mild mania (hypomania): This milder form of mania causes similar but less severe symptoms, which often begin with someone feeling better and more productive than usual, but then usually build into a full-blown mania or crash into depression.

Depression (major depressive episode): To be considered a full-blown "major" depressive episode, a child will feel sad and lack interest for at least two weeks, in addition to exhibiting at least four other symptoms:

- Trouble sleeping or sleeping too much
- Loss of appetite or eating too much
- Problems concentrating or making decisions
- Feeling slow or agitated
- Feeling worthless or guilty
- Loss of energy; fatigue
- Thoughts of suicide or death
- Hallucinations or delusions (in severe cases)

Mixed episode: The most disabling episodes are those that include symptoms of both mania and depression at the same time, or that alternate often during the day. A person in this condition will feel excited or agitated but also feel irritable and depressed.

Types of Episodes

Untreated patients with bipolar disorder may have more than 10 total episodes of mania and depression during their lifetime. Often, five years or more may pass between the first and second episode, but the time periods between subsequent episodes get shorter and shorter. However, people do not all experience bipolar disorder in the same way. Some people have equal numbers of manic and depressive episodes; others have mostly one type or the other.

The average person with bipolar disorder has four episodes during the first 10 years of the illness. Boys are more likely to begin with a manic episode, while girls tend to experience depression first. While a number of years can elapse between the first two or three episodes of mania or depression, without treatment most people eventually have episodes more often. Sometimes these follow a seasonal pattern, but a few people cycle frequently or even continuously through the year.

Episodes can last days, months, or sometimes even years. On average, without treatment, manic or mild manic episodes last a few months, while depressions often last well over six months. Some children recover completely between episodes and may go many years without any symptoms, while others continue to have low-grade but troubling depression or mild swings up and down. There are two main types of bipolar disorder:

- *Bipolar I:* the "classic" form of the condition, which most often involves widely spaced, long-lasting bouts of mania followed by long-lasting bouts of depression
- *Bipolar II:* at least one episode of mild mania (hypomania) and one major depressive episode

Although the shifts from one state to another are usually gradual, they can be quite sudden. In this so-called rapid-cycling form of the disorder, a person could experience four or more complete mood cycles within a year's time. Some rapid cyclers can complete a mood cycle in a matter of days (or more rarely, hours). Rapid cycling occurs in between 5 percent and 15 percent of patients.

While there are a few rare documented cases of mania without depression, the DSM-IV does not currently include a category for "mania." Using DSM-IV to diagnose the condition, a person with symptoms of mania will almost always be diagnosed as bipolar.

Diagnosis

Typically, children with bipolar disorder see three or four doctors over at least eight years before being correctly diagnosed. The earlier the diagnosis and proper treatment, the quicker children can be helped and the more likely they will be able to avoid later problems with suicide attempts, alcohol, and substance abuse. In addition, some research suggests that the earlier the treatment the better the outcome; evidence indicates that the

more mood episodes a person has, the harder it is to treat each subsequent episode and the more frequent episodes may become. This is sometimes referred to as "kindling."

Treatment

While there is no cure for bipolar disorder, a combination of drug treatment and therapy can lessen the frequency, severity, and consequences of symptoms and improve functioning between episodes. The two most important types of medication used to control the symptoms of bipolar disorder are mood stabilizers and antidepressants; other medications can help ease insomnia, anxiety, restlessness, or psychotic symptoms.

Mood stabilizers are used to improve manic symptoms, but they also may sometimes ease depression as well. They are the mainstay of long-term preventive treatment for both mania and depression. Three mood stabilizers are widely used in the United States: lithium, valproate, and carbamazepine. Each of the three affects the body differently, so that if one does not work another may prove to be better. For all three, blood tests determine the correct dose.

Traditionally, lithium has been the primary drug treatment for patients with bipolar disorder. Discovered to be effective in 1949, it has been widely used since the mid-1960s for prevention and treatment. Valproate and carbamazepine are newer drugs used for bipolar disorder since the late 1970s.

Although mood stabilizers (especially lithium) can ease depression, many patients also need a specific antidepressant to treat the depressive episode. However, antidepressants alone can sometimes trigger a manic attack or rapid cycling. For this reason, an antidepressant is given together with a mood stabilizer.

Although electroconvulsive therapy (ECT) has received negative publicity, it can be the safest and most effective treatment for psychotic depression. ECT may also be needed if a patient is severely ill and cannot wait for medicine to work, if there have been several unsuccessful attempts with different antidepressants, or if the patient is pregnant or has a health condition that makes drug therapy less safe. Like all treatments, ECT has potential side effects, including a short-term memory loss.

Hospitalization may be needed but usually lasts only a week or two, and it can prevent self-destructive, impulsive, or aggressive behavior. During a depressed phase, hospitalization may be needed if a person becomes suicidal. Hospitalization is also used for people who have medical complications that make it hard to monitor medication or for those who cannot stop using drugs or alcohol. Early recognition and treatment of manic and depressive episodes can lower the chances of hospitalization.

Side Effects

At least half of those who take medication have side effects, especially if high doses and a combination of medicines are needed. Lower doses and fewer medicines help offset symptoms, but some people may have severe enough side effects to require different medicine. Although side effects tend to be worse early in the treatment, some people who have taken lithium for 20 years or more can suddenly develop side effects as they age. Valproate or carbamazepine make excellent alternatives as long the switch is made gradually. Valproate appears to cause the fewest side effects during long-term treatment.

Prevention

Successful management of bipolar disorder can be challenging, especially if a patient wants to stop medication because he feels better, does not like the side effects, or misses the "highs." A patient who stops medication probably will not have an acute episode right away, but eventually a relapse will likely occur, and each episode runs the risk of making it harder to manage subsequent flare-ups.

Sometimes a diagnosis of bipolar disorder is not clear after just one episode, and medication can be tapered off after about a year. However, if a patient has had only one episode of mania but has a very strong family history, or if the episode was severe, experts believe the patient should probably take medication for several years—or for life. After two or more manic or depressive episodes, experts strongly recommend taking preventive medication indefinitely.

About one in three people with bipolar disorder will be completely free of symptoms by taking lithium, valproate, or carbamazepine for life, and most people become ill much less often and much less severely with each episode.

birth defect An abnormality of structure, function, or body metabolism present at birth that results in physical or mental disability, or death. Birth defects may range from mild to severe, and some may be life threatening; they may leave a child unable to walk, to hear, to think, or to fight off disease.

Birth defects are the leading cause of death in the first year of life. About 150,000 babies are born in the United States each year with birth defects. Birth defects may occur in babies anywhere in the world, to families of any nationality. While the normal risk of birth defects in any pregnancy is about three or four percent, in families with a genetic history of birth defects the risk is much higher.

The rate of birth defects–associated deaths declined over the past decade, which may reflect improvements in medical and surgical care, better prenatal diagnosis and subsequent pregnancy termination, and underreporting of deaths associated with birth defects. Birth defects were the leading cause of infant mortality, accounting for about 20 percent of all infant deaths, but a substantial percentage of deaths of older children were also related to birth defects.

Types

About three or four out of every 100 babies are born with at least one of the more than 4,000 known types of birth defects. Birth defects of the heart and circulatory system affect more infants than any other type; about one in 115 babies born each year has heart or circulatory defects. The next most common type of birth defect include:

- problems with muscles or the skeleton, one of every 130 births
- genital and urinary tract problems, one in 135
- nervous system and eye problems, one in 235
- chromosome syndromes, one in 600
- club foot, one in 735
- Down syndrome, one in 900
- respiratory tract problems, one in 900

- cleft lip or palate, one in 930
- spina bifida, one in 2,000
- metabolic disorders, one in 3,500
- anencephaly, one in 8,000
- PKU, one in 12,000

When a baby has a structural birth defect, some part of the body (internal or external) is missing or malformed. Heart defects are the most common type of structural birth defect. While advances in surgical treatment have dramatically improved the outlook for babies with heart defects, these remain the leading cause of birth defect–related infant deaths. Doctors usually do not know what causes a baby's heart to form abnormally, although genetic and environmental factors are believed to play a role. SPINA BIFIDA affects one in 2,000 babies. Every baby's spine is open when it first forms, but it normally closes by the 29th day after conception. In cases of spina bifida it fails to close. Affected babies suffer varying degrees of paralysis and bladder and bowel problems. Both genetic and nutritional factors appear to play a role in spina bifida.

About one baby in 135 has a structural defect involving the genitals or urinary tract. These range from abnormal placement of the urinary opening in males (hypospadias) to absence of both kidneys. While hypospadias are correctable, babies born without any kidneys die in the first hours or days of life.

Metabolic disorders affect one in 3,500 babies. Most are recessive genetic diseases that can be fatal if unrecognized and untreated. These diseases are caused by the inability of cells to produce an enzyme needed to change certain chemicals into others, or to carry substances from one place to another. For example, babies with TAY-SACHS DISEASE lack an enzyme needed to break down fatty substances in brain and nerve cells. These substances build up and destroy brain and nerve cells, resulting in blindness, paralysis, and death by age five. PKU (PHENYLKETONURIA) is another metabolic disorder in which affected babies cannot process part of a protein that builds up in blood and causes brain damage.

Rubella (GERMAN MEASLES) is probably the best known congenital infection that can cause birth defects. If a pregnant woman is infected in the first trimester, her baby has a one in four chance of being born with one or more symptoms of congenital rubella syndrome (featuring deafness, mental retardation, heart defects, or blindness). It also can cause stillbirth. Fortunately, with widespread vaccination, this syndrome is now rare in this country.

The most common congenital viral infection is CYTOMEGALOVIRUS (CMV). About 40,000 babies a year in this country are infected, though only about 10 percent of them actually have symptoms, including mental retardation, vision and hearing loss. Pregnant women often acquire CMV from young children, who usually have few or no symptoms.

Sexually transmitted infections in the mother also can endanger the fetus and newborn. For example, untreated syphilis can result in stillbirth, newborn death, or birth defects involving the bones. About one baby in 2,000 is born with congenital syphilis.

Other causes of birth defects include FETAL ALCOHOL SYNDROME, which affects one baby in 1,000 with a pattern of mental and physical birth defects common in babies of mothers who drink heavily during pregnancy. Even moderate or light drinking during pregnancy can pose a risk to the baby.

Rh disease of the newborn refers to an incompatibility between the blood of a mother and her fetus, affects about 4,000 infants a year. It can result in JAUNDICE, anemia, brain damage, and death. Rh disease usually can be prevented by giving an Rh-negative woman an injection of a blood product called immunoglobulin at 28 weeks of pregnancy and after the delivery of an Rh-positive baby. However, not all women who can benefit from this treatment get it, and a few cannot benefit from treatment.

Babies of mothers who use cocaine early in pregnancy are at increased risk of birth defects and are five times more likely to be born with urinary tract defects than babies of women who do not use cocaine.

Causes

While birth defects are due to many different factors, the underlying cause is known in only about

40 percent of cases. Some of these known causes are inherited genetic defects, abnormal chromosomes, environmental problems, harmful chemicals, or infections in the pregnant mother.

Hereditary birth defects are not uncommon. A single abnormal gene can cause birth defects. Every human being has about 100,000 genes that determine traits like eye and hair color, as well as growth and development. Genes are packed into each of the 46 chromosomes inside cells. Children get half their genes from each parent. Occasionally, a child may inherit a genetic disease when one parent who has the disease passes along a single faulty gene. This is called dominant inheritance. Examples of birth defects caused by dominant inheritance include achondroplasia, a form of dwarfism, and MARFAN SYNDROME, a connective tissue disease.

More often, a child inherits a genetic disease only if both healthy parents pass along the same faulty gene. This is called recessive inheritance. Examples include Tay-Sachs disease (a fatal disorder seen mainly in people of Eastern European Jewish heritage) and CYSTIC FIBROSIS (a fatal disorder of lungs and other organs affecting mainly Caucasians of northern European lineage). In X-linked inheritance, sons can inherit a genetic disease from a healthy mother who carries the gene. Examples include hemophilia and Duchenne MUSCULAR DYSTROPHY.

Abnormalities in the number or structure of chromosomes can cause numerous birth defects. Due to an error that occurred when an egg or sperm cell was developing, a baby can be born with one too many or one too few chromosomes, or with one or more chromosomes that are broken or rearranged. Down syndrome, in which a baby is born with an extra chromosome 21, is one of the most common chromosomal abnormalities. Babies also can be born with extra copies of chromosome 18 or 13, which causes multiple birth defects that are usual fatal in the first months of life.

In addition, birth defects may be caused by environmental factors such as drug or alcohol abuse, infections such as German measles (rubella) or cytomegalovirus, or exposure to chemicals such as the acne drug Accutane.

Birth defects may appear to be caused by a combination of one or more genes and environmental factors (called multifactorial inheritance), which may result in cleft lip/palate, clubfoot, and some heart defects.

Testing for Birth Defects

The March of Dimes believes that every state should require testing for at least these 10 disorders:

- medium-chain acyl-coa dehydrogenase (M-CAD) deficiency (Incidence: 1 in 15,000)
- phenylketonuria (PKU) (1 in 12,000)
- congenital hypothyroidism (1 in 4,000)
- congenital adrenal hyperplasia (CAH) (1 in 5,000)
- biotinidase deficiency (1 in 70,000)
- maple syrup urine disease (1 in 250,000)
- galactosemia (1 in 50,000)
- homocystinuria (1 in 275,000)
- sickle cell anemia (1 in 400 among African-Americans; 1 in 1,000–30,000 among Hispanics)
- hearing problems

These diseases all have reliable screening and diagnostic tests, and there are effective treatments for all of them. However, if these defects go untreated, the consequence is almost inevitably serious. In most states that require testing, parents are not asked for consent.

Treatments

More and more babies' lives are being saved because of surgery that corrects birth defects before a baby is born, neonatal intensive care units that provide specialized care to rescue babies, and new tests and treatments to make babies healthier.

One of the weapons in the fight against birth defects is gene therapy. Scientists have recently successfully corrected two genetic diseases in mice (HEMOPHILIA and retinitis pigmentosa, a leading cause of blindness). These successes in the laboratory are a first big step toward curing these disorders in humans.

birthmarks An area of discolored skin present at birth; the most common birthmarks are moles which are malformations of pigment cells. A STRAWBERRY BIRTH MARK is bright red, spongy, and protuberant. PORT-WINE STAINS are purple-red, flat, and often cover large areas of a child's body. Both strawberry marks and port-wine stains are malformations of blood vessels.

True strawberry (capillary) HEMANGIOMAS all clear by age seven, although they may leave an unsightly scar. Port-wine stains never clear. In a few cases, port-wine stains are associated with abnormalities in the blood vessels of the brain.

Unattractive moles can be removed in late childhood by plastic surgery. Port-wine stains can be lightened significantly using laser treatments. The pulsed dye laser is highly effective at lightening port-wine stains, and treatment can be started within the first few weeks of life.

birth weight, low   Low birth weight infants are at risk for a wide range of health, behavior, and learning problems. Recent research has suggested that extremely low birth weight children from age seven through adolescence have poorer reading and math skills; children whose birth weight was less than 2 lbs. lagged behind their peers academically and displayed other subtle behavioral characteristics which undermined their efforts at school. Poor motor skills and neurological immaturity were defined in many of the children.

This is becoming more of a concern since modern medicine can now save many infants with very low birth weight who would have died in the 1980s. In fact, infants whose birth weight was as low as 1 lb. 8 ounces, born after 24 weeks of gestation, have survived in neonatal intensive care units.

Many neonatal intensive care units have follow-up programs to assess the development of children and initiate early intervention strategies, as needed. Unfortunately, physicians traditionally have not received much training in the area of child development and disabilities, although pediatric and family practice training programs today include rotations in child development and rehabilitative services for children. Such assessments are vital since some studies have found that middle class, low-birth-weight children may not require special education services if they receive strong parental support. Early childhood educational partnerships between home and school are essential to help keep low birth weight infants on target in their development.

bites, animal   Every 40 seconds, someone in the United States seeks medical care for a dog bite. Each year, 500,000 children get medical treatment for dog bites alone. Less common but more dangerous are bites from skunks, raccoons, bats, and other wild animals.

Interestingly, the bites of these animals are less infectious than a human bite, although there is still a risk of infection.

Most bites from animals result in some bruising, including blue or yellow discoloration in the surrounding skin. Usually there is some swelling, which is worse two days after the bite; after this period, it rapidly returns to normal. If swelling increases after the third day, the child should see a doctor.

When to See a Doctor
Parents should take the child to see a doctor if there is redness or streaking; if there is drainage of yellow, tan, green, or foul fluid; or if the child has a fever above 101°F.

Treatment
All animal bites require treatment based on the type and severity of the wound. Whether the bite is from a family pet or an animal in the wild, scratches and bites can become infected and cause scarring. Animals can also carry diseases that can be transmitted through a bite; about 5 percent of dog bites and 20 to 50 percent of cat bites become infected. Bites that break the skin and bites of the scalp, face, hand, wrist, or foot are more likely to become infected. In addition, cat scratches can carry CAT SCRATCH DISEASE, a bacterial infection.

Other animals can transmit rabies and tetanus. Rodents such as mice, rats, squirrels, chipmunks, hamsters, guinea pigs, gerbils, and rabbits are at low risk to carry rabies. If the skin has been broken, treatment depends on the depth and location, and on what is known about the animal. The area is first cleaned with an antiseptic, followed by an antibiotic. Stitches may be required, but it is usually best for these wounds to heal without being sewn up to prevent any dangerous organism from getting trapped in the body. Bites on the face, however, will probably need to be stitched to prevent disfiguration.

Most animal bites will not require antibiotics unless evidence of an infection is found.

bites, snake   While there are about 3,000 species of snakes in the world, only 10 percent of them are poisonous. Venomous snakes come in all sizes, from the tiny desert vipers to the king cobra, growing up to 16 feet long; a king cobra, when angered, can rear up and stand as tall as an adult. While there are many folk methods to quickly determine if a snake is poisonous, such as counting the rows of scales, there is no practical way to tell the poisonous from the harmless.

The highest death rates from snakebite in the United States are reported from Arizona, Florida, Georgia, Texas, and Alabama, in that order. There are only four varieties of snakes in the United States that are poisonous: the rattlesnake, copperhead, water moccasin, and coral snake, but they are found throughout the country. Of the 115 species of snakes in this country, only 20 are dangerous, including 16 species of rattlesnakes. Rattlers account for about 65 percent of the venomous snakebites that occur in this country each year, and for nearly all of the nine to 15 deaths.

The water moccasin is found throughout the southwest, the Gulf states, and the Mississippi valley as far north as southern Illinois. The copperhead is found throughout the country, especially in North and South Carolina, West Virginia, Pennsylvania, Missouri, Oklahoma, Arkansas, and Illinois. Rattlesnakes are found throughout the continental United States. The coral snake is associated with the South.

Treatment

Despite the long history of snakebites and their treatment, the problem of how to deal with snakebites remains controversial. More than 200 different first aid procedures for snakebite have been recommended by various experts, but the emphasis on treating snakebite should be to get prompt medical care. First aid should never be considered to be a substitute for antivenin.

Medical experts disagree about the best way to manage poisonous snakebites. Some physicians hold off on immediate treatment to observe the child to gauge a bite's seriousness. Some doctors prefer to surgically treat tissue around the bite. But most often, doctors turn to antivenin as a reliable treatment for serious snakebites.

Antivenin is derived from antibodies created in a horse's blood after the animal is injected with snake venom. Rapid treatment with an antivenin can help a snakebite patient regardless of whether or not the bite would have been fatal. Without antivenin treatment, hospital stays for venomous snake bites last about twice as long.

The venom of all snakes in the Crotalidae family (rattlesnakes, copperheads, and water moccasins) contains similar poisons, and all can be treated with antivenin. The bite from the eastern coral snake requires a separate antivenin, and there is no antivenin for the western coral snake.

In humans, antivenin is administered either through the veins or injected into muscle. Because antivenin is obtained from horses, snakebite patients sensitive to horse products must be carefully managed. The danger is that a child could develop an adverse reaction to the antivenin or even a potentially fatal allergic condition called anaphylactic shock.

First aid   In recent years, fewer experts have been recommending invasive types of first aid such as making incisions over the bite wound. Many health-care professionals embrace just a few basic first-aid techniques. According to the American Red Cross, these steps should be taken:

1. Wash the bite with soap and water.

2. Immobilize the bitten area and keep it lower than the heart.

3. Get medical help without delay.

Some medical professionals, along with the American Red Cross, cautiously recommend two other measures:

4. If a snakebite patient cannot reach medical care within 30 minutes, a bandage wrapped two to four inches above the bite may help slow venom. The bandage should not cut off blood flow from a vein or artery. It should be loose enough that a finger can slip under it.

5. A suction device may be placed over the bite to help draw venom out of the wound without

making cuts. Suction instruments often are included in commercial snakebite kits.

Treatment Drawbacks

Antivenins have been used for decades and are the only effective treatment for some bites. While they have a fairly good safety record, they sometimes cause life-threatening reactions.

Children previously treated with antivenin for snakebites probably will develop a lifelong sensitivity to horse products. To identify these and other sensitive patients, hospitals typically obtain a record of the child's experience with snakebites or horse products. But some people with no history of such exposures may have become sensitive through contact with horses, or possibly exposure to horse dander, and not know they are sensitive. Others may be sensitive without any known or remembered contact with horses.

This is why hospitals also perform a skin test that quickly shows any sensitivity. Some hypersensitive patients may even react severely to the small amount of antivenin used in the skin test. Some children with positive skin tests can be desensitized by gradually administering small amounts of antivenin.

Newer kinds of antivenins derived from sheep are under study now and show some promise, according to the U.S. Food and Drug Administration. Progress has been slow due to low demand and the small number of venomous bites a year.

Prevention

By taking a few precautions, it's possible to lower the risk of being bitten. Children should:

- leave snakes alone. Many people are bitten because they try to kill a snake or get a closer look at it.
- stay out of tall grass unless they wear thick leather boots, and remain on hiking paths as much as possible.
- keep hands and feet out of areas they cannot see. A snake can strike half its length.
- be cautious and alert when climbing rocks.
- walk at least six feet around a snake they encounter when hiking or picnicking.

bites and stings, insect   A fly, tick, or mosquito bite may cause swelling and itching for several days and may lead to infection if a child scratches it open. Most of the time an insect bite or sting is not serious, and discomfort is limited to the sting or bite area.

However, some children may experience an extreme allergic reaction that requires immediate medical attention. The severity of the response can be caused by a child's sensitivity to the particular toxin, such as bee venom. In addition, mosquito bites may rarely transmit disease, such as WEST NILE VIRUS or ENCEPHALITIS. Tick bites may transmit a variety of infectious diseases such as LYME DISEASE or ROCKY MOUNTAIN SPOTTED FEVER.

Symptoms

Children who are bitten or stung experience either a localized or a generalized reaction. A localized reaction is the typical swelling, itching, and redness that is normally limited to the bite site. A generalized (systemic) reaction is far more serious and can be life-threatening, including wheezing, tightness in the throat, shortness of breath, hives, swollen eyes, slurred speech, nausea and vomiting, mental confusion, and loss of consciousness. Emergency medical assistance is imperative in this case.

Consult a Doctor

A doctor should be consulted immediately if the child:

- is bitten by a scorpion, black widow spider, or brown recluse spider.
- has a rash with a distinct "bull's-eye" appearance and flu-like symptoms (signs of LYME DISEASE).
- has a localized reaction that does not improve within 72 hours.
- shows signs of infection after a localized reaction subsides (usually after 24 hours): fever, redness and swelling, and pus.

Treatment

Because flies, ticks, and mosquitoes can spread disease, the bite area should be washed with soap and water, followed by the application of an antiseptic. The stinger can be removed by gently scraping it out with a clean fingernail or knife blade so no more venom is released. Cold compresses should be applied immediately following a bite or sting. Ticks should be carefully removed by grasping the body with tweezers and pulling.

To control itching, a nonprescription antihistamine, calamine lotion, ice packs, or oatmeal bath may help. Alternatively, itching may be controlled by applying a paste to the skin made up of any of the following:

- salt and water
- baking soda and water
- epsom salts (1 tbs. in 1 quart of water, chilled)

In the event of a generalized reaction, the child should rest immediately to slow the movement of venom through the body.

Prevention
DEET (N1N-diethyl-m-toluamide) is the most effective of all bug repellants, and it may be used on children—but not on infants. DEET should be kept out of the eyes. New preparations combine sunscreen and a bug repellant in one cream. To avoid attracting insects or bugs, children should avoid wearing brightly colored clothes or applying a scented lotion to the skin.

Any child who has experienced generalized allergic reactions after a bee sting or insect bite should always carry a kit containing epinephrine, especially when outdoors. A child who has experienced generalized reactions to bites or stings should wear a medic alert bracelet or necklace.

black eye
A discoloration and swelling over the eye usually caused by trauma, bruising the tissue around the eye. Most black eyes heal completely and do not cause any damage to the eye.

Treatment may include cold compresses for the first 24 hours, followed by warm compresses after the first 24 hours until the swelling stops. The child's head should be raised to help decrease the amount of swelling. It is normal for the swelling and bruising to spread down the cheek or to the other eye.

bladder infection
See URINARY TRACT INFECTION.

bleeding, nose
See NOSEBLEED.

blepharitis
Inflamed eyelids characterized by red, irritated scaly skin at the edges of the lids.

Cause
This common eyelid infection is associated with dandruff, allergy, or eczema of the scalp. Ulcerative blepharitis is caused by a bacterial infection.

Symptoms
Burning and discomfort in the eyes, with flakes or crusts on lashes. Sometimes the surface of the eye may also be inflamed and red, and sometimes even the roots of the eyelashes may be affected.

Treatment
Scales can be removed with cotton moistened with warm water. The inflammation often recurs, which requires more treatment. Ulcerated eyelids must be treated by a physician, since severe cases can lead to problems with the cornea.

blister
A raised oval or round collection of fluid within or beneath the outer layer of the skin. Blisters larger than a half inch in diameter are sometimes called "bullae"; small blisters are also called vesicles. Blisters that have been inadvertently pierced may be susceptible to infection, which is indicated by redness, swelling, an odor, or cloudy fluid.

Cause
A blister appears after minor skin damage when serum leaks from blood vessels in underlying skin. The serum is usually sterile, and the blister provides valuable protection to the damaged tissue. Blisters often appear after BURNS, SUNBURN, or friction (such as damage to the heel from wearing a poorly fitting shoe).

In addition, small blisters develop in the early stages of many viral infections, including CHICKEN POX, SHINGLES, and HERPES simplex; these blisters contain infectious particles capable of spreading the infection.

Treatment
A blister should not be disturbed but should be left to heal on its own. It may be pierced at the edge using a sterile needle, allowing the fluid to slowly seep out. However, a blister should never be unroofed, as the top flap of skin protects against

infection. Children with large, troublesome, or unexplained blisters should be seen by a doctor.

To protect the blister, a moleskin pad (available at drug stores) can be cut to resemble a doughnut, with the blister in the middle; the moleskin will absorb the friction of daily activity.

If a blister inadvertently bursts or gets pierced, the skin should not be removed over the top. Left intact even after the blister has drained, this skin flap will act as a type of bandage; it will eventually harden and fall off by itself.

Triple topical antibiotics (such as Neosporin) may eliminate bacterial contamination, but iodine or camphor-phenol will slow down healing.

Prevention

Children should always wear socks with shoes, and gloves on hands when using tools. Feet should be powdered when wearing new shoes. Children at risk for getting a blister on the foot should try coating blister-prone areas with petroleum jelly or diaper rash ointment (such as A&D ointment) to cut down friction.

Experts do not agree on the type of sock that best protects against blisters, but current research suggests that acrylic spun fibers may be better than cotton in the presence of water. Wearing two sets of different sock materials on each foot with properly fitted shoes helps prevent blistering.

blood poisoning   See SEPTICEMIA.

blood transfusions   The injection of blood from a healthy person into the circulation of a child whose blood is deficient in quality or quantity. Several different components of blood can be transfused into a child, but red blood cells are the most common type of blood product transfusion.

There are several reasons why a child may require a blood transfusion, including a sudden loss of blood; low hemoglobin count before, during, or after surgery; severe heart or lung disease; bone marrow failure or anemia.

Most of the body's blood cells are produced in the bone marrow, the spongy material in the center of the bones. Blood is made of plasma that carries red and white blood cells and platelets. Red blood cells carry oxygen from the lungs to other body organs and carry carbon dioxide back to the lungs. Bleeding after an accident, surgery, or disease may lower the red blood cell count. White blood cells fight infections by destroying bacteria, viruses, and other germs. White blood cell transfusions are rarely given and are usually reserved for children with a low white cell count and severe infection that does not respond to antibiotic therapy.

Platelets help control bleeding by plugging blood vessels damaged by injury or surgery. Platelet count might be low because of bone marrow disorders, increased destruction of platelets, or medications. Platelets may be transfused before a surgical procedure that could trigger bleeding in a child with a low platelet count.

Plasma carries blood cells throughout the body and contains proteins, vitamins, and minerals, some of which help the blood to clot. Plasma or fresh frozen plasma can be transfused in children who have a severe deficiency of certain clotting components of the blood.

The blood used at most hospitals is from volunteer donors who are not paid for giving blood or blood products. Each blood donor must answer medical history questions and be given a limited physical examination before being accepted as a donor. All donated blood is tested for HEPATITIS, SYPHILIS, and antibodies to immunodeficiency viruses including the AIDS virus. These tests decrease the chances of transfusion-related infections.

Blood is collected and stored in sterile bags which are used once and then thrown away. Before blood is given to a child, it is cross-matched with the child's own blood to make sure it is compatible. The blood is given through a needle in the vein.

Because of concerns over possible contaminants in blood, some patients prefer to use blood donated from people they know. A directed (or designated) blood donation is one in which a person donates blood that is reserved at the time of donation for the transfusion of a specific patient at a later date. The donor is usually a family member or a close friend who has been chosen by the patient's family. There is no proof that directed donors are safer than volunteer donors, and not all directed donor blood will be compatible with the patient's blood.

Risks

Risks

Most transfusions do not cause any problems, but mild side effects may include symptoms of an allergic reaction such as headache, fever, itching, increased breathing effort, or rash. This type of reaction can usually be treated with medication if the child needs more transfusions in the future. Serious reactions are rare. The most common serious side effect is serum hepatitis, an infection of the liver.

boil An inflamed pus-filled section of skin (usually an infected hair follicle) found often on the back of the neck or moist areas such as the armpits and groin. A very large boil is called a CARBUNCLE.

Cause

Boils are usually caused by infection with the bacterium *Staphylococcus aureus,* which invades the body through a break in the skin, where it infects a blocked oil gland or hair follicle. When the body's immune system sends in white blood cells to kill the germs, the resulting inflammation produces pus.

Symptoms

A boil begins with a red, painful lump that swells as it fills with pus, until it becomes rounded with a yellowish tip. It may either continue to grow until it erupts, drains, and fades away, or it can be reabsorbed by the body. Recurrent boils may occur in people with known or unrecognized diabetes mellitus or other diseases involving lowered body resistance.

Treatment

Bursting a boil might spread the infection. Instead, apply a hot compress for 20 minutes every two hours to relieve discomfort and hasten drainage and healing. After treating a boil, wash hands thoroughly before cooking to guard against staph infection getting into food.

It may take up to a week for the boil to break on its own. To further reduce chance of infection, showers, not baths should be taken. If the boil is large and painful, a physician may prescribe an antibiotic or open the boil with a sterile needle to drain the pus. Occasionally, large boils must be lanced with a surgical knife; this is usually done using a local anesthetic.

Complications

More seriously, bacteria from a boil may find its way into the blood, causing blood poisoning; for this reason, doctors advise against squeezing boils that appear around the lips or nose, since the infection can be carried to the brain. (Other danger areas include the groin, armpit, and breast of a nursing woman.) Signs of a spreading infection include generalized symptoms of fever and chills, swelling lymph nodes, or red lines radiating from the boil.

Prevention

Some experts note that boils are usually infected cysts and recommend leaving cysts untouched, or having them lanced by a physician. For patients prone to boils, some experts recommend washing the skin with an antiseptic soap.

Keep skin around a boil clean while drainage is occurring and take showers to lessen the chance of spreading the infection.

borderline intellectual functioning An IQ between 70 and 85 in the absence of functional or adaptive problems, sometimes considered in the "slow learner" educational category. Earlier classifications referred to this IQ range as borderline MENTAL RETARDATION. Neither term is linked to borderline personality disorder.

borderline personality disorder A pervasive pattern of instability in interpersonal relationships and self-image, with marked impulsivity, beginning by early adulthood.

Because the impulsivity and inappropriate behavior of this condition may mimic symptoms of ATTENTION DEFICIT HYPERACTIVITY DISORDER, a diagnosis by an experienced clinician is important.

Borderline personality disorder (BPD) affects one in 50 children in the United States. The name "borderline personality disorder" was given because experts once thought the condition fell somewhere between neurosis and psychosis on the mental illness continuum. Professionals who are educated about the BPD all agree that the name should be changed as it does in no way describe the disorder.

Symptoms

This type of personality disorder leads to intense feelings of abandonment, poor self-image, and unrealistic expectations of others. Moodiness and angry outbursts may be common, and the individual may seem depressed or suicidal. The hallmark of the disorder is chronic instability, affecting relationships with family members or colleagues, and a lack of close, long-term interpersonal relationships that can add to the sense of isolation and abandonment.

Cause

Although some experts believe the condition is a true personality disorder acquired from childhood trauma, research does not support this theory. While the exact cause is still unknown, more and more research has discovered that the BPD is genetic. Mothers who have the condition are five times more likely to give birth to an affected child than a mother without the BPD.

Treatment

Recent research has shown that medications can significantly relieve the suffering of borderline patients when used in combination with psychotherapy. Treatment may be some combination of antipsychotic or antianxiety drugs, antidepressants, and psychotherapy. Due to their suicide attempts or brief psychotic episodes, borderline patients frequently are hospitalized.

botulism The most common type of the infectious disease known as "botulism" is a food-borne illness involving the toxin *Clostridium botulinum*, which is both rare and very deadly (two-thirds of those afflicted die). Another type is known as "infant botulism," an uncommon illness that strikes infants under the age of one. Because botulism is technically an intoxication, not an infection, the patient cannot infect others even though the toxin and bacteria will be excreted in feces for months after the illness.

Botulism is more common in the United States than anywhere else in the world owing to the popularity of home canning; there are about 20 cases of food-borne botulism poisoning each year. Botulism got its name during the 1800s from *botulus*,

the Latin word for "sausage," because of a wave of poisoning from contaminated sausages.

Cause

Botulism toxins are a type of neurotoxin that attaches to the nerves, blocking the messages that are sent to the muscles. The *C. botulinum* spores (latent form of the bacteria) are found in air, water, and food; they are harmless until deprived of oxygen (such as inside a sealed can or jar). If conditions are favorable, the spores will start to generate and multiply, producing one of the most deadly toxins known—seven million times more deadly than cobra venom.

Cases of botulism from commercially canned food are rare because of strict health standards enforced by the U.S. Food and Drug Administration, although some people have gotten botulism from eating improperly handled commercial pot pies. In Canada cases have been reported from seal meat, smoked salmon, and fermented salmon eggs. Most cases occur during home canning.

Canned foods that are highly susceptible to contamination include green beans, beets, peppers, corn, and meat. Although the spores can survive boiling, the ideal temperature for their growth is between 78°F and 96°F. They can also survive freezing.

Even though botulism spores are invisible, it is possible to tell if food is spoiled by noticing if jars have lost their vacuum seal; when the spores grow, they give off gas that makes cans and jars lose the seal. Jars will burst or cans will swell. Any food that is spoiled or whose color or odor does not seem right inside a home-canned jar or can should be thrown away without tasting or even sniffing, since botulism can be fatal in extremely small amounts.

Botulism can also occur if the *C. botulinum* bacteria in the soil enters the body through an open wound, although this is extremely rare.

Symptoms

Onset of symptoms may be as soon as three hours or as late as 14 days after ingestion, although most symptoms usually appear between 12 and 26 hours. The first sign is usually muscle weakness beginning with the head, often leading to double vision. This is followed by problems in swallowing or speaking, followed by the paralysis of the muscles needed to breathe. Other symptoms can include nausea, vomiting, diarrhea, and stomach cramps. The earlier the onset of symptoms, the more severe the reaction. Symptoms generally lasts between three to six days; death occurs in about 70 percent of untreated cases, usually from suffocation as a result of respiratory muscle paralysis. In infants, symptoms may go unrecognized by parents for some time until the poisoning has reached a critical stage.

Diagnosis

Large commercial labs or state health labs can test for the toxin in food, blood, or stool; it is also possible to grow the bacteria from food or stool in a special culture.

Treatment

Prompt administration of the antitoxin (type ABE botulinus) lowers the risk of death to 10 percent. Most untreated victims will die. The Centers for Disease Control is the only agency with the antitoxin, and it makes the decision to treat. Local health departments should be called first for this information. While induced vomiting may help following ingestion of food known to contain botulism toxin, it may not eliminate the toxin completely. The disease can occur with only a small amount of toxin, thus botulism may still develop. Enemas may be necessary. Patients are usually put on a respirator to ease breathing.

Prevention

Botulism is easy to prevent, since it is killed when canned food is boiled at 100°C for one minute, or if the food is first sterilized by pressure cooking at 250°F for 30 minutes.

While the tightly fitted lids of home-canned food will provide the anaerobic environment necessary for the growth of botulism toxins, the spores will not grow if the food is very acidic, sweet, or salty (such as canned fruit juice, jams and jellies, sauerkraut, tomatoes, and heavily salted hams).

botulism, infant Unlike BOTULISM in adults, which occurs after eating contaminated food, infant botulism occurs in babies under one year of age and is less serious. While all botulism is caused by toxins given off by *Clostridium botulinum* bacteria, in infant botulism the baby does not ingest the toxin. Instead, the spores from botulism bacteria reproduce the toxin in the baby's digestive tract, which then travels to the baby's nerve cells. Fortunately, most babies will recover with prompt hospital treatment.

Some experts believe that infant botulism may be responsible for up to 5 percent of all cases of SUDDEN INFANT DEATH SYNDROME.

Cause

This rare disease may be difficult to trace, since the spores may survive for a long time in the environment. It is clear that about 10 percent of commercial honey contains botulism spores, and occasionally light and dark corn syrup also harbors the bacteria. For this reason, parents are advised not to feed either food to infants under a year of age. The illness is found in all races, in North and South America, in Asia and Europe. In 1993 there were only 65 reported cases in the United States.

Although an infected baby will excrete toxin for weeks in feces, the baby cannot pass on the infection to others.

Symptoms

Infant botulism symptoms include constipation, facial muscle flaccidity, sucking problems, irritability, lethargy, and floppy arms and legs.

Treatment

The antitoxin used to treat adults with botulism is not safe for infants. Antibiotics may be used to treat secondary infections. In severe cases, the baby may need breathing assistance; while recovery may be slow, most completely recover.

Prevention

Babies under age one should not be fed honey or corn syrup. They should be kept away from dust (both from vacuum cleaners and from the outdoors), especially around construction sites.

bovine spongiform encephalopathy The medical name for mad cow disease, a chronic, degenerative disease affecting the central nervous system of cattle. It is one of a group of fatal brain diseases called transmissible spongiform encephalopathies (TSEs). These infectious diseases, which are always fatal, create holes throughout the brain, making it look like a sponge. The first known TSE appeared in sheep, but now people, cows, elk, deer, mink, rats, mice, hamsters, and possibly monkeys all get various types of the disease.

BSE was first identified in Britain in 1986, and was thought to be transmitted to humans via contaminated meat and bonemeal. The human version of BSE is called new variant Creutzfeldt-Jakob disease.

As of November 2000 more than 177,500 cases of mad cow disease were confirmed in the United Kingdom alone in more than 35,000 herds; it had peaked in January 1993 at almost 1,000 new cases a week. The outbreak was caused by feeding tainted sheep meat and bonemeal to cattle, amplified by feeding rendered cow meat-and-bone meal to young calves. Since the feeding of bovine offal to cows was stopped in Britain, the incidence of the disease has declined significantly.

Worldwide there have been more than 180,000 cases since the disease was first diagnosed in 1986. While there is a decline in the number of cases of BSE in the United Kingdom, confirmed cases of BSE have risen in other European countries, including Belgium, Czech Republic, Denmark, France, Germany, Greece, Ireland, Italy, Luxembourg, Liechtenstein, the Netherlands, Northern Ireland, Portugal, Spain, and Switzerland. More than 90 percent of all BSE cases have occurred in the United Kingdom. In the United States, officials restricted imports of live cattle and meat from countries with BSE in 1989. In December 2003 the first cases of mad cow disease was identified in a herd in Washington. No human cases in the United States have yet been diagnosed.

The cause of BSE has been linked to three main theories: an unconventional virus, an abnormal prion, or a virino ("incomplete" virus) composed of naked nucleic acid protected by host proteins. What scientists do know is that the BSE agent is smaller than most viral particles and is highly resistant to heat, ultraviolet light, ionizing radiation, and common disinfectants that normally inactivate viruses or bacteria. They also know that it causes no detectable immune or inflammatory response and has not been observed microscopically. At present, most scientists blame prions as the most likely cause.

There is no test to detect the disease in a live animal, but two lab methods can confirm a diagnosis of BSE on autopsy: microscopic examination of the brain tissue to identify characteristic changes or techniques that detect the prion.

bowed legs   Abnormal appearance of the legs, curving outward and resulting in a gap between the knees when standing. Some degree of bowing is normal in small children. If a doctor has determined by observation or X-ray examination that a child has bowed legs, this condition might require treatment to prevent future problems.

In the first 18 months of life, the legs naturally bow outward, straightening as the baby grows. By age four, many children are knock-kneed, but by age seven through 10 the legs again become straight.

Cause

Children with bowed legs often have a family history of the condition. In other cases, bowing may be caused by infection or an abnormality of the growth plate at the top of the shinbone. Early walking does not always cause bowed legs.

Treatment

If the bowing is not equal in both legs or if a child is older than 24 months, the doctor may want to take a X ray of the legs to help determine if treatment is necessary. Treatment may involve wearing braces or surgery when the child is older. In untreated, severe cases, arthritis or an awkward gait may occur in later life.

broken bones   A broken or fractured bone requires emergency care. However, it is not always clear if a child has broken a bone or just sprained a ligament. A broken bone should be suspected if the child heard or felt a bone snap, has trouble moving the injured part, or if the injured part moves in an unnatural way or is very painful to the touch.

Treatment

If the injury involves a child's neck or back, he should not be moved unless he is in imminent danger, because movement can cause serious nerve damage. If the child must be moved, the neck and back must be completely immobilized first. To keep the child's head, neck, and back in alignment, the child must be moved as a unit.

If the child has a compound fracture (an open break in which the bone protrudes through the skin) and there is severe bleeding, pressure should be applied to the bleeding area with a gauze pad. However, the wound should not be washed, nor should anyone try to push back the part of the bone that may be sticking out.

If a child must be moved, splints should be applied around the injured limb to prevent further injury. The limb should be left in the original position. The splints should be applied in that position. Splints can be made by using boards, brooms, a stack of newspapers, cardboard, or anything firm, and can be padded with pillows, shirts, towels, or anything soft. Splints must be long enough to extend beyond the joints above and below the fracture. Cold packs or a bag of ice wrapped in cloth should be placed on the injured area. Keep the child lying down until medical help arrives.

bronchiolitis   Acute viral infection of the lungs that primarily affects infants and young children. Winter epidemics tend to occur every two or three years, affecting thousands of children in the United States. A virus that may induce only a mild head or chest infection in an adult can cause severe bronchiolitis in an infant. However, with prompt treatment, even the sickest infants usually recover completely within a few days. Infants at greatest risk are those who were born prematurely or those with certain lung diseases.

Cause

The smaller airways that branch off the bronchial tubes become inflamed, usually because of the RES-PIRATORY SYNCYTIAL VIRUS (RSV), although other viruses may be responsible. Adult attacks may follow BRONCHITIS brought on by INFLUENZA. The viruses may be transmitted from person to person through airborne drops.

Symptoms

Cough, shortness of breath, and (in severe cases) blue-purple skin color. A physician can hear bubbling noises in the lungs. A baby or young child with a cold and cough that suddenly gets worse should see a physician.

Treatment

Sometimes no treatment is needed. In severe cases the child may need to be hospitalized for oxygen and receive respiratory therapy to clear the mucus. Antibiotics and corticosteroid drugs will not work against this viral infection, although antibiotics may be prescribed anyway to prevent a secondary bacterial infection. Sometimes a child may need to be placed on an artificial ventilator until normal breathing returns.

bronchitis   Sudden inflammation of the airways that connect the windpipe (trachea) to the lungs that produces a persistent cough with quantities of sputum. Attacks usually occur in the winter among smokers, babies, the elderly, and those with lung disease.

Cause

Acute bronchitis is usually a complication of a viral infection (such as a cold or the flu), although it can also be caused by air pollution. A bacterial infection also may lead to acute bronchitis, or it may follow an attack of acute bronchitis brought on by other causes.

Symptoms

As the bronchial tubes swell and become congested with pus, symptoms include wheezing, breathlessness, and a persistent cough that produces yellow or green phlegm. There also may be pain behind the breastbone and a fever.

Treatment

Humidifying the lungs will ease symptoms, either by using a humidifier or by inhaling steam. Drinking plenty of fluids also helps bring up phlegm. Most acute bronchitis clears up on its own without further treatment. If there is a suspicion of an underlying bacterial infection, antibiotics will be prescribed.

Complications

Pleurisy or PNEUMONIA may rarely occur. A physician should be consulted if any of the following symptoms appear:

- severe breathlessness
- no improvement after three days
- blood is coughed up
- fever rises above 101°F
- patient has underlying lung disease

bronchopneumonia   See PNEUMONIA.

bulimia   A destructive pattern of overeating followed by vomiting or other purging behaviors in order to control weight.

Unlike girls with ANOREXIA, those with bulimia eat large amounts of food and then get rid of the excess calories by vomiting, abusing laxatives or diuretics, taking enemas, or exercising obsessively. Some use a combination of all of these. Because many girls with bulimia binge and purge in secret and maintain normal or above-normal body weight, they often can successfully hide their problem from others for years.

Bulimia becomes a serious problem when a girl is bingeing and purging at least twice a week for three months, while becoming excessively worried about her body shape and weight. Dieting heavily between episodes of bingeing and purging is common; eventually, half of girls with anorexia will develop bulimia.

About 2 percent to 3 percent of young girls develop bulimia.

Cause

Certain personality characteristics seem to be associated with bulimia, including a fear of losing control, inflexible thinking, perfectionism, dissatisfaction with body shape, and an overwhelming desire to be thin. Bulimia has also been linked to mood disturbances such as DEPRESSION or social anxiety.

As with anorexia, bulimia typically begins during adolescence and occurs most often among girls. Girls with bulimia deny their hunger and restrict their food intake for several days or weeks at a time, but sooner or later, they begin to eat and cannot stop eating until they have stuffed themselves. Experts think this overeating compensates for the prior calorie restriction. Binge eating may also be related to problems with feeling satisfied after meals, since many bulimics report that they have trouble feeling full unless they eat large amounts of food.

Symptoms

Even bulimia patients at normal weight can severely damage their bodies by frequent binge eating and purging. In rare instances, binge eating causes the stomach to rupture; purging may lead to heart failure because of loss of vital minerals, such as potassium. Constant vomiting causes other less deadly, but serious problems; the acid in vomit wears down the outer layer of the teeth, the esophagus becomes inflamed, and glands near the cheeks become swollen. As with anorexia, bulimia may lead to irregular menstrual periods.

Some girls with bulimia also struggle with addictions, including abuse of drugs and alcohol, or compulsive stealing. Many suffer from clinical depression, anxiety, obsessive-compulsive disorder, and other mental health problems. These problems, combined with impulsive tendencies, place them at increase risk for suicide.

Treatment

In treating bulimia, doctors must first deal with any serious physical complications. In some cases the binge-purge cycle is so severe that the girl cannot stop on her own and hospitalization may be necessary, followed by individual counseling, sometimes combined with medication.

Counseling may last for about four to six months; group therapy is also very helpful for bulimics. Antidepressants may also be effective in treating girls with bulimia. In outpatient treatment, bulimic patients are often asked to keep a food intake diary, making sure they eat three meals a day of moderate caloric intake, even if they are still binge eating. Exercise is limited, and if the girl becomes compulsive about it, is not permitted at all.

Bulimia is a chronic disorder that comes and goes. Of those girls who are treated, three years later less than a third will be fully recovered; more than one-third will show some improvement in symptoms, and the final third will have relapsed. (See BINGE EATING DISORDER; EATING DISORDERS.)

bullying Bullying is an all-too-common experience for many children and adolescents, affecting as many as half of all children at some time during their school years. At least 10 percent of all children are bullied on a regular basis.

Bullying behavior can be physical or verbal, and can occur anywhere—at home, at school, on the playground, and even in online chat rooms and through e-mail.

Victims of this torment experience real suffering that can interfere with social and emotional development, as well as school performance. Some victims of bullying have even attempted suicide rather than continue to endure such harassment and punishment.

A bully thrives on controlling or dominating others and often has been the victim of physical abuse or bullying himself. Bullies also may be depressed, angry, or upset about events at school or at home.

Children who are bullied also tend to fit a particular profile of being passive, easily intimidated, and having few friends. Victims may be smaller or younger than the bully.

Parents who suspect their child is bullying others should seek help as soon as possible. Without intervention, bullying can lead to serious academic, social, emotional, and legal problems. A comprehensive evaluation by a mental health professional can help parents and child understand what is causing the bullying, and how to stop the destructive behavior.

Parents who think their child may be the victim of a bully should provide opportunities to talk in an open and honest way. It is also important to respond in a positive and accepting manner. Parents should ask the child what should be done and seek help from the child's teacher or school guidance counselor. Most bullying occurs on playgrounds, in lunchrooms, in bathrooms, on school buses, or in unsupervised halls. Parents can explore ways to stop bullying, such as peer mediation, conflict resolution, anger management training, and increased adult supervision.

burns Every year thousands of children are burned or scalded badly enough to require medical attention. Burns and scalds are a major cause of serious injury in children from infancy through age 14. Children from birth to four years of age are at greatest risk.

The skin is a living tissue, and temperatures that even briefly reach 120°F will destroy its cells. Young children have thinner skin than that of older children and adults, thus their skin burns at lower temperatures and more deeply. A child exposed to hot tap water at 140°F for three seconds will sustain a third-degree burn. Moreover, children under age four may not perceive danger, may have less control of their environment, may lack the ability to escape a life-threatening burn situation, and may not be able to tolerate the physical stress of a post-burn injury.

In 1998, 608 children aged 14 and under died due to fire- and burn-related injuries. In 1999 an estimated 99,500 children aged 14 and under were treated in hospital emergency rooms for burn-related injuries. Of these injuries, 62,580 were thermal burns, 23,620 were scald burns, 9,430 were chemical burns, and 2,250 were electrical burns.

Burns and scalds are usually due to preventable accidents at home. Burns can be caused by contact with hot substances, flames, chemicals, or radiation (as in sunlight, X rays, or ionizing radiation). While most accidental burns are visible almost immediately after the accident, burns from SUNBURN may appear several hours to a day later. It may be 10 to 30 days before the full effects of ionizing X-ray irradiation burns appear.

The severity of burns depends on two factors: how deep the tissue destruction has penetrated, and the amount of body surface that has been affected. Burn recovery is also influenced by the age and general health of the child, the location of the burn, and any other associated injuries.

Traditionally, doctors have characterized burns as first, second, or third degree, depending on the depth of skin damage. By accurately estimating the extent of damage, the doctor can best determine appropriate treatment.

First-Degree Burns

This type of minor burn affects only the top layer of skin (epidermis), causing reddening but no blisters or swelling. Typically, pain ebbs within 48 to

72 hours, and the burn heals quickly without scars, although the damaged skin might peel off in a day or two. A sunburn is an example of a first-degree burn.

Second-Degree Burns

This type of burn destroys the skin on a deeper level, creating redness and blisters; the deeper the burn, the more blisters, which increase in size within a few hours after the injury. Second-degree burns may be extremely painful. Because some of the deep layer of skin remains, this type of burn can usually heal without scarring as long as there has been no accompanying infection and the burn has not penetrated too deeply into the skin. How well a second-degree burn heals depends on the amount of damaged skin. In very deep second-degree burns, the healed skin may resemble the severe scars from a third-degree burn. These deeper burns take longer to heal (often up to a month or more), and the healing top skin layer is very fragile.

Third-Degree Burns

This is the most serious type of burn, which destroys all the layers of the skin and may expose muscles and bones. The affected area will look white or charred, and even if the burned area is small, it will require special treatment and skin grafts to help prevent serious scarring.

There is no pain in this type of burn because the pain receptors have been destroyed along with the rest of the skin and blood vessels, sweat glands, sebaceous glands, and hair follicles. Fluid loss and metabolic problems in these injuries can be profound. These burns always heal with scars. Extensive third-degree burns require aggressive treatment in a hospital burn unit, and the death rate (usually from infection) is significant.

Fourth-Degree Burns

Occasionally, burns even deeper than a full thickness of skin occur, such as in an electrical burn, or when a part of the body is trapped in flame. These deep burns enter the muscle and bone and are also called "black" or "char" burns. If a fourth-degree burn involves more than a very small area of the body, the prognosis is very grave, since these deep burns can release toxic substances into the blood-stream. If the burn involves a small area, it should be cut away down to healthy tissue; a charred large area on an arm or leg usually requires amputation.

Electrical Burns

Electrical accidents can cause several different types of burns, including flame burns caused by ignited clothing, electrical current injury, or electrothermal burns from arcing current. Sometimes all three types will be found on the same child. Nearly two-thirds of electrical burn injuries among children aged 12 and under are associated with household electrical cords and extension cords. Wall outlets are associated with an additional 14 percent of these injuries. Among children aged 14 and under, hair curlers and curling irons, room heaters, ovens and ranges, irons, gasoline, and fireworks are the most common causes of product-related thermal burn injuries.

An electric current injury is characterized by focal burns at the point where the current entered and left through the skin. Once an electric current enters the body, its path within the body is determined by tissues with the least resistance. Bone offers the most resistance to electrical current, followed in descending order by fat, tendon, skin, muscle, blood, and nerve. The path the current takes determines whether the child will survive, since current passing through the heart or the brainstem will result in almost instantaneous death from a disturbed heart rhythm. As current passes through muscle, it can set off severe spasms that can fracture or dislocate bones. Although bone does not conduct current well, it stores the heat from the electricity and can damage surrounding muscles.

Electrothermal burns are heat injuries to the skin that occur when high-tension electrical current touches the skin, causing intense, deep damage. Damage is severe because the arc carries temperature of about 2,500°C (hot enough to melt bone). Skin at both entry and exit of the current is usually gray, yellow, and depressed; there may be some charring. All of these wounds must be debrided, which is the removal of ruined or dead tissue.

Chemical Burns

A burn caused by a chemical can be just as destructive as an injury caused by an open flame. If a chemical burns the skin, the chemical should be flushed off the skin surface with cool, running water for 20 minutes or more. If the burning chemical is a powderlike substance such as lime, it should be brushed off the skin before flushing. Clothing or jewelry contaminated by the chemical should be removed. A lotion, such as one containing aloe vera, may be used to prevent drying and to make the skin feel more comfortable. The burned area should be wrapped with a dry, sterile dressing or a clean cloth. The burn should be rinsed again for several more minutes if the child complains of increased burning after the initial washing.

Minor chemical burns usually heal without further treatment. Medical care is required if the child has symptoms of shock (fainting, pale skin, shallow breathing); if the chemical burned through the first layer of skin and the burn covers an area more than two or three inches in diameter, or if the chemical burn occurred on the eyes, hands, feet, face, groin, or buttocks, or over a major joint.

Extent of Burns

When a health care worker estimates a burned patient's injuries in a percentage ("a burn over 60 percent of the body") the percentage is not simply a guess. Health care workers use a "rule of nines" to estimate the amount of body area affected by a burn. The percentage figure is computed by dividing the body into sections: nine percent for the head and neck, nine percent for each arm, 18 percent for each foot and leg, and 18 percent each for the front and back of the trunk. The remaining one percent makes up the perineum (the region between the anus and the urethral opening). This rule is less reliable in children, whose body proportions are different from adults.

Effects

Because a burn destroys a large area of skin, it also disrupts fluid balance, metabolism, temperature, and immune response. Fluid is lost in part by oozing from blisters (called a "weeping burn") and also from dilation of blood vessels that leak fluid into the area beneath the burned skin 36 to 48 hours after the injury. After this period, the fluid is slowly reabsorbed by the body. This fluid and salt loss can be significant, depending on the percentage of the burn.

While there is not much weeping from second- and third-degree burns, the underlying fluid loss is extensive; there may even be fluid loss from remote capillaries in unburned tissue, such as the lungs. If fluid loss is not reversed within an hour after the burn, the fluid loss begins to interfere with organ function and shock sets in. Once the fluid loss reaches a critical level, the circulatory shock becomes irreversible and nothing can be done to save the child's life.

Burn patients also experience an increase in their metabolic and oxygen use rates. This metabolic change is at first fueled by glycogen stored in the liver and muscles, but when these stores are depleted, the body begins to break down its own protein structures. This reaches a maximum level in burns of more than 40 percent.

Most burn patients die from infections of the skin, blood, and lungs, in part due to a weakened immune system.

First/Second-Degree Burn Treatment

Generally, first-degree burns can be treated effectively with first aid. Second-degree burns covering more than 10 percent of a child's body, or burns to the face, hands, or feet, require prompt medical attention. All children with third-degree burns should seek immediate medical help.

First, burns should be flushed with plenty of cold water for 15 to 30 minutes; if the burn was caused by hot grease or acid, the saturated clothing should be removed. The grease should then be washed off the skin and the burn should be soaked in cold water. If clothing sticks to the skin, it should not be pulled off. Instead, the child should be taken to the emergency room.

After rinsing with cold water, the burn should be wrapped in clean dry gauze and left alone for 24 hours. Antiseptics or other irritating substances should not be applied.

A good way to remember how to treat these burns is not to put any substance on the burn that the patient would not put in an eye. If a first- or second-degree burn is smaller than a quarter on a child, the burn can be treated at home. Any burn on an infant, or any large burn, should be treated by a doctor. Butter, an old folk remedy, should never be placed on a burn, since the fat can hold in heat and worsen the injury, possibly causing infection. Ice should never be used to treat a burn in children, who can become seriously chilled with this type of treatment.

Third-Degree Burn Treatment

A third-degree burn should be seen by a doctor as soon as possible. These wounds should not be plunged into water, since cool water may worsen the shock that often accompanies a severe burn. Instead, the injury should be covered with a bulky sterile dressing or with freshly laundered bed linens. Clothing stuck to the wound should not be removed, and no ointments, salves, or sprays should be applied. Burned feet and legs should be elevated; burned hands should be raised above the level of the heart. Breathing should be closely monitored.

The doctor will either lightly dress these burns with an antibacterial dressing, or leave them exposed to enhance healing. Every effort is made to keep the skin germ free by reverse isolation nursing. Reverse isolation nursing protects the patient from the hospital environment by having personnel follow strict gown, glove, and hand-washing procedures. If necessary, painkillers and antibiotics are prescribed, and intravenous fluids are given to offset fluid loss.

Extensive second-degree and all third-degree burns are treated with skin grafts or artificial skin to minimize scars. Extensive burns may need repeated plastic surgery.

Complications

Despite the widespread use of antibacterial drugs, infection remains one of the most serious complications of burn wounds. Children are also prone to developing post-burn seizures, probably from electrolyte imbalances, low oxygen levels in the blood, or infection. Another complication in children is high blood pressure after a burn, probably related to the release of stress hormones after the injury.

Common complications of burn grafts are the formation of fibrous masses of scar tissue called "keloid" or hypertrophic scars, especially in children with dark skin. Direct pressure on inflamed tissue reduces its blood supply and collagen content, which can head off the development of these scars. This pressure can be provided by wearing a variety

of special burn splints, sleeves, stockings, and jackets. Some children may require body traction.

Prognosis

Scars are most common after serious burns and may require years of additional plastic surgery after grafting to release the contractures over joints. Unfortunately, despite modern cosmetic surgical techniques, burn scars are almost always unsightly and the results are almost never as good as the child's pre-burn condition.

Burn scars should be carefully treated, even after they have completely healed. They should not be exposed to sunlight, and those areas of the skin exposed to the sun should be covered by sunscreen. Since deep burns destroy oil and sweat glands, the child may need to apply emollients and lotions to prevent drying and cracking.

Recovery from serious burns may take many years. Children may require extensive psychological counseling in order to adjust to disfigurement, and physical therapy to regain or maintain mobility in damaged joints.

Prevention

About 75 percent of all burn injuries in children are preventable. Most common are scalding injuries that take place in the home, both in the bathroom from too-hot tub water and in the kitchen. An average of nine children aged 14 and under die from scald burn-related injuries each year; children aged four and under account for nearly all of these deaths. And yet more than 75 percent of all scald burn-related injuries among children aged two and under could be prevented through behavioral and environmental modifications.

Water heater safety To reduce the risk of injury to children from hot water scalds, which are the most common type of burn injuries in children, the hot water heater should be turned down to no more than 120°F, which should provide plenty of hot water for normal household activities. At 130°F, a serious burn can occur in 30 seconds. At 140°F, only five seconds are required. The time may be reduced by 50 percent or more for children under age five.

Gas water heaters can be adjusted easily, but electric water heaters need to be disconnected from the electricity and have the cover plates removed in order to adjust the thermostat. After the thermostat is turned down, the temperature should be checked 24 hours later by running the hot water to make sure the temperature is low enough to be safe.

Many communities have established local ordinances or building codes which require the installation of anti-scald plumbing devices in all new construction. Such legislation has been effective in reducing the number of scald burn deaths and injuries associated with hot tap water.

Bathroom Hot tap water accounts for nearly one-fourth of all scald burns among children and is associated with more deaths and hospitalizations than other hot liquid burns. Tap-water burns most often occur in the bathroom and tend to be more severe and cover a larger portion of the body than other scald burns.

The water in a child's bath should never be warmer than 100°F. Parents should run cold water into the tub first, adding hot water later to reach a safe temperature. This will prevent a scald burn if the child should fall into the tub while it is being filled. Before placing a child into the bathtub, parents should check the temperature of the water by moving a hand through the water for a few seconds. If the water feels hot, it is too hot for the child. The child should be faced away from the faucets at the other end of the tub. Most hot tap water scalds happen in the bathroom, so even with the water turned down, parents should never leave a small child unsupervised in the tub.

Pressure balancing, thermostatically controlled shower and tub valves that reduce the water temperature to 115°F or less can help prevent scalding injuries. These valves can be attached to the bathtub fixtures, installed in the wall at the bathtub, or connected at the water heater. Temperature-controlling valves vary in cost and installation requirements and can be purchased at some hardware stores or through plumbers.

Kitchen safety The second most common place for burn and scald injuries is the kitchen. There are a number of safety measures parents should take to protect their children:

- Saucepan handles should be turned toward the back of the stove.

- Hot drinks should be kept away from the edge of the table; a drink heated to 140°F can cause a burn in five seconds and at 160°F, a burn will occur in one second.

- Back burners should be used whenever possible.

- Tablecloths should be avoided if toddlers are in the home. If a child tries to pull himself up by the tablecloth, a heavy object or hot liquid on the table could fall on the child.

- All hot items should be kept near the center of the table to prevent a young child from reaching them.

- While someone is cooking, young children should be kept in a high chair or playpen, at a safe distance from hot surfaces, hot liquids, and other kitchen hazards.

- Deep fat (oil) cookers/fryers should be used with caution when young children are present. The fat or oil may reach temperatures over 400°F, hot enough to instantly cause a very serious burn.

- Ground fault circuit interrupter receptacles should be placed near sinks and other wet areas.

- Appliance cords should be kept away from the edge of counters and unplugged when not in use. A dangling cord is dangerous because it can get caught in a cabinet door or be pulled on by a curious child.

- Snack foods should be stored away from the stove area so children will not be tempted to reach across a hot burner.

- Parents should establish a "safe area" in the kitchen where a child can be placed away from risk but under continuous supervision. Parents should establish a "no zone" directly in front of the stove marked with yellow tape or a piece of bright carpet and teach children to avoid this area.

Microwave safety The vast majority (95 percent) of microwave burns among children are scald burns. Microwave burns are typically caused by spilling hot liquids or food, and injuries are primarily associated with the trunk or the face. Children should be careful when removing a wrapper or cover from a hot item, since hot steam escaping from the container as the covering is lifted can cause a burn. When liquids are heated in the microwave, the containers may feel only warm rather than hot. Cooking some foods in the microwave is more likely to result in scald burns unless very specific precautions are taken. Children should check the microwave oven manual for specific instructions for cooking eggs, squash, potatoes, and eggplant.

In addition, food can heat unevenly in a microwave oven, which can cause serious mouth burns. For example, the jelly in a jelly-filled pastry may be scalding while the pastry itself is only warm. Frozen foods may be cold or only warm in one spot and scalding in another. Children should use caution and follow directions when popping popcorn in the microwave, since the vapor produced in the bag may exceed 180°F.

When heating foods for a young child, parents should check the temperature by sampling the food before allowing the child to eat it. Heating baby formula or milk in bottles with disposable plastic liners may be risky, because the liner may burst. Using a baby bottle warmer is a safer way to heat baby bottles. Parents should not hold a child while removing items from the microwave. Children should be kept at a safe distance from the microwave oven.

As a general rule, only those who have read and understand the directions should use the microwave oven. This means that children under age seven may be at risk, unless they are closely supervised. Even children over seven must be properly supervised and taught microwave safety. A child's height is important to consider when allowing microwave use. Children should be tall enough that their faces are not directly in front of the microwave heating chamber when the door is open.

Smoke alarms Smoke alarms are extremely effective at preventing fire-related death and injury; the chances of dying in a residential fire are cut in half if a smoke alarm is present. In fact, smoke alarms and sprinkler systems combined could reduce fire-related deaths by 82 percent and injuries by 46 percent. For this reason, many states have laws requiring smoke alarms in new and existing dwellings.

Smoke alarms should be installed in the home on every level and in every sleeping area. They should be tested monthly, and batteries should be replaced at least once a year (or at the beginning and end of daylight savings time). The alarms themselves should be replaced every 10 years. Ten-year lithium alarms are also available and do not require an annual battery change.

Flammable sleepwear To prevent burn injuries, the U.S. Consumer Product Safety Commission (CPSC) recommends that parents make sure their children's sleepwear is either flame-resistant or snug-fitting. Loose-fitting T-shirts and other clothing made of cotton or cotton blends should not be used for children's sleepwear, since these garments can catch fire easily, burn rapidly, and are associated with nearly 300 emergency-room-treated burn injuries to children each year.

Children are most at risk for burn injuries from playing with fire (matches, lighters, candles, or burners on stoves) just before bedtime and just after getting up in the morning. For this reason, CPSC requires hangtags and permanent labels on snug-fitting children's sleepwear made of cotton or cotton blends to remind consumers that because the garment is not flame-resistant, it must fit snugly for safety. Parents should look for tags that say the garment is flame-resistant or snug-fitting.

Flame-resistant garments are made from inherently flame-resistant fabrics or are treated with flame retardants and do not continue to burn when removed from a small flame. Snug-fitting sleepwear is made of stretchy cotton or cotton blends that fit closely against a child's body. Snug-fitting sleepwear is less likely than loose T-shirts to come into contact with a flame and does not ignite as easily or burn as rapidly because there is little air under the garment to feed a fire.

CPSC sets national safety standards for children's sleepwear flammability to protect children from serious burn injuries if they come in contact with a small flame. Under federal safety rules, garments sold as children's sleepwear for sizes larger than nine months must be either flame-resistant or snug-fitting.

Fireworks More than 40 percent of people injured in fireworks accidents each year are under 14 years of age. In 1999 nearly 3,800 children aged

14 and under were treated in hospital emergency rooms for fireworks-related injuries. Boys are injured three times as often as girls, and boys between five and 14 years of age have the highest fireworks-related injury rate of all. Not surprisingly, those who are actively participating in fireworks-related activities are more often and more severely injured than are bystanders.

Most injuries occur at home during the July Fourth festivities. Fireworks-related injuries most frequently involve hands and fingers (40 percent), the head and face (20 percent), and eyes (18 percent), and more than half of the injuries are burns. In addition, fireworks can cause life-threatening residential fires.

Nearly two-thirds of fireworks-related injuries are caused by backyard, "class C" fireworks such as firecrackers, bottle rockets, Roman candles, fountains, and sparklers that are legal in many states. However, the most severe injuries are typically caused by "class B" fireworks, such as rockets, cherry bombs, and M-80s, which are federally banned from public sale. In spite of federal regulations and varying state prohibitions, class B and C fireworks are often accessible by the public. It is not uncommon to find fireworks distributors near state borders, where residents of states with strict fireworks regulations can take advantage of another state's more lenient laws.

Among class C fireworks, bottle rockets can fly into the face and cause eye injuries; sparklers can ignite clothing (sparklers burn at more than 1,000°F); and firecrackers can injure hands or face if they explode at close range. Children aged four and under are at the highest risk for sparkler-related injuries.

Injuries may occur if the child is too close to fireworks when they explode; for example, when a child bends over to look more closely at a firework that has been ignited, or when a misguided bottle rocket hits a nearby person.

One study estimates that children are 11 times more likely to be injured by fireworks if they are unsupervised. Younger children often lack the physical coordination to handle fireworks safely, and they are often excited and curious around fireworks, which can increase their chances of being injured. Homemade fireworks can lead to dangerous explosions.

Cigarette lighters Disposable and novelty cigarette lighters were required to be made child-resistant in a 1994 mandatory safety standard by the CPSC. Since this standard has been in effect, the number of child-play lighter fires has dropped 42 percent, and the number of deaths and injuries associated with these fires has declined 31 percent and 26 percent, respectively.

Burns United Support Group   A support group for BURN survivors and their families that provides support services and information on burn care and prevention. The group conducts educational programs and children's services and operates a speaker's bureau.

calamine lotion A pink compound of ferric oxide and zinc oxide that is applied as a lotion, ointment, or dusting powder to cool, dry, and protect the skin. Calamine lotion is used to ease the itch or irritation of DERMATITIS, ECZEMA, CHICKEN POX, POISON IVY, insect bites, or SUNBURN. It may also be combined with a topical local anesthetic such as benzocaine, or with corticosteroids or ANTIHISTAMINES, which reduce inflammation.

California encephalitis See ENCEPHALITIS, CALIFORNIA.

campylobacteriosis A form of food-borne illness first recognized in the 1970s that causes gastroenteritis or "traveler's diarrhea." Much more common than either SALMONELLA POISONING or SHIGELLOSIS, campylobacteriosis is responsible for between 5 and 14 percent of all diarrheal infections in the world. It may affect between two and four million Americans each year.

The *Campylobacter* organism is actually a group of spiral-shaped bacteria. Most human illness is caused by one species, called *Campylobacter jejuni*, but 1 percent of human campylobacteriosis cases are caused by other species. *C. jejuni* grows best at the body temperature of a bird and seems to be well adapted to birds, who carry it without becoming ill.

The bacterium is fragile; it cannot tolerate dryness and can be killed by oxygen. It grows only if there is less than the atmospheric amount of oxygen present. Freezing reduces the number of *Campylobacter* bacteria present on raw meat.

In the 1980s, more than 3,000 residents in Bennington, Vermont, became ill with diarrhea when their town's water supply was contaminated with the rod-shaped bacterium *C. jejuni*.

Without treatment, the stool is infectious for several weeks, but three days of antibiotics will eliminate the bacteria from the stool. While the illness can be uncomfortable and even disabling, deaths among otherwise healthy patients are rare.

Cause

While there are several different forms of *Campylobacter*, the most common is *C. jejuni*, which accounts for 99 percent of all *Campylobacter* infections. Campylobacteriosis is caused by eating or drinking food or water contaminated with the bacteria; only a small amount is necessary to cause illness. It can survive in undercooked food such as chicken, lamb, beef, or pork, and in water and raw milk. The disease may also be spread by the diarrhea of affected young dogs or cats.

The most common source of *Campylobacter* infection is in contaminated poultry (one-third to half of all raw chicken on the market is contaminated). Consumers get sick when they eat undercooked chicken, or when the organisms are transferred to the mouth from the raw meat or raw meat drippings. The bacteria is common among healthy chickens on chicken farms, where it may spread undetected among the flocks (perhaps through drinking water supplies). When the birds are slaughtered, the bacteria is transferred from the intestines to the meat.

Other forms of *Campylobacter* are harder to diagnose and appear to be much more rare than *C. jejuni;* it is not yet clear what the source of those infections are.

Symptoms

Symptoms begin from two to 10 days after tainted food is eaten and may last up to 10 days. They include nausea and vomiting, abdominal pain, followed by watery or bloody diarrhea. Other symptoms may include headaches, fatigue, and body aches.

Diagnosis

The infection is diagnosed when a stool is sent to the lab and cultured using special techniques.

Treatment

Unless antibiotics are taken at the very beginning of the illness they will not affect symptoms, although they will shorten the infectious period. For mild cases, rest and fluids should be sufficient. Young children are usually given antibiotics (usually erythromycin) as a way of reducing the risk of passing the infection on to other children via infected stool.

Prevention

Hands should be washed after using the toilet. Anyone with diarrhea should use a separate towel and washcloth and should not prepare food (especially food consumed uncooked).

Complications

Infection with *Campylobacter* may provoke a paralyzing neurologic illness called Guillain-Barré syndrome in a small percentage of patients. Guillain-Barré syndrome occurs when a person's immune system attacks the body's own nerves, and it can lead to paralysis that lasts several weeks. It is estimated that approximately one in every 1,000 reported campylobacteriosis cases leads to Guillain-Barré syndrome. As many as 40 percent of Guillain-Barré syndrome cases in this country may be triggered by campylobacteriosis. Most people who get campylobacteriosis recover completely within two to five days, although recovery may take up to 10 days.

cancer   See CHILDHOOD CANCERS.

candidiasis   See THRUSH; DIAPER RASH; VAGINITIS; YEAST INFECTIONS.

Candlelighter's Childhood Cancer Foundation

A nonprofit foundation that offers a voice for pediatric cancer families and survivors to the general public, the medical community, government, schools, employers, and the media. Candlelighter's Childhood Cancer Foundation (CCCF) was founded in 1970 by concerned parents of children with cancer. The current 43,000 members include parents of children who are being treated or have been treated for cancer; children with cancer; survivors of childhood cancer; immediate or extended family members; bereaved families; health care professionals; and educators. CCCF's information clearinghouse can provide information on many aspects of childhood cancer, including quarterly publications, newsletters, and informative brochures.

The group has a network of parent support groups in all states and on every continent, providing meetings, speakers, parent-to-parent visitation, summer camps, transportation, emergency funding, and publications. In addition, the foundation works with other cancer patient advocacy groups for better funding for pediatric cancer research and on legislative issues which impact members. Candlelighters provides referrals to volunteers who can help families and survivors in the areas of employment, insurance, education, the military, and government benefits. It can also help obtain second medical opinions.

canker sore   A small painful ulcer on the inside of the mouth, lip, or underneath the tongue that heals without treatment. About 20 percent of Americans at any one time experience a canker sore, which are most common between ages 10 and 40. The most severely affected people have almost continuous sores, while others have just one or two per year.

Cause

Because hemolytic streptococcus bacteria have so often been isolated from canker sores, experts believe they may be caused by a hypersensitive reaction to the bacteria. Other factors often associated with a flare-up include trauma (such as biting the inside of the cheek), acute stress and allergies, or chemical irritants in toothpaste or mouthwash. More women than men experience canker sores, which are more likely to occur during the premenstrual period and are more likely to occur if other members of the family suffer from them. Interestingly, the older a person gets the less likely they are to suffer a canker sore. Some experts believe canker sores may be connected to an underlying immune system defect similar to an allergy.

Symptoms

A canker sore is usually a small oval ulcer with a gray center surrounded by a red, inflamed halo, which usually lasts for one or two weeks. They are similar but not identical to COLD SORES (or "fever blisters)", which also appear on the mouth. Both usually cause small sores that heal within two weeks. However, canker sores are not usually preceded by a blister. Canker sores are usually larger than fever blisters, but they do not usually merge to form one large sore as fever blisters do. Finally, canker sores usually erupt on movable parts of the mouth (such as the tongue and the cheek or lip linings), whereas cold sores usually appear on the gums, roof of the mouth, lips, or nostrils.

Treatment

While the ulcers will heal themselves, topical painkillers may ease the pain; healing may be speeded up by using a corticosteroid ointment or a tetracycline mouthwash. Victims may also cover the sore with a waterproof ointment to protect it. A canker sore should heal within two weeks; if it persists, or if the sufferer cannot eat, speak, or sleep, seek medical help.

Over-the-counter medication containing carbamide peroxide (Cankaid, Glyoxide, and Amosan) may be effective in treating the sore. Other possibilities include medications that include liquid or gel forms of benzocaine, menthol, camphor, eucalyptol and/or alcohol, or pastes (such as Orabase) that form a protective "bandage" over the sore. For short-term pain relief, rinse with a prescription mouthwash containing viscous lidocaine, an anesthetic.

Prevention

Children prone to canker sores should avoid coffee, spices, citrus fruits, walnuts, strawberries, and chocolates. Instead, eating at least four tablespoons of plain yogurt containing *Lactobacillus acidophilus* daily introduces helpful bacteria into the mouth to fight canker sore bacteria. To prevent outbreaks and to heal severe ones, a prescription anti-inflammatory steroid may help.

Children should avoid commercial toothpastes and mouthwashes and brush teeth with baking soda for a month or two. The mouth should be rinsed with warm salt water. Specifically, scientists found that toothpaste with the detergent sodium lauryl sulfate (SLS) was linked to canker sores in susceptible children. In a study of 10 people prone to sores, brushing with SLS-free paste for three months led to a 70 percent decrease in the number of canker sores. Scientists suggest that SLS may dry out the mucous layer of the mouth, leaving gums and cheeks vulnerable to irritants.

carbon monoxide poisoning A colorless, poisonous gas that is produced by the incomplete combustion of solid, liquid, and gaseous fuels. Nearly 5,000 people in the United States are treated each year in the hospital for carbon monoxide poisoning; this number may be quite low, since many people mistake the symptoms of poisoning for the flu and never get treated. Unborn babies, infants, and children with anemia are especially sensitive to carbon monoxide poisoning.

Cause

Appliances fueled with gas, oil, kerosene, or wood may produce carbon dioxide. If these appliances are not installed, maintained, and used properly, carbon monoxide may build up to dangerous levels. Common sources include gas cooking ranges, hot water heaters and dryers, wood- or coal-burning stoves and fireplaces, oil burners, and kerosene heaters. Gas water heaters and dryers and oil burners must have stacks that direct the carbon monoxide outside. Wood-burning stoves and fireplaces must have chimneys that vent the gas outside. Unvented kerosene heaters spread carbon monoxide gas indoors; therefore, a window must always be open slightly when a kerosene heater is being used. Carbon monoxide is also found in the exhaust of internal combustion car engines.

Symptoms

Breathing carbon monoxide causes headaches, dizziness, weakness, sleepiness, nausea and vomiting, confusion, and disorientation. At very high levels, the gas in the blood rises, leaving the child confused and clumsy. Loss of consciousness and death soon follow.

Symptoms are particularly dangerous because the effects often are not recognized, since the gas is odorless and some of the symptoms are similar to other common illnesses.

Breathing low levels of the chemical can cause fatigue and increase chest pain in people with chronic heart disease and may cause fatal heart attacks.

Treatment

The child must be removed to fresh air immediately. If the child is not breathing (or is breathing irregularly), artificial respiration must be performed. The child should be kept warm and quiet to prevent shock. Medical personnel can give oxygen (often with 5 percent carbon dioxide) and a doctor should be consulted to check for long-term effects, even if the child appears to have recovered.

Prevention

Although carbon monoxide cannot be seen or smelled, there are signs that might indicate a problem, such as visible rust or stains on vents and chimneys, appliances that make unusual sounds or smells, or an appliance that keeps shutting off.

Dangerous levels of carbon monoxide can be prevented by proper appliance use, maintenance, and installation. A qualified service technician should check a home's central and room heating appliances each year. The technician should look at the electrical and mechanical components of appliances, such as thermostat controls and automatic safety devices. In addition,

- Chimneys and flues should be checked for blockages, corrosion, and loose connections
- Individual appliances should be serviced regularly
- Kerosene and gas space heaters should be cleaned and inspected
- New appliances should be installed and vented properly
- The room where an unvented gas or kerosene space heater is used should be well ventilated, and doors leading to another room should be open to ensure proper ventilation
- An unvented combustion heater should never be used overnight or in a room where someone is sleeping

One of the best ways to prevent carbon monoxide poisoning is to install detectors that meet the requirements of Underwriters Laboratories (UL) standard 2034. Detectors that meet the UL standard measure both high carbon monoxide concentrations over short periods of time, and low concentrations over long periods of time. Detectors sound an alarm before the level of carbon monoxide in a person's blood becomes dangerous. Since carbon monoxide gases move evenly and fairly quickly throughout the house, a CO detector should be installed on the wall or ceiling in sleeping areas, but outside individual bedrooms.

carbuncle A cluster of boils (pus-filled inflamed hair roots) infected with bacteria, commonly found on the back of the neck and the buttocks.

Cause

Carbuncles are usually caused by the bacterium *Staphylococcus aureus*.

Symptoms

Carbuncles usually begin as single boils that spread, but they are less common than single boils. They primarily affect patients with lowered resistance to infection.

Treatment

Carbuncles are treated with oral and topical antibiotics and hot compresses or plasters. These may relieve the pain by causing the pus-filled heads to burst; if this occurs, the carbuncle should be covered with a dressing until it has healed completely. Once the inflammation has been controlled, the lesion may be cut and drained. The cavity may then need packing with a petroleum jelly or iodoform dressing.

In some cases, draining is not necessary if a 10-day course of antibiotics and topical antibiotics cures the infection.

Prevention

Recurrent carbuncles usually mean that patients are constantly reinfecting themselves. Regular washing with antibacterial soap (especially around rashes, irritations, shaving, or areas of heavy sweating) can help get rid of the infection. Also, hands and bedding should be washed often.

car seats   Child safety seats can reduce the risk of a potentially fatal injury by 69 percent for babies younger than one year old, and by 47 percent for one- to four-year-old children. Yet despite laws in all 50 states requiring the use of car safety seats or child restraint devices for young children, many continue to be killed each year while riding unrestrained or improperly restrained in motor vehicles. In 1994, 673 children younger than five years of age died while riding in motor vehicles; 362 were unrestrained, and many more were restrained improperly. Unfortunately, 80 percent of all safety seats are used incorrectly, according to the National Highway Traffic Safety Administration (NHTSA).

As of September 1, 2002, all new cars and child safety seats must have attachments designed to make them fit together like a key in a lock. The new system, called LATCH (Lower Anchors and Tethers for Children), is designed to make it easier to fit the child seat tightly in the vehicle. By law, every new car must be made with six-millimeter bars (or anchors) in the backseat where the cushions meet, and every child seat must be built with clips that connect to the anchors for a secure fit.

The second feature of LATCH is a tether behind the backseat that connects to a strap on top of the child seat. The tethers, which have been required since 2000, are designed to keep the child from whipping forward during an accident.

The LATCH system works only with forward- and rear-facing child seats; it is not used with booster seats recommended for children aged four to eight.

Reaction to the system has been largely positive among manufacturers, safety advocates, and parents, although some safety advocates complain that LATCH anchors can be hard to find in the seat upholstery and may not be strong enough for toddlers weighing more than 50 pounds. Also, automakers are required to put the anchors only at the two outboard seats; many parents prefer to put their children in the middle of the backseat to avoid injuries in side impact accidents. Although many vehicles already have the LATCH system, it has not been available in many car seats until recently because of the cost. Car seats with a rigid metal attachment can add $34 to $44 to the cost, while those with the more common flexible strap connectors cost $10 to $21 more.

Some car seat manufacturers sell retrofit kits averaging around $25 that allow the seat to work with a car's LATCH system, but they are not necessary if a seat is tightly secured with a seat belt. Retrofits will not be available for the lower anchors for most vehicles, although Volkswagen and Audi are offering to install the hardware for free in 1993 and newer models.

In addition, the American Academy of Pediatrics recommends that:

- Children should face the rear of the car until they weigh at least 20 pounds and are one year old to reduce the risk of cervical spine injury in the event of a crash. Infants who weigh 20 pounds before one year should ride facing the rear in a convertible seat or infant seat approved for higher weights until one year of age.

- A rear-facing car safety seat must not be placed in the front passenger seat of any car equipped with a passenger-side front air bag.

- Premature and small infants should not be placed in car safety seats with shields, abdominal pads, or arm rests that could directly contact an infant's face and neck during an impact.

- In rear-facing car safety seats for infants, shoulder straps must be in the lowest slots until the infant's shoulders are above the slots; the harness must be snug; and the car safety seat's retainer clip should be positioned at the midpoint of the infant's chest, not on the abdomen or in the neck area.

- If the vehicle seat slopes so that the infant's head flops forward, the car safety seat should be reclined halfway back, at a 45 degree angle. A firm roll of cloth or newspaper can be wedged under the car safety seat below the infant's feet to achieve this angle.

- A convertible safety seat (that is positioned reclined and rear facing for a child until age one and 20 pounds, and semi-upright and forward facing for a child over age one who weighs 20 to 40 pounds) should be used as long as the child's ears are below the top of the back of the seat and shoulders are below the seat strap slots.

- A booster seat should be used when the child has outgrown a convertible safety seat but is too small to fit properly in a car safety belt. A belt-positioning booster seat with a combination lap/shoulder belt is better than a booster seat with a small shield, which can be used when only a lap belt is available.

Older Children

Companies across the United States have responded to the problem of older children who do not fit well in seat belts by designing add-on devices that try to make the shoulder portion of the safety belt fit correctly. These products vary in design, yet all claim to solve the problem of poorly fitting shoulder harnesses. However, some of these products actually seem to interfere with proper lap and shoulder harness fit by positioning the lap belt too high on the abdomen and the shoulder harness too low across the shoulder and by allowing too much slack in the shoulder harness. Although in some cases these products may help shoulder harnesses fit as they were designed, the add-on products are usually tested only by their manufacturers, which allows manufacturers to make claims that cannot be substantiated by independent means.

Parents should read their car owner's manual and child restraint device instructions carefully and test the car safety seat for a safe, snug fit in the vehicle to avoid potentially life-threatening incompatibility problems between the design of the car safety seat, vehicle seat, and seat belt system.

Choosing a Seat

When choosing any car seat, there are important general guidelines to follow in order to ensure the child's safety. According to the American Academy of Pediatrics (AAP), the best car seat is the one that best fits a child's weight, size, and age, as well as the car. Once a seat has been chosen, it should be tried out, since store displays and illustrations might not show correct the usage. It is up to the adult to learn how to install a car safety seat properly and strap in the child. Parents should:

- choose a seat whose label states that it meets or exceeds Federal Motor Vehicle Safety Standard 213

- accept a used seat with caution and never accept a seat that is more than 10 years old or one that was in a crash (it could be structurally unsound)

- avoid seats that are missing parts or are not labeled with the manufacture date and model number (there is no way to know about recalls)

- check the seat for the manufacturer's recommended "expiration date"

- call the manufacturer of a used seat to find out if the seat was ever recalled. The manufacturer may be able to provide a replacement part or new model.

carsickness   A type of motion sickness caused by the movement of a car, characterized by vertigo, sweating, salivation, nausea, and vomiting. Car sickness is caused by the motion associated with travel and can occur not just in the car but also in a boat, airplane, or any activity accompanied by irregular motion.

Carsickness begins not in the stomach but in the inner ear, when irregular motion (such as in a car, plane, or boat) causes fluid changes in the semicircular canals of the inner ear, making it unable to maintain a state of equilibrium. The result is the symptoms of car sickness.

Prevention

Unfortunately, there are not any drugs that children can take to prevent carsickness. Those that are available for adults such as scopalamine are not safe for children.

Children who tend to get car sick may feel better if they can sit high enough to see out of the car and look out the window. Scheduling a trip during naptime may help, as can scheduling as many rest stops as possible. Carsickness is often partly a conditioned response because of a prior experience—if children had a bad car ride in the past, this may trigger a queasy feeling every time they get in the car. Distraction can help, including toys and snacks youngsters normally do not get at home. (However, if the child tends to vomit on a car trip, a snack might not be a good idea.) The window should be cracked open, since fresh air will help ease discomfort.

A queasy child should pick out a landmark on the horizon and keep watching that spot. Looking out into the distance will give the brain input about the fact that the car is moving and should help resolve some of the carsickness. Above all, children who get carsick should not read in the car. While it may be a distraction, it will only make children sicker because when they focus on a still page while moving, the brain gets the mixed signals that cause motion sickness.

cat-scratch disease (CSD) A mild illness following the scratch or bite of a kitten or cat that may involve a rash, caused by a small bacterium recently identified as *Bartonella* (formerly *Rochalimaea*) *henselae*. There are about 22,000 cases of cat-scratch disease (CSD) in the United States each year; three-quarters of the cases occur in children, more often in fall and winter. While the disease causes few problems in healthy youngsters, those with a weakened immune system can develop a life-threatening infection.

Cause
The disease was first recognized in the 1950s, but the organism that causes it has only been recently discovered. The bacteria are transmitted between cats by the common cat flea. The animal itself does not appear to be ill, and about 90 percent of cases are caused by kittens; the rest result from grown cats, dogs, and other animals.

Researchers still do not understand how the bacteria can live in the bloodstream, since blood is normally sterile and bacteria are usually killed by the immune system. While cats with the disease are not ill, many have large numbers of organisms in their blood.

The disease cannot be transmitted from one person to another, and it is not clear if one episode confers immunity.

Symptoms
About two weeks after a bite or scratch, the victim reports a red round lump at the site of infection and one or more swollen lymph nodes near the scratch, which may become painful and tender and occasionally discharge. Occasionally there is fever, rash, malaise, and headache. In most cases, symptoms disappear on their own.

Diagnosis
CSD can be diagnosed by symptoms, history, and negative tests for other diseases that cause swollen lymph glands. In 1992 the Centers for Disease Control developed a blood test that detects antibodies to the bacteria. The test is available free to doctors and state health departments. Biopsy of a small sample of the swollen lymph node is not necessary unless there is an unusual symptom.

Treatment
There are no antibiotics effective against CSD, although they are often prescribed for children with severe pain or swelling. A severely affected lymph node or blister may have to be drained, and a heating pad may help swollen, tender lymph glands. Acetaminophen may relieve pain, aches, and fever over 101°F. In most cases, the illness fades after one or two months, and the cat does not need to be destroyed.

A rare complication is ENCEPHALITIS, or cat-scratch disease of the brain, which appears about one or two weeks after the first symptoms of CSD. This usually resolves on its own without treatment. Signs of complications include: unusual spots or bruises on the skin, eye infections, unusual pain, high fever (over 103°F), stiff neck, severe headache, or severe vomiting.

Prevention
Other than avoiding cats, there is no way to avoid the disease. However, cats only carry the infecting organism for a few weeks during their lifetimes, so the likelihood of being reinfected, or infected by just one pet in the home, is minimal. Children with weakened immune systems do not need to get rid of their cats, but they should try to avoid getting scratched. If a scratch does occur, it should be washed thoroughly with soap and water.

cefaclor (Ceclor) A common cephalosporin-type antibiotic used to treat EAR INFECTIONS, upper and lower respiratory tract infections, URINARY TRACT INFECTIONS, skin infections, sore throat, and TONSILLITIS. The drug should be used with caution in patients who are allergic to penicillin.

Side Effects
Severe diarrhea, nausea and vomiting, or skin rash.

celiac disease A condition in which the small intestine cannot absorb and digest food, caused by

GLUTEN SENSITIVITY. Although an estimated one in 4,700 Americans have been diagnosed with this disease, a study from the Red Cross suggests it may be far more common: one in every 250 Americans.

For those who cannot tolerate gluten, the substance damages the lining of the intestines and flattens the villi—small hair-like projections that normally protrude from the intestinal surfaces that help absorb nutrients.

Permanent intolerance to gluten that damages the small intestine can be reversed by avoiding gluten in the diet. As the villi become damaged, they are unable to absorb water and nutrients, which causes the child to be susceptible to a variety of other conditions related to malabsorption.

Celiac disease is hereditary and primarily affects whites of northwestern European ancestry, rarely affecting blacks, Jews, Asians, or people of Mediterranean ancestry. It affects twice as many girls as boys and usually affects more children than adults.

There are many names for celiac disease, all of which refer to the inability to tolerate gluten. These include celiac sprue, coeliac disease, Gee-Herter's disease (or syndrome), gluten intolerance, gluten sensitive enteropathy (GSE), gluten sensitivity, idiopathic steatorrhea, intestinal infantilism, malabsorption syndrome, nontropical sprue, or celiac syndrome.

Symptoms

The symptoms of celiac disease vary, ranging from no symptoms at all to severe gas, bloating, diarrhea, and abdominal pain. It can be triggered by overexposure to wheat, severe stress, emotional or physical trauma, surgery, or a viral infection. Symptoms may include irritability, depression, muscle cramps, joint pain, fatigue, and menstrual irregularities. Reactions to ingestion of gluten can be immediate or delayed for weeks or even months.

Diagnosis

There is no test that can directly identify celiac disease, but blood antibody tests can measure levels of antibodies to gluten. If the antibodies in the blood are higher than normal, a biopsy of the small intestine can check for damage to the villi. If the villi appear damaged, the child is given a gluten-free diet and then rebiopsied after another six months.

Symptoms or an abnormal intestinal biopsy that improves after a gluten-free diet provide the most convincing evidence that a child has celiac disease or gluten sensitivity.

Treatment

The only acceptable treatment for celiac disease requires a lifelong avoidance of all products that contain gluten, which can prevent almost all complications caused by the disease. If untreated, the child can become malnourished and eventually risk life-threatening complications such as cancer, osteoporosis, anemia, and seizures.

Terms to avoid   Gluten masquerades under many different names, and children with celiac disease must also avoid ingredients including durum flour, rye, oats and barley, couscous, semolina, spelt, kamut, bulgur, triticale, caramel coloring, enriched flour, cereal, MSG, emulsifiers, stabilizers, and distilled vinegar. Other terms to watch out for include dextrin, malt, maltodextrin, modified food starch, fillers, natural flavoring, hydrolyzed vegetable protein (HVP), and hydrolyzed plant protein (HPP)—any of these may also contain gluten. In addition, products labeled "wheat-free" are not necessarily gluten-free. The term "starch" can refer to "cornstarch" or "wheat starch"—the first is allowed, but the second is not. Gluten is often used as a thickener, and so it may be included in canned soups, catsups, mustards, soy sauce, and other condiments.

Products to avoid   Most cereals, grains, pastas, breads, and processed foods contain some type of gluten, unless they are specifically made to be gluten-free. Vegetable cooking sprays, tomato pastes, spaghetti sauces, and veined cheeses like Roquefort and bleu cheese also may contain gluten. In addition to foods, many vitamins and medications may contain gluten as additives.

Simply avoiding foods with gluten is not enough, however. It is also important to make sure safe foods have not come in contact with gluten-containing products or cooking utensils and containers previously used. A cross-contaminated item might be a toaster, deep fryer, griddle, butter, or jelly. Imitation seafood and instant or flavored coffees and teas may also be hidden sources of gluten. Because the glues used on envelopes and postage stamps contain gluten, children should use a moistened cloth or sponge to seal or attach these items.

Some health and beauty aids contain gluten, so all labels on lotions, creams, and cosmetics should be checked. Likewise, chewing gum may also contain gluten since it might be dusted with wheat flour to keep it from being sticky.

Safe foods Still, children with gluten intolerance can eat a well-balanced diet with a variety of foods, including bread and pasta made with special flours. Many types of food do not contain gluten, including all fresh vegetables and fruits, fresh meat, fish, aged cheeses, dried beans and peas, rice, and many canned and processed foods.

Wheat flour substitutes Gluten-free mixes and flours are available from a variety of sources, including health food stores. Many types of flour can be substituted in place of regular flour when baking gluten-free products:

- Amaranth flour adds flavor but since it does not stick together well when used on its own, it should be combined with other flours to make cakes, biscuits, and pancakes.

- Buckwheat flour should be used in small amounts only because it has a very strong flavor and is sometimes difficult to digest.

- Carob flour can be used in cakes, biscuits, drinks, desserts, and sweets.

- Corn flour can be blended with cornmeal when making corn breads or muffins.

- Millet flour tends to make breads dry and coarse, so it should be mixed in with other flours.

- Nut or legume flours can be used in small portions to enhance the taste of puddings, cookies, or homemade pasta.

- Potato starch flour is excellent for baking and thickening cream soups when combined with other flours.

- Quinoa flour makes excellent biscuits and pancakes, although it can taste a bit bitter.

- Rice flour (brown or white) is good for thickening gravies, sauces, and cream pies.

- Sorghum flour is the best general purpose gluten-free flour, and it is excellent for baking.

- Soy flour has a nutty flavor and should be combined with other flours in baked products containing nuts, chocolate, or fruit.

- Tapioca flour can make baked goods chewy and is an excellent choice in small amounts.

Related Disorders

Celiac disease is linked to many immune-related disorders, including diabetes mellitus, chronic active HEPATITIS, chronic fatigue syndrome, and inflammatory bowel disease. Some researchers believe that gluten intolerance can impair mental functioning in some individuals, and that it may cause or aggravate AUTISM, ATTENTION DEFICIT HYPERACTIVITY DISORDER (ADHD), or SCHIZOPHRENIA. Many children with celiac disease also suffer from LACTOSE INTOLERANCE.

cellulitis A bacterial infection of loose connective tissue (particularly subcutaneous tissue). Untreated, the disease may lead to bacteremia, blood infection, or gangrene; facial infections may spread to the eye socket.

Cause

Cellulitis is usually caused by B-hemolytic streptococci bacteria. Very rarely, cellulitis develops after childbirth and may spread to the pelvic organs. Before the development of antibiotics, cellulitis was occasionally fatal. Today any form of cellulitis is likely to be more serious in those with compromised immune systems.

Symptoms

The affected area (usually the face, neck, or legs) is usually hot, tender, and red; other symptoms include fever and chills.

Treatment

Antibiotics (penicillin, erythromycin, or clindamycin) must be taken for up to two weeks to clear the infection.

Center to Prevent Handgun Violence The legal action, research, and education affiliate of Handgun Control. Founded in 1983, the Center builds bridges to law enforcement, educators, legal scholars, public health officials, and health care providers, uniting diverse experts in a search for solutions to the gun violence epidemic.

cephalexin (Keflex, Biocef) A cephalosporin antibacterial prescribed to treat skin, bone, ear, and respiratory tract infections.

Side Effects

Cephalexin may cause nausea, diarrhea, or allergic reactions, especially in children sensitive to penicillin.

cerebral palsy A condition caused by injury to the parts of the brain that control the ability to use muscles. Most often the injury happens before or during birth or soon afterward. A child can have mild, moderate, or severe cerebral palsy (CP). In mild cases, a child simply may be clumsy. With moderate CP, a child might walk with a limp and require a special leg brace or a cane. More severe CP can affect all parts of a child's physical abilities and require use of a wheelchair and other special equipment.

Sometimes children with CP can also have learning problems, problems with hearing or vision, or MENTAL RETARDATION. Usually, the greater the injury to the brain, the more severe the CP, but the condition does not worsen over time, and most children with CP have a normal life span.

About 500,000 Americans have some form of CP; each year 8,000 infants and nearly 1,500 preschoolage children are diagnosed with the condition.

Symptoms

There are three main types of cerebral palsy: spastic, athetoid, and a combination of these two types known as "mixed."

Spastic CP is the most common form and is characterized by extremely tight muscles, with stiff movements of the legs, arms, or back. Children with this form of CP move their legs awkwardly, turning in or scissoring their legs as they try to walk.

Athetoid CP (also called *dyskinetic CP*) can affect movements of the entire body. Typically, this involves slow, uncontrolled body movements and low muscle tone that make it hard for the person to sit straight and walk.

Mixed CP is a combination of the symptoms listed above. A child with this form has some muscles that are too tight and others that are too loose, creating a mix of stiffness and involuntary movements.

In some cases of cerebral palsy, only the legs are affected (diplegia) or only half the body (hemiplegia).

Treatment

With early and ongoing treatment the effects can be reduced. Children younger than age three benefit from early intervention; older children can get special education services through the public school. Typically, children with CP may need different kinds of therapy, including:

- *Physical therapy* to help develop stronger muscles, with emphasis on walking, sitting, and keeping his or her balance
- *Occupational therapy* to help develop fine motor skills such as dressing, feeding, writing, and other daily living tasks
- *Speech-language pathology* to help develop communication skills

A variety of special equipment may help. This may include braces to hold the foot in place when the child stands or walks or custom splints to help a child use the hands. A variety of therapy equipment and adapted toys can help children play, and activities such as swimming or horseback riding can help strengthen weaker muscles and relax the tighter ones. Surgery, Botox injections, or other medications can help lessen the effects of CP, but there is no cure for the condition.

Education

A child with CP can face many challenges in school and is likely to need individualized help. For children up to age three, services are provided through an early intervention system. Schools work with the child's family to develop an individualized family services plan that describes the child's unique needs and required services. The plan also emphasizes the unique needs of the family, so that parents and other family members will know how to help their young child.

For school-aged children (including preschoolers), special education and services will be provided through the school. School staff will work with the child's parents to develop an individualized education program (IEP), which describes the child's unique needs and necessary services. Special education and related services, which can include physical and occupational therapy and speech-language pathology, are provided free.

In addition to therapy services and special equipment, children with CP may need communication devices like voice synthesizers, or communication boards with pictures, symbols, letters, or words attached. The child communicates by pointing to or gazing at the pictures. Other types of technology may include electronic toys with special switches or a sophisticated computer.

cerebrospinal fluid analysis   See SPINAL TAP.

cereus   A type of food poisoning caused by the *Bacillus cereus* bacteria, which multiplies in raw foods at room temperature. The *B. cereus* bacteria produces toxins most often found in steamed or refried rice. It is believed that poisoning with *B. cereus* is underreported because its symptoms are so similar to other types of food poisoning (especially staphylococcal and *Clostridium perfringens* poisoning).

A wide variety of foods including meats, milk, vegetables, and fish have been associated with the diarrheal type of cereus food poisoning. The vomiting-type outbreaks have generally been associated with rice products, but other starchy foods such as potatoes, pasta, and cheese products have also been implicated. Food mixtures such as sauces, puddings, soups, casseroles, pastries, and salads have often been linked to food poisoning outbreaks.

Nine outbreaks were reported to the Centers for Disease Control in 1980 related to such foods as beef, turkey, and Mexican foods. In 1981 eight outbreaks primarily involved rice and shellfish. Other outbreaks go unreported or are misdiagnosed because symptoms are so similar to *Staphylococcus aureus* intoxication (*B. cereus* vomiting-type) or *C. perfringens* food poisoning (*B. cereus* diarrheal type).

Symptoms
This bacteria produces two distinct types of food poisoning: The first features a short incubation period after eating tainted food (usually less than six hours), causing cramps and vomiting and occasionally a short bout with diarrhea. Almost 80 percent of patients with these symptoms who test positive for *B. cereus* poisoning have eaten steamed or refried rice at Chinese restaurants.

The second type of *B. cereus* poisoning is very similar to *C. perfringens* poisoning; it appears within eight to 24 hours after ingestion of tainted food and causes abdominal cramps and diarrhea with very little vomiting.

Treatment
Treatment of both types of the disease is aimed at making the child comfortable. There are no medications that will shorten the course of the disease.

chancroid   A sexually transmitted disease rarely seen in the past 30 years but making a comeback since the early 1980s. There have been outbreaks in the United States in large cities in California and parts of the South over the past 15 years.

Those most at risk are teens with multiple sex partners or those with other STDs (especially syphilis). However, any sexually active person can be infected with chancroid.

Cause
Chancroid is caused by *Hemophilus ducreyi,* a rod-shaped bacterium that grows only in the absence of oxygen (much like GONORRHEA bacteria). The bacteria is transmitted from the draining sores of an infected person during sex. It is more likely to be transmitted to another person with a small cut or scratch in the genital area. The chances of transmission are greater if a person is very active sexually and does not practice personal hygiene.

Symptoms
Symptoms usually appear within a week of infection. In girls, there will be a small pimple with a reddish base that will gradually fill with pus, opening and hollowing. Eventually, several ulcers usually appear that are very painful and soft. About a week later, the pelvic lymph gland on one side of

the groin may become enlarged and painful. Other girls do not notice sores but have pain during sex or while urinating. Still others never notice any symptoms, especially if the sores are on the vaginal walls or cervix.

Boys experience painful sores under the foreskin or on the underside of the penis that fill with pus and turn into ulcers. About 50 percent of infected boys will go on to develop painful, enlarged lymph glands in the groin.

Both boys and girls are infectious until the lesions are completely healed, which may take up to a week. It is not possible to become immune.

Diagnosis

The disease is diagnosed by symptoms and negative test results for other more common causes of genital ulcers (such as syphilis or HERPES). About half the time, a gram stain from a draining ulcer will correctly diagnose the infection; a culture of the drainage will provide a correct diagnosis but the bacteria are not easy to grow and many labs are not equipped to do the test.

Treatment

Antibiotics for both partners, such as azithromycin or erythromycin, or a shot of ceftriaxone, will cure the disease in about a week. Lesions and ulcers will heal in about two weeks.

Complications

Untreated chancroid often causes ulcers on the genitals that may persist for weeks or months. The infection does not harm the fetus of a pregnant girl. However, the lesion does increase the chances of contracting HIV if a person has sex with an HIV-infected partner.

chicken pox (varicella) This is a common childhood infectious disease characterized by a rash and slight fever affecting about four million children each year in the United States. About 90 percent of cases occur in children under age 10, primarily in winter and spring. Chicken pox is also known as varicella, after the virus that causes the disease (varicella-zoster, or VZV). The name "varicella" dates to the 1700s, where it comes from the Latin term for SMALLPOX.

Most people throughout the world have had the disease by age 10, and chicken pox is rare in adults. When it does occur after childhood, it is a far more serious illness.

Cause

VZV is a member of the family of herpes viruses similar to the herpes simplex virus (HSV); the same virus that causes chicken pox also causes SHINGLES. Having chicken pox creates a lifelong immunity, but the virus stays in the body in a latent stage, hiding in the nerves of the lower spinal cord for the rest of the person's life. In old age or during times of stress the virus can reactivate and lead to shingles.

Symptoms

The VZV virus, which is spread by airborne droplets, is extremely contagious. The incubation period ranges from 10 to 23 days. One to three weeks after exposure, a rash appears on the torso, face, armpits, upper arms and legs, inside the mouth, and sometimes in the windpipe and bronchial tubes, causing a dry cough.

The rash is made up of small, red, itchy spots that grow into fluid-filled blisters within a few hours. After several days, the blisters dry out and form scabs. New spots usually continue to form over four to seven days. Children usually have only a slight fever, but an adult may experience fever with severe pneumonia and breathing problems. Adults usually have higher fevers, more intense rash, and more complications than children.

The average child will have between 250 and 500 blisters over about five days; the more blisters the child has, the harder the body has to fight to make enough antibodies to destroy the virus. The fight between the virus and the immune system causes fevers, fatigue, and poor appetite. Those who catch the disease from a sibling instead of a classmate usually have a more severe illness, from 300 to 5,000 blisters. This is because the close contact at home causes a much larger amount of virus to enter the system.

The patient is infectious from five days before the rash erupts until all the blisters are completely healed, dried, and scabbed over. This can take from six to 10 days after the rash appears.

Complications

In children, complications may include bacterial infection and, rarely, REYE'S SYNDROME or encephalitis (an inflammation of the brain). Immunocompromised patients who are susceptible to VZV are at high risk for having severe varicella infections with widespread lesions.

Between 40 and 200 people die every year in the United States due to VZV infections; half are previously healthy people and the other half are those with impaired immune systems. Death occurs more often in adults than children.

Treatment

In most cases, rest is all that is needed for children, who usually recover within 10 days. Acetaminophen may reduce the fever, and calamine lotion, baking soda baths, and oral antihistamines ease the itch. Compresses can dry weeping lesions. *Aspirin should never be given to a child who has flu-like symptoms or has been exposed to (or has recently recovered from) chicken pox;* giving aspirin in these cases has been linked to Reye's syndrome.

The drug acyclovir may be prescribed for a chicken pox patient over age 13 within the first 24 hours after the rash appears if the child is not pregnant and who have any of the following: chronic skin or lung disorders, required regular administration of aspirin or steroids, severe case of chicken pox, a compromised immune system. Unlike the herpes viruses, VZV is relatively resistant to acyclovir, and doses required for treatment are much larger and must be administered intravenously. While the drug may shorten the length of the illness and lessen symptoms, its high cost and marginal effectiveness have prompted the American Academy of Pediatrics not to recommend it as a routine treatment. Scratching should be avoided, as it may lead to secondary bacterial infection and increase the chance of scarring.

If possible, parents should not take a child with suspected chicken pox into the doctor's office where others will be exposed to the disease; it can be very dangerous to newborns or those with suppressed immune systems. The virus can be spread both through the air and by direct contact with an infected individual. Instead, parents should call the physician on the phone and describe the symptoms.

Prevention

A chicken pox vaccine was tested in more than 9,400 healthy children and more than 1,600 adults in the United States before it was licensed in 1995. Several million doses of vaccine have since been given to children in the United States. Studies continue to show the vaccine to be safe and effective. Rarely (in less than one person out of 1,000) there may be seizure caused by fever. Very rarely, pneumonia may result. Other serious problems, including severe brain reactions and low blood count, have been reported after chicken pox vaccination. These happen so rarely that experts cannot tell whether the vaccine causes them or not.

An infected child should not play with anyone at risk for serious disease from chicken pox and should be kept away from infants younger than six weeks of age. They should also stay away from crowded public places where high-risk people might congregate.

Passive immunity that offers only temporary protection is available for high-risk, susceptible patients, who are given varicella-zoster immune globulin. This can abort or modify infection if administered within three days of exposure. Passive immunization is the administration of antibodies from donor's blood; since a person's blood is completely replaced every three months, the immunity lasts only that long.

Passive immunity may be offered to high-risk children and women who may be pregnant if they have been exposed to chicken pox. The shot must be given within 48 hours after exposure and no later than 96 hours. There is some disagreement about the value of giving passive immunity to a susceptible pregnant women in the first trimester; some fear that while it may prevent symptoms, the virus may still be in the mother's blood and thereby infect the fetus.

Anyone who has ever had a blood transfusion will also have gotten whatever antibodies the donor had.

Vaccine

Active immunization is provided by a vaccination that stimulates the immune system to make protective antibodies that protect you for life. The chicken pox vaccine—Varivax—is made from a live, weakened virus that works by creating a mild infection similar to natural chicken pox but without the related problems. The mild infection spurs the body to develop an immune response to the disease. These defenses are then ready when the body encounters the natural virus.

The development of a vaccine against the disease has been studied and used in clinical trials with children and adults in the United States since the early 1980s; it has been used in Japan for some time. It protects 70 to 90 percent of children but does not work well on adults.

In March 1995 the U.S. Food and Drug Administration licensed the vaccine for general use; the American Academy of Pediatrics has recommended the vaccine for all children and teenagers. Children younger than 12 require one dose; children 13 and over require two shots four to eight weeks apart.

Not all physicians agree on the benefits of the vaccine for healthy children, however. While proponents of the vaccine point out that suffering children and parents' considerable lost work time are good reasons to use the vaccine, some researchers are uncertain about how long the vaccine confers immunity. Critics warn that if the vaccine wears off in later life, the adult could then be vulnerable to infection at an age when chicken pox can be serious.

Other experts are concerned about possible side effects of the vaccine. Since the chicken pox virus belongs to the herpes virus group, there were concerns that the vaccine might cause periodic reactivation of the varicella zoster virus, causing shingles. However, research indicates the vaccine causes fewer or no more cases of shingles than naturally-contracted chicken pox.

Recent reports also note that the vaccine may cause birth defects when given to pregnant women, or to women who conceive within three months after vaccination. Doctors already know that having chicken pox while pregnant increases the risk of bearing a child with birth defects. To determine the link (if any) between birth defects and Varivax immunization of mothers, the U.S. Centers for Disease Control and Merck (the company that makes the vaccine) have set up a registry of women who receive the vaccine while pregnant

or in the three months before conception. Patients and health care workers should report Varivax vaccinations to this group at (800) 986-8999. Reports may also be mailed to: Merck Research Labs, Worldwide Product Safety & Epidemiology, BLA-31, West Point, PA 19486.

The chicken pox vaccine is recommended for children 15 months of age and older.

chigger bites   Chiggers are mites whose larvae live outdoors throughout the southeastern United States, and they are especially active in the grass near trees in summer. They attach themselves to their victims' legs where they feed on blood. The swelling may progress to form a blister, and the itching can last for weeks. Secondary infection may occur as a result of scratching.

A bite from the chigger causes an intense, itchy swelling up to half an inch across the skin, usually fading without treatment in between three days and a week. The female mites are attracted to warm moist areas of the body, such as the skin underneath sweat bands, where they burrow under the skin's surface. Chigger bites may be prevented by wearing close-fitting clothing with shirts tucked in and pants tucked into socks.

child abuse   Anything that endangers or impairs a child's physical or emotional health and development. Child abuse includes any damage done to a child that cannot be reasonably explained and that is often represented by an injury or pattern of injuries that do not appear to be accidental. Child abuse may include emotional abuse, physical abuse, sexual abuse, or neglect.

Each day in the United States, more than three children die as a result of child abuse in the home—most are younger than six years of age. In 2001 an estimated 1,300 children died of abuse and neglect, according to the U.S. Administration for Children and Families, which releases its most current child abuse statistics in April of each year. Statistics for 2001 were released in 2003. More than 2.67 million reports of possible maltreatment involving 3 million children were made to child protective service agencies in calendar year 2001. However, the actual incidence of abuse and neglect is estimated to be three times higher than the cases reported to authorities. Child abuse is reported on average every 10 seconds.

More children age four and younger die from child abuse and neglect than from any other single leading cause of death from injury for infants and young children. This includes falls, choking on food, suffocation, drowning, residential fires, and motor vehicle accidents.

Child abuse has a direct effect on a youngster's mental health. It should come as no surprise that men and women in the nation's prisons and jails report a higher incidence of abuse as children than the general population. In fact, more than a third of women in the nation's prisons and jails reported abuse as children, compared with 12 to 17 percent for women in the general population. About 14 percent of male inmates reported abuse as children, compared with 5 to 8 percent of men in the general population.

In addition, research has found that repeated sexual abuse affects the function of a key brain region related to substance abuse, which may cause an individual to be particularly irritable and to seek relief from drugs or alcohol. While researchers have known for a long time that a history of child abuse increases the risk for substance abuse in adults, a clear developmental mechanism by which this phenomenon occurs had been unclear until now.

Help for Parents

Most parents want to do a good job of raising their children, but life stresses may interfere with effective parenting. Parents who feel overwhelmed can call helplines for assistance, such as the Childhelp USA National Child Abuse Hotline at 1-800-4-A-CHILD (1-800-422-4453); parents can press 1 to talk to a hotline counselor or press 2 to have information sent by mail. The hotline is staffed by professional counselors available 24 hours a day, every day of the year. All calls are anonymous and toll-free. The hotline counselors can help parents with a child's problem behaviors by identifying the situations that trigger a child's problem behavior and helping parents choose appropriate ways of responding. They can also recommend parenting books, suggest ways to improve communication with children, and discuss how to discipline in a fair manner.

Counselors also can help parents to understand what constitutes normal behavior at a particular stage, for example, that babies sometimes cry for no reason and that two- and three-year-olds have tantrums. These behaviors, while frustrating to deal with, are not necessarily indications of bad parenting. Counselors are trained to provide nonjudgmental emotional support, which can help parents find a safe outlet for stress and anger. In addition, hotline counselors can refer parents to local groups by using a database of thousands of emergency, social service, and support resources.

Emotional Abuse

Any attitude or behavior that interferes with a child's mental health or social development can be considered emotional abuse, including yelling, name-calling, shaming, negative comparisons to others, labeling as "bad" or "worthless." Emotional abuse also includes the failure to provide the affection and support necessary for the development of a child's emotional, social, physical, and intellectual well-being. This includes ignoring, lack of appropriate physical affection, not saying "I love you," withdrawal of attention, lack of praise, and lack of positive reinforcement.

Physical Abuse

Any intentional injury to a child can be considered physical abuse, including hitting, kicking, slapping, shaking, burning, pinching, hair pulling, biting, choking, throwing, shoving, whipping, and paddling.

Sexual Abuse

Any sexual act between an adult and child is considered to be sexual abuse, including fondling, penetration, intercourse, exploitation, pornography, exhibitionism, child prostitution, group sex, oral sex, or forced observation of sexual acts.

Neglect

Neglect is defined as any failure to provide for a child's physical needs, including lack of supervision, inappropriate housing, malnourishment, inappropriate clothing for season or weather, abandonment, denial of medical care, and poor hygiene.

Reporting Abuse

Certain people are legally required to report suspected cases of abuse; typically, a report must be made when the reporter suspects or has reasons to suspect that a child has been abused or neglected. Mandated reporters include health-care workers, school personnel, child-care providers, social workers, law enforcement officers, and mental-health professionals.

Some states also require others to report suspected abuse or neglect, including animal control officers, veterinarians, commercial film or photograph processors, substance abuse counselors, and firefighters. Four states—Alaska, Arkansas, Connecticut, and South Dakota—include domestic violence workers on the list of mandated reporters. About 18 states require all citizens to report suspected abuse or neglect, regardless of profession.

Privileged communications About 34 states and territories specify in their reporting laws when a "communication" is privileged and therefore exempt from mandated reporting. Privileged communications, those a state recognizes as falling under the right to maintain the confidentiality of communications between professionals and their clients or patients, are exempt from mandatory reporting laws.

The privilege most widely recognized by the states is that of attorney-client. The privilege pertaining to clergy-penitent also is frequently recognized, but it is limited to situations in which a member of the clergy becomes aware of child abuse through a confession or in the capacity of spiritual adviser. However, five states—New Hampshire, North Carolina, Rhode Island, Texas, and West Virginia—deny the clergy-penitent privilege. Very few states recognize physician-patient and mental-health professional–patient privileges as exempt from mandatory reporting laws.

child and adolescent psychiatrist A physician who specializes in the diagnosis and treatment of disorders of thinking, feeling, and behaving affecting children and adolescents. Unlike psychologists, psychiatrists can prescribe medication.

The child and adolescent psychiatrist uses knowledge of biological, psychological, and social factors in working with patients. After a comprehensive examination, the child and adolescent psychiatrist arrives at a diagnosis and designs a treatment plan. An integrated approach may involve individual, group, or family psychotherapy; medication or consultation with other physicians or professionals from schools, juvenile courts, social agencies, or other community organizations. The child psychiatrist is prepared and expected to act as an advocate for the best interests of children and adolescents.

Child and adolescent psychiatric training requires four years of medical school, at least three years of approved residency training in medicine, neurology, and general psychiatry with adults, and two years of training in psychiatric work with children, adolescents, and their families in an accredited residency in child and adolescent psychiatry. The trainee acquires a thorough knowledge of normal child and family development, psychopathology, and treatment. Special importance is given to disorders that appear in childhood, such as pervasive developmental disorder, ATTENTION DEFICIT HYPERACTIVITY DISORDER (ADHD), LEARNING DISABILITY, MENTAL RETARDATION, mood disorders, DEPRESSION, ANXIETY DISORDERS, drug dependency, and CONDUCT DISORDER. After completing residency and successfully passing a certification exam in general psychiatry given by the American Board of Psychiatry and Neurology (ABPN), the child and adolescent psychiatrist is eligible to take the certification exam in the subspecialty of child and adolescent psychiatry. Although the ABPN examinations are not required for practice, they are a further assurance that the child and adolescent psychiatrist can diagnose and treat all psychiatric conditions in patients of any age and contribute in many ways to serve the welfare and interests of children and their families.

Child and adolescent psychiatrists can be found through local medical and psychiatric societies, local mental health associations, local hospitals or medical centers, departments of psychiatry in medical schools, and national organizations like the AMERICAN ACADEMY OF CHILD AND ADOLESCENT PSYCHIATRY and the American Psychiatric Association. In addition, pediatricians, family physicians, school counselors, and employee assistance programs can help identify child and adolescent psychiatrists.

child care centers and infectious disease Since young children are often vulnerable targets for infectious disease due to their immature immune systems, grouping many infants and preschoolers together in day-care centers contributes to the spread of infectious disease. The problem is exacerbated by the fact that young children are not particularly concerned with good hygiene, and many day-care centers care for children who are not yet toilet trained.

Still, there are ways to lessen the risk. In fact, recent research indicates that after the first year, children in child care get sick at about half the rate as do those who are cared for at home. This is because youngsters in day care are exposed to germs sooner, and their immune systems learn to cope with the onslaught of exposure.

Many studies have shown that if the center staff understand the risks and are supervised and educated about infection control, there is much less infectious illness among the children in their care. Simply by emphasizing hand washing, some centers have managed to cut diarrhea in half.

Before child-care facilities can be licensed, they must meet certain hygiene standards in a variety of areas, as set by local and state licensing authorities. Among other things, centers should clean all surfaces with a safe disinfectant. Surfaces should be dried with paper towels after being sprayed. Adequate ventilation and sanitation are necessary. Chemical air fresheners should not be used, because many children are allergic to them.

Many infections in child-care centers are spread by fecal contamination. When diapers are changed, tiny amounts of feces on hands can be transferred to countertops, toys, and door handles, so that if one child is shedding an infection in the feces, it is not long before the infection spreads. Some infectious viruses will appear in feces before diarrhea starts and will remain in feces for more than a week after symptoms disappear.

To prevent these problems, diapers should be checked every hour. Diaper-changing areas should not be located where food is prepared, stored, or served. The changing table should be cleaned after each use. Soiled diapers should be thrown away in separate covered containers. Staffers should wash hands before and after changing diapers. If a child has diarrhea, staff should wear disposable gloves before changing diapers.

Hands should be washed after using the toilet or handling diapers; after helping a child at the toilet; before preparing, handling, or serving food; before feeding an infant; before setting the table; after wiping or blowing noses; after touching blood, vomit, saliva, or eye secretions; after handling pets; and before and after eating.

Children can catch infectious diseases in a variety of ways. Airborne germs may transmit CHICKEN POX, the COMMON COLD, FIFTH DISEASE, INFLUENZA, MENINGITIS, and TUBERCULOSIS. Germs can be transmitted by direct contact to cause COLD SORES, CYTOMEGALOVIRUS, head LICE, SCABIES, and STREPTOCOCCAL INFECTIONS. Germs can be spread via the fecal-oral route to cause diarrheal diseases or HEPATITIS A.

childhood cancers Cancer is the number-one disease killer of children—more than genetic problems, CYSTIC FIBROSIS, and AIDS combined. About 8,600 children in the United States were diagnosed with cancer in 2001, and about 1,500 of them died from the disease that year. Still, cancer is relatively rare in this age group, with only about one or two children developing the disease each year for every 10,000 children in the United States.

Since the 1980s, there has been an increase in the incidence of children diagnosed with all forms of invasive cancer; from 11.4 cases per 100,000 children in 1975 to 15.2 per 100,000 children in 1998. During this same time, however, death rates declined dramatically and survival increased for most childhood cancers. For example, the five-year survival rates for all childhood cancers combined increased from 55.7 percent in 1974 to 76, to 77.1 percent in 1992 to 1997. This improvement in survival rates is due to significant advances in treatment, resulting in cure or long-term remission for a substantial proportion of children with cancer.

Over the last half of the 20th century, progress in childhood cancer diagnosis and treatment has transformed a once uniformly fatal disease into a group of malignancies that are now curable in most children. For example, LEUKEMIA survival rates have increased from just over 60 percent in the mid-1970s to near 80 percent in the mid-90s.

Causes

The causes of childhood cancers are largely unknown. A few conditions, such as DOWN SYNDROME, genetic problems, and ionizing radiation exposures explain a small percentage of cases. Environmental causes of childhood cancer have long been suspected by many scientists but have been difficult to identify, partly because cancer in children is rare and partly because it is so difficult to identify past exposure levels in children. In addition, each of the distinctive types of childhood cancers develops differently, with a potentially wide variety of causes.

Scientists do know that children treated with chemotherapy and radiation therapy for certain forms of childhood and adolescent cancers, such as Hodgkin's disease, brain tumors, sarcomas, and others, may develop a second primary malignancy. They also know what does not cause childhood cancers: low levels of radiation exposure from radon are not significantly associated with childhood leukemias, nor is ultrasound use during pregnancy. Residential magnetic field exposure from power lines is not significantly associated with childhood leukemias, nor is on-the-job exposure of parents.

Although pesticides have been suspected to be involved in the development of certain forms of childhood cancer, results have been inconsistent and have not yet been validated by physical evidence of pesticides in the child's body or environment.

Several studies have found no link between maternal cigarette smoking before pregnancy and childhood cancers, but increased risks were related to the father's prenatal smoking habits in studies in the United Kingdom and China.

Little evidence has been found to link specific viruses or other infectious agents to the development of most types of childhood cancers, although scientists are exploring the role of exposure of very young children to some common infectious agents that may protect children from, or put them at risk for, certain leukemias.

Recent research has shown that children with AIDS have an increased risk of developing certain cancers, predominantly non-Hodgkin's lymphoma and Kaposi's sarcoma, and leiomyosarcoma (a type of muscle cancer).

Specific genetic syndromes, such as the Li-Fraumeni syndrome or NEUROFIBROMATOSIS, have been linked to an increased risk of specific childhood cancers.

The role of a mother's exposure to birth control pills, fertility drugs, and diethylstilbestrol (DES) is being studied in several ongoing trials.

Types of Childhood Cancers

Among the 12 major types of childhood cancers, leukemia and brain cancer account for more than half of the new cases.

Leukemia About a third of childhood cancers are leukemias (cancer of the bone marrow and tissues that make the blood cells). About 2,700 children younger than 15 years were diagnosed with leukemia in 2001. Leukemia triggers the production of too many abnormal white cells that invade the marrow and crowd out normal healthy blood cells, making the patient susceptible to anemia, infection, and bruising. The most common type of leukemia in children is acute lymphoblastic (ALL), which is highly treatable; today, about 70 percent of affected children are cured.

Brain cancer Tumors of the brain and spinal cord are the most common types of solid tumors in children. Some tumors are benign, and some children can be cured by surgery, but because of the difficulty in diagnosing and treating brain tumors, there has been less dramatic progress in treating them than other childhood malignancies. Today, 20 percent of all primary brain tumors occur in children younger than 15, with a peak in incidence between the ages of five and 10 years. Brain tumors are more common in boys than girls.

Bone cancers Cancer usually spreads to the bones from other sites, but some types originate in the skeleton. The most common bone cancer in children is osteogenic sarcoma. Bone cancer in children occurs most often during adolescent growth spurts; 85 percent of affected teenagers have tumors on their legs or arms, half of them around the knee. Ewing's sarcoma differs from osteosarcoma in that it affects the bone shaft, and tends to be found in bones other than the long bones of the arm and the leg, such as the ribs. Child deaths from bone cancer during 1950 to 1980 dropped by 50 percent.

Lymphomas This type of cancer begins in the lymph system, the body's circulatory network designed to filter out impurities. There are two general types of lymphomas: Hodgkin's disease and non-Hodgkin's lymphoma. Non-Hodgkin's lymphoma is more common in children; it can occur in the tonsils, thymus, bone, small intestine, spleen, or in lymph glands. The disease can spread to the central nervous system and the bone marrow. Today, treatments can cure many children, and promising treatments are being developed.

Neuroblastoma This type of tumor is found only in children and begins in the adrenal glands near the kidneys. Neuroblastoma usually appears in very young children.

Rhabdomyosarcoma The most common soft tissue sarcoma in children, this extremely malignant tumor originates in muscles, usually in the head and neck area (including the eyes), the genitourinary tract, or arms and legs. Although rhabdomyosarcoma tends to spread quickly, its symptoms are easy to spot compared to other forms of childhood cancer.

Wilms' tumor This rapidly developing tumor of the kidney most often appears in children between the ages of two and four. Wilms' tumor in children acts differently than does kidney cancer in adults. In children, the disease often spreads to the lungs; in the past, the death rate from this cancer was extremely high. However, treatment combining surgery, radiation therapy, and chemotherapy has been very effective in controlling the disease. As a result, cure rates for Wilms' tumor have improved.

Retinoblastoma This hereditary malignant eye tumor occurs in infants and young children, accounting for just 2 percent of childhood cancer. This disease is the first cancer for which researchers identified a tumor suppressor gene.

Other Other rare forms of childhood cancers include germ cell tumors, thyroid cancer, malignant melanoma (a type of skin cancer), testicular cancer, and primary cancers in the kidney, liver, and lung.

Child vs. Adult Cancers

When cancer strikes children and young people, it affects them differently than it does adults. For example, young patients often have a more advanced stage of cancer when first diagnosed. While only about 20 percent of adults with cancer have evidence that the disease has already spread when it is diagnosed, 80 percent of children's cancer has already invaded distant sites at diagnosis. While most adult cancers are linked to lifestyle factors such as smoking, diet, or exposure to cancer-causing agents, the causes of most childhood cancers are unknown.

Adult cancers primarily affect the lung, colon, breast, prostate and pancreas, while childhood cancers usually affect the white blood cells (leukemias), brain, bone, the lymphatic system, muscles, kidneys, and nervous system.

While most adult cancer patients are treated in their local community, cancers in children are rarely treated by family physicians or pediatricians. A child with cancer must be diagnosed precisely and treated by physicians and clinical and laboratory scientists who have special expertise in managing the care of children with cancer. Such teams are found only in major children's hospitals, university medical centers, and cancer centers.

child psychologist A mental-health professional with a Ph.D. who conducts scientific research and/or provides psychological services to infants, toddlers, children, and adolescents. Child psychology is focused on understanding, preventing, diagnosing and treating children's psychological, cognitive, emotional, developmental, behavioral, and family problems.

Child psychologists work in a variety of settings including private practice, hospitals, schools, and within the justice system. They do therapy, testing, evaluation, consultation, teaching, and research, depending on where they work and their specific job requirements.

Child psychologists must have a bachelor's degree in psychology or a related field, a master's degree (another two years) in psychology, and a doctorate in psychology, which may take up to five years after that, including internships and writing a dissertation. In most states a doctorate is required to practice independently as a child psychologist.

Children and Adults with Attention Deficit Hyperactivity Disorder (CHADD)   A nonprofit organization founded in 1987 in response to the frustration and sense of isolation experienced by parents and their children with ADHD. At that time, there were very few places for support or information, and people misunderstood ADHD. Many clinicians and educators knew little about the disability, and individuals with ADHD were often mistakenly labeled a behavior problem, unmotivated, or unintelligent.

From one parent support group in Florida, the organization grew dramatically to become the leading nonprofit national organization for children and adults with ADHD. Today the organization continues to be run by volunteers, with the support of a small national staff, and offers education, advocacy, and support. (For contact information, see Appendix I.)

Children's Brain Tumor Foundation, The   A nonprofit organization established in 1988 by parents, physicians, and friends dedicated to improving the treatment, quality of life, and long-term outlook for children with brain and spinal cord tumors. The foundation funds research for basic, clinical, and psychosocial research on pediatric brain and spinal cord tumors and their consequences. If offers support services and a parent-to-parent network and publishes a free resource guide on pediatric brain and spinal cord tumors for families. The foundation also cosponsors conferences on pediatric brain tumors. (For contact information, see Appendix I.)

Children's Craniofacial Association (CCA)   A national nonprofit organization dedicated to improving the quality of life for children with facial differences and their families.

Headquartered in Dallas, the Children's Craniofacial Association (CCA) addresses the medical, financial, psychosocial, emotional, and educational concerns relating to CRANIOFACIAL CONDITIONS. CCA's mission is to empower and give hope to facially disfigured children and their families. (For contact information, see Appendix I.)

Children's Defense Fund   A national nonprofit organization that works to ensure that every child has a "Healthy Start, a Head Start, a Fair Start, a Safe Start, and a Moral Start" in life with the help of caring families and communities. The Children's Defense Fund (CDF) provides a strong, effective voice for all the children of America who cannot vote, lobby, or speak for themselves, paying particular attention to the needs of poor and minority children and those with disabilities. The CDF educates the nation about the needs of children and encourages preventive investment before they get sick or into trouble, drop out of school, or suffer family breakdown.

The organization began in 1973 and is supported by foundations, corporation grants, and individual donations. The group has never accepted government funds. (For contact information, see Appendix I.)

Children's Health Act of 2000   A law enacted in November 2000 that includes a lengthy list of provisions to improve the health of America's children, including establishment of the NATIONAL CENTER ON BIRTH DEFECTS AND DEVELOPMENTAL DISABILITIES. It also improved newborn screening, boosted autism research and pediatric research in general, and authorized the development of a national surveillance program designed to monitor maternal and infant health.

National Center on Birth Defects and Developmental Disabilities

The act created a seventh center at the Centers for Disease Control and Prevention (CDC) that will improve policy development regarding birth defects and developmental disabilities. The center collects, analyzes, and distributes data on birth defects and developmental disabilities, including information on causes, incidence, and prevalence. The center conducts research on preventing defects and disabilities and provides information on prevention activities.

Newborn Screening Initiative

The act authorized grants to states to improve and expand newborn screening programs and created an advisory committee to provide recommendations to the secretary of the U.S. Department of Health and Human Services (HHS).

Folic Acid Awareness Campaign

The act expanded CDC's folic acid education and public awareness campaign and authorized research to identify ways to increase folic acid consumption by women of reproductive age. Finally, it enabled CDC to conduct research to increase the understanding of the effects of folic acid in preventing birth defects.

Autism Research and Surveillance

The act authorized the expansion of federal research on autism and established three CDC regional centers of excellence in autism and pervasive developmental disabilities to analyze information on autism and related developmental disabilities. Additionally, it called for establishing a program to provide information on autism to health professionals and the general public and established a committee to coordinate all autism-related activities within HHS.

Pediatric Research at the National Institutes of Health

The act authorized a "Pediatric Research Initiative" at the National Institutes of Health (NIH) to enhance collaborative efforts among NIH institutes and provide increased support for pediatric biomedical research.

Safe Motherhood Monitoring and Infant Health Promotion

The act authorized the development of a national surveillance program designed to improve the understanding of maternal complications and mortality, authorized research into risk factors and prevention, and authorized public education campaigns to promote healthy pregnancies. Finally, it authorized funding for research initiatives and programs to prevent drug, alcohol, and tobacco use among pregnant women.

Children's Hospice International (CHI) A nonprofit HOSPICE organization that ensures emotional, spiritual, and medical support for children with life-threatening conditions and their families. The hospice group tries to carry the children and families through the time of illness and dying in a way that minimizes pain, fear, and uncertainty, to dignify the meaning of life and death, and to support them during bereavement. The group also provides advocacy and outreach services to create public awareness of the needs of children with life-threatening conditions and their families, and of what children's hospice care can do to meet those needs. The group provides ongoing research, education, training, and technical assistance programs to include hospice perspectives in all areas of pediatric care and education.

Children's Hospice International (CHI) was founded in 1983 to provide a network of support and care for children using a team effort that provides medical, psychological, social, and spiritual expertise and information. CHI is committed to the hospice concept of care that recognizes the right and need for children and their families to choose health care and support whether in their own home, hospital, or hospice care facility.

The crusade for children's hospice care was triggered when an eight-year-old boy was denied hospice support in 1977 because he was a child. This denial set off the crusade for children's hospice care and the official development of CHI.

In 1983 only four hospice programs of 1,400 in the United States were able to accept children. CHI has worked effectively to dramatically change these numbers, so that by 1989, 447 programs include children as patients, and almost all of the existing 2,000 hospice programs will consider accepting a child.

Headquartered in Alexandria, Virginia, the organization works closely with medical professionals as a research and resource bank, providing medical and technical assistance, research, and education.

The goal of hospice care for children is enhancement of the quality of life each day. The child and family are included to the fullest degree possible in the decision process about treatment and choices. CHI ensures continuity and consistency of care through the coordination of a team of volunteer support professionals from medical, nursing, psychological, and spiritual fields, along with other services as appropriate. CHI's hospice care for children and their families is also attentive to needs related to loss and grieving.

In 1988 Children's Hospice International initiated a national outreach service, the first national telephone hotline, "1-800-2-4-CHILD," for the needs of terminally ill children and teens. Funded by the Cancer Research Foundation of America, CHI's hotline number allows CHI staff to respond quickly and directly to these special children, their families, and health care providers.

Each year, approximately 100,000 children die in the United States, many after a lengthy illness lasting years, without the benefit of pediatric hospice support in the areas of pain and symptom management and counseling. Today, approximately one million children have life-threatening conditions in the United States. With the number of children contracting cancer and AIDS rising dramatically, more families are confronted daily with the emotional and medical needs of their children. CHI's hotline puts qualified professionals in touch with these children no matter where they are.

In addition, CHI has also been instrumental in helping health care providers better understand the needs of dying children. CHI has developed and directed educational programs, seminars, and workshops; it has provided for technical assistance to pediatricians, nurses, psychologists, teachers, and volunteers throughout the United States and abroad. The group also offers a series of publications devoted to home care and pain and symptom management, as well as other related subjects.

CHI works closely with other organizations including the AMERICAN ACADEMY OF PEDIATRICS, National Association of Children's Hospitals, National Hospice Organization, Hospice Association of America, and World Health Organization.

children's hospitals   Pediatric hospitals designed exclusively for the care and treatment of children. Within their walls and outpatient clinics, children with the most challenging medical needs are treated by practitioners of medicine, nursing, therapy, and social work.

Although children's hospitals represent only 1 percent of all hospitals in the United States, freestanding and self-governing children's hospitals serve about 12 percent of all hospitalized children and train about 25 percent of all pediatricians. In addition, outpatient services at children's hospitals aid more than 8.3 million children each year.

Children's hospitals are expert in the most basic health care needs of all children and provide medical care, education, and research for children with special needs. In most states, they serve a disproportionate share of children who are uninsured and those who rely on the Medicaid program to pay for their health care. Almost half of all care in children's hospitals is provided to the poor. The percentage of Medicaid patients in children's hospitals fell slightly in 1995.

In addition, children's hospitals are centers of medical education and research, pioneering new approaches to organ transplants, open heart surgery, and the treatment of trauma. Founded more than a century ago as charitable refuges for sick and abandoned children, these special hospitals today continue to fight against social problems threatening America's children, including violence, tobacco and drug use, inadequate parenting skills, and lack of access to appropriate health care.

Child Welfare League of America (CWLA)   A nonprofit association of more than 1,100 public and private nonprofit agencies that help more than 3.5 million abused and neglected children and their families each year. The League is the nation's oldest and largest membership-based child welfare organization. Working with and through its member agencies, the Child Welfare League of America (CWLA) is committed to activities such as developing practice standards for high-quality services that protect children and youths and strengthen families and neighborhoods; providing consultation, conferences, publications, and other membership services; promoting public policies that contribute to the well-being of children; and making sure that all child welfare services are provided with respect for cultural and ethnic diversity. (For contact information, see Appendix I.)

chlamydia   The most common sexually transmitted disease (STD) in the United States, infecting more than 4.5 million people each year. It is a serious but easily cured disease that is three times more common than GONORRHEA, six times more common than genital HERPES, and 30 times more common than SYPHILIS. Between 1988 and 1992, the rate of reported cases of chlamydia more than doubled. Sexually active teens have high rates of chlamydia infections.

The organism that causes chlamydia *(Chlamydia trachomatis)* is classified as a bacterium, even though it is similar to a virus. It is a parasite that—like a virus—cannot reproduce outside living cells, but it is enough like bacteria to be vulnerable to antibiotics.

Those at highest risk for contracting the disease are women under age 24, women who take birth control pills, men and women who have had more than one sex partner, and people with other STDs (especially gonorrhea).

In girls the bacteria centers on the cervix, where it causes an inflammation known as mucopurulent cervicitis, which can cause a yellow thick discharge, white blood cells, or bleeding from the cervix that a doctor can diagnosis during a pelvic exam.

Cause

A person becomes infected during sexual intercourse with a partner infected with *C. trachomatis.* A baby can contract the disease from an infected mother during birth; the disease can be transmitted as the baby passes through the infected birth canal, not during the previous nine months of the pregnancy.

The disease does not confer immunity; some studies suggest that if a child has ever had chlamydia, he or she is more likely to be reinfected sometime in the future.

Symptoms

Most girls experience no symptoms at all; but even if a girl has no symptoms, she can infect her sex partner. About 20 percent notice a heavy, yellow vaginal discharge. If chlamydia affects the urinary tract, there may be pain, burning, or a frequent urge to urinate.

Many boys have symptoms that are so mild they are ignored. The rest experience burning or pain during urination or notice a watery, milky, or thick discharge from the penis. This is caused by an inflamed urethra.

Some studies suggest that a person can become infected from one to two weeks after exposure. The person remains infectious until the complete course of antibiotics has been taken. Untreated infected people may be infectious for years.

Diagnosis

The most reliable test in girls is a culture taken from the cervical cells. the best current test (90 percent accurate) can identify antibodies in 24 hours. For boys, doctors assume that any boy with the above symptoms who does not have gonorrhea has chlamydia. Some doctors may try to identify white blood cells in the discharge. A boy should be treated for chlamydia if his sex partner has a positive chlamydia test, whether or not he has symptoms. Tests using urine samples have also recently been developed.

Complications

Untreated girls may go on to develop infected tubes (salpingitis) or an infected uterus lining (endometritis). PELVIC INFLAMMATORY DISEASE (PID) can lead to a buildup of scar tissue that will block the fallopian tubes, causing infertility or tubal pregnancy. Some studies have linked chlamydia with a higher risk of premature birth or a low birth weight baby.

About two-thirds of babies born to infected mothers go on to develop CONJUNCTIVITIS within two weeks of birth, although permanent damage to the baby's eyes is rare. A treated baby is in no risk of permanent damage. About 10 to 20 percent of exposed newborns may develop chlamydia pneumonia in the first three to four months of age. While it is usually mild, some babies may be quite ill and are at risk for developing lung problems later in childhood.

Treatment

The disease can be cured by taking antibiotics (doxycycline) for seven days or a one-gram single dose of azithromycin. Pregnant women can take erythromycin for seven days. Penicillin is not effective against chlamydia.

Prevention

All sexually active girls should be tested for chlamydia; many college health services and family planning clinics routinely test for chlamydia during physical exams. From 5 to 10 percent of female college students have the disease. Anyone who is treated for any STD should also be tested for chlamydia. (In some areas of the United States, half of the patients with gonorrhea also have chlamydia). The sex partner of anyone with chlamydia must also be treated at the same time; otherwise, reinfection will occur. Condoms reduce the risk of transmission, but they do not provide complete protection.

chlamydial pneumonia   See PNEUMONIA.

cholera   An infection of the small intestine characterized by profuse, painless, watery diarrhea. If untreated, severe cases can cause rapid dehydration and death within a few hours. There has been a dramatic increase in cholera in the United States and its territories, and many cases may go undetected by physicians who are not familiar with the disease, according to the National Center for Infectious Diseases.

The disease thrives in places without running water or treated sewage disposal. This is why cholera does not spread from one person to the next in the United States and Canada. Any cholera organisms in infected feces are killed by sewage treatment and chlorinated water.

For centuries cholera thrived only in northeast India, where outbreaks still occur regularly, but as the world trade routes opened in the 1800s, cholera became pandemic, spreading throughout the world and killing millions of people in a series of epidemics. It was London physician John Snow who correctly identified sewage-contaminated drinking water as the source of the epidemic of 1853–54. In his research, he compared the incidence of cholera in a neighborhood with two different sources of water, one of which was contaminated with sewage.

Thirty years later, German microbiologist Robert Koch identified the "comma bacilli" (now called *Vibrio cholerae*) under the microscope as the actual cause of cholera.

For the first half of the 20th century, cholera was confined to Asia, and not a single case was reported anywhere in the entire Western Hemisphere between 1911 and 1973. Then between 1974 and 1988, a few cases appeared in states bordering the Gulf of Mexico (Florida, Louisiana, and Texas). In 1989 no cases were reported.

Unexpectedly, in 1991 a cholera epidemic began in Peru when a ship from the Far East dumped cholera-infected bilgewater into the Lima harbor. The bacteria contaminated the fish and shellfish, which Peruvians ate raw; from there the bacteria got into the sewers and from there into the water supply. The disease then spread throughout South and Central America where the epidemic continues to this day. The particular bacterium responsible for the pandemic—"El tor" *(V. cholerae 01)*—can survive in water for long periods. By September 1994 more than one million people in 20 countries had contracted the disease, and more than 9,000 had died.

In most years, there are a handful of cases in the United States, usually among people who have traveled to Asia or Africa. A few cases appear in areas bordering the Gulf of Mexico and around the Mediterranean. Usually, the victim has eaten tainted shellfish. From 1961 to 1991 there was an average of five cases per year in the United States, 31 percent acquired abroad. From 1992 to 1994 there were 160 cholera cases reported in the United States (about 53 per year); this is compared to a total of 136 cases reported in the previous 26 years. Experts suggest the reported cases are probably only a fraction of the actual incident of cholera, since as many as 90 percent sufferers have only mild diarrhea.

If patients can be given enough fluids, most will recover. The death rate soars in pandemics when there is not enough clean water, or if so many people become ill that there are not enough healthy people to care for the sick. After one infection, resulting antibodies will protect the patient from reinfection with the same strain.

Cause

Cholera is caused by the comma-shaped bacterium *Vibrio cholerae* that is acquired by swallowing food or water contaminated with human feces. A person may also contract cholera from eating fruits or vegetables washed in tainted water, from eating raw or undercooked shellfish harvested from contaminated water, or from eating food prepared by someone with contaminated hands. Sometimes flies can carry the bacteria to food.

The rapid fluid loss that is the primary symptom of cholera occurs because of the action of a toxin produced by the bacterium that boosts the passage of fluid from the blood into the large and small intestines.

Symptoms

Between a few hours and five days after infection, symptoms appear suddenly, beginning with diarrhea and often vomiting. More than a pint of fluid may be lost hourly, and if this is not replaced, death will occur within a few hours. Because the bacteria is inhibited by gastric acid, those with lots of gastric acid will have only a mild infection. Those who are poorly nourished have less gastric acid and therefore may have a more severe diarrhea. Many people, especially those living in areas where cholera is rampant, may have no symptoms, but they can still spread the disease to others.

If the diarrhea is very bloody, the cause is probably not cholera but may be SHIGELLOSIS, *E. coli*, or CAMPYLOBACTER.

Treatment

Cholera is treated by quickly replacing the lost fluids with water containing salts and sugar. Intravenous fluids may sometimes be needed. Antibiotics (such as tetracycline hydrochloride) may shorten both the period of diarrhea and the infectiousness. While it is usually taken by mouth, IV tetracycline may be needed for very sick patients. Antidiarrheal medicine should not be taken without a prescription.

As soon as vomiting stops, the patient should eat a bland diet rich in carbohydrates and low in protein and fats. Airlines are required to carry onboard packets of oral rehydration solution if they carry passengers to and from cholera-infected areas so that anyone developing severe diarrhea on a long flight will not get dehydrated.

With proper treatment, most patients will recover with no permanent damage.

Diagnosis

A positive stool culture will confirm the diagnosis. Stool specimens must be cultured on special culture media designed to find cholera. A blood test taken a few weeks after the illness begins will show antibodies to cholera.

Complications

A few patients will experience profuse watery diarrhea; without prompt treatment, half the people with severe cholera will die from profound dehydration within a few hours. The patient will become extremely thirsty, have no urine, will be cramped, have wrinkled skin, sunken eyes, and weakness. Because there will not be enough fluid in the body to maintain circulation, shock, coma, and death can follow.

Prevention

A cholera vaccine is available for those traveling to Africa and the Middle and Far East, but it is no longer recommended because it is only 50 percent effective and protects for only three to six months. The vaccine is no help against controlling epidemics. A new, more effective oral vaccine is being tested, but it is not yet licensed.

The bacteria are killed by chlorine and boiling. Contaminated shellfish must be boiled or steamed for 10 minutes to kill all bacteria. The core temperatures of cooked food should be 158°F. Unless all the bacteria are killed by cooking, they will multiply rapidly at room temperature in cooked shellfish.

Cholera can be controlled by improved sanitation, especially by maintaining untainted water supplies. Travelers to high-risk areas—affected areas in Latin America, Africa, and Asia—must:

- not bring perishable seafood back to the United States
- not eat unboiled or untreated water or ice
- not eat food or beverages from street vendors
- not eat raw or partially cooked fish or shellfish
- not eat raw vegetables or salads
- treat unbottled water with chlorine or iodine tablets
- drink carbonated bottled water or bottled soft drinks (the carbonation destroys the bacteria)
- drink tea and coffee made only with boiled water
- eat only fruits with a peel
- eat only foods that are cooked and hot

ciguatera poisoning   The most common clinical syndrome caused by eating certain tropical marine reef fish, mostly barracuda, red snapper, amberjack, surgeon fish, sea bass, and grouper. The fish are toxic at certain times of the year when they ingest a type of dinoflagellate called *Gambierdiscus* *toxicus*, which contains "ciguatoxin," an odorless, tasteless poison that cannot be destroyed by either heating or freezing.

Ciguatera poisoning occurs most often in the Caribbean Islands, Florida, Hawaii, and the Pacific Islands. Recent reports documented 129 cases over a two-year period in Dade County alone. It appears to be occurring more often, probably because of the increased demand for seafood around the world.

Ciguatera poisoning usually goes away on its own, and symptoms often subside within several days. However, in severe cases the neurological symptoms can persist for months. In a few isolated cases neurological symptoms have persisted for several years, and in other cases recovered patients have experienced recurrence of neurological symptoms years after recovery. Such relapses are most often associated with changes in diet or with drinking alcohol.

Cause

Ciguatera poisoning occurs after eating any of more than 300 species of fish that may contain ciguatoxin, which is found in greatest concentration in internal organs, but it cannot be detected by inspection, taste, or smell. Ciguatoxin more common among larger, predatory coral reef fish.

Symptoms

Eating a fish contaminated with ciguatoxin produces both stomach ailments and neurologic symptoms. Patients often report a curious type of sensory reversal, so that picking up a cold glass would cause a burning hot sensation. Other symptoms include a tingling sensation in the lips and mouth followed by numbness, nausea, vomiting, abdominal cramps, weakness, headache, vertigo, paralysis, convulsions, and skin rash. Coma and death from respiratory paralysis occur in about 12 percent of cases. Subsequent episodes of ciguatera may be more severe.

Treatment

Ciguatera has been successfully treated with IV mannitol, which appears to abbreviate (if not stop) the symptoms of ciguatera fish poisoning. Preliminary evidence suggests that the earlier a victim is diagnosed and treated with IV mannitol, the more likely the success. Mannitol has been shown to be safe and effective in children as young as four years of age.

Untreated, ciguatera is usually a self-limited disease lasting one to two months, but symptoms can persist for months to years.

circumcision Surgical removal of the foreskin of the penis. This operation is usually performed for religious and ethnic reasons. Widespread infant circumcision is a relatively recent phenomenon in the United States. Prior to the 1930s when babies were often born at home, infant boys were rarely circumcised except for religious reasons. After World War II, however, nearly all babies were born in hospitals, and for a number of reasons almost all baby boys were circumcised, often immediately after birth. The United States is the only country in the world that routinely circumcises most of its male infants for nonreligious reasons; more than 80 percent of the world's males are not circumcised.

However, in the past 25 years, major cultural changes have altered the birth experience, with a movement toward natural childbirth and improvements in pain control. Likewise, cultural changes have begun to alter American attitudes on circumcision as well. Until recently, circumcision was the most frequently performed surgery in the United States. Even today, infant circumcision in the United States costs about $200 million a year.

Experts, including the AMERICAN ACADEMY OF PEDIATRICS, believe there are no medical reasons to recommend routine and universal newborn circumcision, because circumcision does not prevent sexually transmitted diseases, it does not appear to prevent cancer of the penis, and it does not prevent cancer of the cervix in women. There is a slightly higher chance that an uncircumcised boy will have a urinary tract infection in the first six months of life, but since only 1 percent of uncircumcised baby boys develop these infections, it is hard to justify universal circumcision on that basis alone. Today, most experts believe that infants do indeed feel pain, and that the pain of circumcision is considerable.

In the end the decision to circumcise is a religious, cultural, or personal decision. Boys who are not circumcised do not require any special care for the penis and foreskin until the foreskin is completely retractable, which occurs any time from four months to five years of age or later. No one—not even the baby's doctor—should ever pull the foreskin back forcibly. Once the child grows, the foreskin will begin to retract easily with gentle manipulation. When the boy is old enough to bathe himself, he can be taught to pull back the foreskin and wash gently in the shower or bath. Until then, the flow of urine under the foreskin and a gentle swish of the penis in the bath is enough to keep the penis and foreskin clean.

Most experts believe that parents who want to have their baby circumcised should find a doctor who uses local anesthesia.

cleft lip and palate   A fissure in the midline of the lip and/or palate caused by a failure of the two sides to fuse together before birth. Facial clefts affect nearly one of 800 births in the United States, making it one of the most common BIRTH DEFECTS in the nation.

In the early weeks of fetal development, the right and left sides of the lip and the roof of the mouth normally grow together. Occasionally, those sections do not quite meet. A child born with a separation in the upper lip is said to have a cleft lip. A similar birth defect in the roof of the mouth, or palate, is called a cleft palate. Since the lip and the palate develop separately, it is possible for a child to have a cleft lip, a cleft palate, or variations of both.

A cleft lip can range in severity from a slight notch in the red part of the upper lip to a complete separation of the lip extending into the nose, and can occur on one or both sides of the upper lip. In some children, a cleft palate may involve only a tiny portion at the back of the roof of the mouth; for others, it can mean a complete separation that extends from front to back. Just as in cleft lip, cleft palate may appear on one or both sides of the upper mouth.

Clefts of the lip and palate are complex conditions that affect not only the child's appearance and self-esteem, but also how well a child can speak, hear, and eat. Many children with cleft lip or palate develop hearing problems as a result of chronic ear infections, which, if left untreated, will create speech and language problems.

An immediate problem after birth is feeding, but special nipples and prostheses are available to ensure that children with oral clefts receive adequate nutrition until surgical treatment is provided.

Cause
The causes of cleft lip/palate are not well understood. Studies suggest that a number of genes, as well as environmental factors such as drugs (including antiseizure drugs), infections, maternal illnesses, maternal alcohol use, and possibly, B vitamin folic acid deficiency may be involved. Clefts are more common in Asian, Latino, and Native American ethnic groups. In most cases, however, there is no identifiable cause or risk factor.

Up to 13 percent of babies with cleft lip/palate have other birth defects. Some cases involve genetic syndromes which may pose other specific problems for the baby. For this reason, babies with cleft lip/palate should be thoroughly examined by a doctor soon after birth.

The causes of isolated cleft palate are not well understood either, although a number of genes as well as environmental factors also may play a role. In the case of cleft palate alone, however, neither antiseizure drugs nor maternal alcohol use appear to contribute to the problem, though deficiency of folic acid may do so. Isolated cleft palate appears to be associated with genetic syndromes more often than the combined cleft lip/palate. Babies with isolated cleft palate are more likely than babies with cleft lip/palate to have other birth defects; in fact, up to half of babies with isolated cleft palate may have other birth defects.

If normal parents have a child with a cleft, the chance that a subsequent baby will have a cleft is 2 to 4 percent. These risk figures are the same for cleft lip/palate and isolated cleft palate. However, a second baby is at risk for only the same type of cleft that affected the first child.

If either parent has an oral-facial cleft but no affected children, the risk of the same type of cleft in any subsequent pregnancy is about 3 to 4 percent. If more than one of the parents and/or children are affected, the risk for future offspring is higher.

Treatment

A plastic surgeon can repair a cleft lip shortly after birth (usually at two to three months of age). The cleft palate can be repaired by 12 months of age, before the child's first spoken words. At the time of the cleft repairs, tubes may also be placed in the child's ears to help treat ear infections and maximize hearing sensitivity. In cleft palate surgery, the goal is to close the opening in the roof of the mouth so the child can eat and learn to speak properly. Occasionally, poor healing in the palate or poor speech may require a second operation.

Surgery is generally done when the child is about 10 weeks old. To repair a cleft lip, the surgeon will make an incision on either side of the cleft from the mouth into the nostril. The surgeon turns the dark pink outer portion of the cleft down and pulls the muscle and the skin of the lip together to close the separation. Muscle function and the normal "cupid's bow" shape of the mouth are restored. The nostril deformity often associated with cleft lip may also be improved at the time of lip repair or in a later surgery.

The child may be restless after surgery, but medication can relieve any discomfort. Elbow restraints may be necessary for a few weeks to prevent the baby from rubbing the stitched area. If dressings have been used, they will be removed within a day or two, and the stitches will either dissolve or be removed within five days.

It is normal for the surgical scar to appear to get bigger and redder for a few weeks after surgery. This will gradually fade, although the scar will never totally disappear. In many children, however, it is barely noticeable because of the shadows formed by the nose and upper lip.

Repairing a cleft palate involves more extensive surgery than repairing a cleft lip. This surgery is usually done when the child is nine to 18 months old, so the baby is bigger and better able to tolerate surgery. To repair a cleft palate, the surgeon makes an incision on both sides of the separation, moving tissue from each side of the cleft to the center or midline of the roof of the mouth. This rebuilds the palate, joining muscle together and providing enough length in the palate so that the child can eat and learn to speak properly.

For a day or two, the child will feel some soreness and pain that is easily controlled by medication. Because a child will not eat or drink as much as usual during recovery, an intravenous line will be used to maintain fluid levels. Elbow restraints may be used to prevent the baby from rubbing the repaired area.

At about age three, the child's speech is assessed by a speech/language pathologist. If treatment is needed, the speech pathologist works with the parent and the child. In about 20 percent of cases, children with cleft palate will require a second operation on the palate to improve speech. The need for extra surgery cannot be predicted at the time of the original palate surgery. This surgery may be needed if speech therapy alone cannot improve the child's ability to speak normally. Surgery involves improving the function of the palate and throat where the air needed for sound is directed.

Before the child begins school, any significant residual cleft deformities involving the lip and nose are surgically corrected to help lessen the psychological effects of the problem.

Pediatric dental and orthodontic services begin to play a more important role as the teeth develop during the later years in childhood. Surgery to restore the residual cleft in the dental arch is frequently done at this time.

While nearly all cleft children will need braces as they enter adolescence, some will also need jaw surgery. For these children, the growth of the upper jaw lags behind the lower jaw and the face develops a sunken appearance. The surgery repositions the jaws to improve the child's bite and appearance. Once the facial bones are in correct relationship to each other, the final nose and lip surgery can be completed.

Many children with clefts involving the gum line need an operation called an alveolar bone graft to put extra bone in the gum, which allows the permanent teeth to come in better. This operation is done sometime between the ages of six and 10, depending on how fast the permanent teeth are developing.

Children with clefts of the lip may need or want another operation to improve the appearance of the scars. As teenagers, some need nasal surgery to improve breathing or appearance. In some children with clefts, the jaws are not in good alignment. In these cases, surgery can be done to align the bite.

Complications

In cleft lip surgery, the most common problem is asymmetry, when one side of the mouth and nose does not match the other side. The goal of cleft lip surgery is to close the separation in the first operation. Occasionally, a second operation may be needed.

Most children with clefts do not have other birth defects or any problems with intelligence or abilities. However, some children with clefts do have a higher chance of fluid in the ear because the cleft can interfere with the function of the middle ear. If untreated, frequent ear infections and even hearing loss can result. To permit proper drainage and air circulation, a small plastic ventilation tube may be inserted in the eardrum. This relatively minor operation may be done later or at the time of the cleft repair.

Cleft Palate Foundation, The (CPF)   A nonprofit organization dedicated to helping children with birth defects of the head and neck, and their families. It was founded by a parent group, the American Cleft Palate–Craniofacial Association (ACPA) in 1973 to be the public service arm of the professional association. The Cleft Palate Foundation's (CPF) primary purpose is to enhance the quality of life for individuals with congenital facial deformities and their families through education, research support, and the facilitation of family-centered care.

CPF's major activities include the operation of CLEFTLINE—(800) 24-CLEFT—and the dissemination of publications. The CLEFTLINE is a toll-free service providing information to callers about clefts and other craniofacial anomalies. Callers can request information about cleft palate/craniofacial teams and parent-patient support groups in their local region. Brochures and fact sheets on various aspects of cleft lip and palate and other craniofacial birth defects are distributed free to families. The CLEFTLINE is supported entirely by tax-deductible contributions.

CPF also conducts public education activities and awards annual research grants to junior and senior investigators. CPF is supported solely through tax-deductible contributions. The foundation is governed by a seven-member Board of Directors and supported by seven committees. (For contact information, see Appendix I.)

Clostridium perfringens infection   A mild food-borne illness caused by multiplying toxins found in *Clostridium perfringens* type A bacteria in human and animal feces, in soil and water, and in meat that has not been properly cooked. This type of food poisoning is among the most widely occurring in the United States, with an estimated 10,000 cases each year, according to the U.S. Centers for Disease Control. Most cases go unreported.

Cause

The bacteria is found in undercooked meat (such as rare beef, meat pies, burritos, tacos, enchiladas, or reheated meats or gravies made from beef, turkey, or chicken). The bacteria multiply quickly in reheated foods. Once ingested, the bacteria produce a toxin in the digestive tract about six hours later. A large amount of the bacteria must be ingested in order to cause illness. Outbreaks have been often traced to restaurants, caterers, and cafeterias that do not have adequate refrigeration facilities.

The bacteria produce spores, a dormant form of bacteria that is not killed by cooking; the spores cannot reproduce into bacteria at temperatures below 40°F or above 140°F.

Symptoms

The illness appears within nine to 15 hours after eating, causing severe colic or cramps and abdominal gas pains followed by a 24-hour bout of watery diarrhea. There may be nausea but usually not vomiting or fever. While usually a mild illness, it can be dangerous to infants and the elderly, who may become dehydrated. The disease does not confer immunity, but patients are not infectious.

When present in wounds or injuries, this type of bacteria causes potentially fatal gangrene.

Diagnosis

Recently scientists at the University of Illinois at Urbana-Champaign produced a test that can detect the presence of the bacterium. The bacteria will also grow on a culture plate in a lab from either the food or a stool sample.

Treatment

Because this is technically not an infection but an intoxication, no antibiotic will cure it. Patients should drink small sips of clear fluids and electrolytes to replace what is lost. If dehydration is suspected, seek medical help. If food poisoning is suspected, local health departments should be notified.

clubfoot   A congenital deformity of one or both feet that affects the bones, muscles, tendons, and blood vessels. The foot is usually short and broad in appearance, with the heel pointing downward while the front half of the foot turns inward. The Achilles tendon is tight, the heel looks narrow, and the muscles in the calf are smaller compared to a normal lower leg.

Clubfoot occurs in about one in every 1,000 live births and affects boys twice as often as girls. Half the time, both feet are affected.

Cause

Clubfoot is considered a multifactorial trait, which means that it involves both genetic and environmental factors. While experts do not really know what causes clubfoot, it may occur when a baby's foot stops growing at a certain point before birth, there is pressure on the baby's foot in the mother's womb, one of the bones in the foot does not form right, so that the rest of the foot grows crooked, or some of the muscles in the foot do not form normally and cause the bones to grow crooked.

Risk factors include a family history of clubfoot, position of the baby in the uterus, neuromuscular disorders such as CEREBRAL PALSY (CP) and SPINA BIFIDA, and a decreased amount of amniotic fluid surrounding the fetus during pregnancy. If a family has one or more relatives who have clubfoot, then the chances are higher that the baby may have one also. If a couple already has one child with clubfoot, then the chances of having another child with the same condition are about one in 50.

Complications

Babies born with clubfoot may have a higher risk of having an associated hip condition known as developmental dysplasia of the hip, a condition of the hip joint in which the top of the thigh bone slips in and out of its socket because the socket is too shallow to keep the joint intact.

Symptoms

The symptoms of clubfoot may resemble other medical conditions of the foot. If the affected foot is flexible, it is known as a "positional clubfoot." This flexible type of clubfoot is caused by the baby's position in the uterus. Positional clubfoot can easily be positioned into a normal position by hand. A true clubfoot, however, is rigid and very hard to manipulate.

In addition to the foot problem, the muscles in the lower leg are not as large as usual, and the joints in the ankle are not normal and do not move as much as a normal ankle. The affected foot and leg is usually smaller, and the child may need to wear a smaller shoe on the clubfoot.

Treatment

Ideally, the foot should be straightened so that it can grow and develop normally. Treatment options for infants include serial manipulation and casting, a type of treatment that begins with stretching of the foot by hand right after diagnosis. Soon after birth, the baby's foot is encased in a cast to help stretch the soft tissues of the foot so that the position of the foot can be held in place. The doctor changes the plaster casts every week for the first month, then every two weeks until the foot is straight (usually from six to 12 weeks). The foot usually responds to this type of treatment within the first few months; half of all children with clubfeet are successfully treated with serial manipulation and casting alone.

Surgery   If the position of the foot does not respond to serial manipulation and casting, then surgery may be considered. Sometimes percutaneous heel cord lengthening is used to augment casting.

Ideally, surgery is performed on children six to nine months of age. During surgery, the foot is aligned in a more normal position and a pin is implanted to hold the bones in place while they heal. The pin can be seen between the big and second toes. Following surgery, plaster long leg casts are applied to hold the foot in place as it heals. The usual hospital stay is three to five days. The first cast may be changed 10 days after surgery, and the cast and pin are removed usually three to six weeks after surgery. Short leg casts will continue to be used for at least three more months to continue to hold the foot in place and allow the tissues and bones to heal.

After the cast is removed regular shoes may be worn or a brace may be needed, depending on the child's diagnosis. Regular doctor visits are important after surgery. An X ray may be made every other year to see that the bones are in the corrected position. Occasionally a foot will begin to grow crooked again, and another surgery may be needed. If the doctor thinks the foot is starting to turn in again, the child will need to come back to the clinic more often. Sometimes special shoes or a brace must be worn at night to help the foot stay straight.

CMV See CYTOMEGALOVIRUS.

cold, common An upper respiratory infection caused by one of at least 200 different types of viruses. Colds are most likely to occur during "cold season," which begins in the fall and continues throughout the spring. After one bout with a particular virus, the child will develop an immunity to that precise virus. This is why adults have fewer colds than children.

A child who lives in a polluted environment, or who is exposed to secondhand smoke, has a higher chance of coming down with a cold. This is because air pollution and the nicotine and tars in tobacco smoke can irritate the lining of the nose and throat, making it easier for a cold virus to enter the cells and cause an infection. This irritation can also prolong the length of the infection.

Cause

Different types of viruses proliferate at different times; in the fall and late spring, a cold may be caused by one of the more than 100 types of rhinoviruses. Infection with these common germs occurs more often during this time because of crowding indoors and school openings. Between December and May several types of coronaviruses are responsible for most cases of the common cold. Besides these two types of viruses, colds may also be caused by parainfluenza, ADENOVIRUS, ENTEROVIRUSES, and INFLUENZA. All of these viruses seem to be able to change their characteristics from one season to the next.

A child does not catch a cold because he sits in a draft, has wet feet, or goes outside without a jacket. Because the cold viruses are so specific, a child can only get a cold if the virus travels high up inside the nose, into the nasopharynx. A cold virus can only reach this area by touch or, less often, through the air. One study found that while saliva did not pass on germs, even a very brief contact with a contaminated hand—as quick as a 10-second touch—led to transmission of viruses in 20 of 28 subjects.

While cold temperatures do not seem to bring on a cold, fatigue, stress, or anything else that weakens the body's immune system can influence a child's likelihood of getting sick. It is possible to catch a cold from other people who have colds, or from the things they use or touch, such as faucets, phones, doorknobs, light switches, or toys. A virus can survive for many hours on these objects, unless someone washes it off with alcohol, a household disinfectant, or hot sudsy water. Any child who touches one of these contaminated objects and then touches the nose, eyes, or mouth can get the virus. Once the virus is on the hands, others can be exposed by shaking hands or by touching other things that they touch.

Cold viruses are not carried very far through the air. If a child with a cold sneezes across the room, neighbors will not come down with the cold. However, if a child should cough or sneeze right into someone else's face, that person could get sick.

Healthy children have a film of mucus lining the nose and throat; tiny hairs called cilia move this mucus from sinuses and throat to the stomach. As the mucus is moved along, it traps harmful bacteria and viruses and carries them along to the stomach, where they are broken down by acids. A healthy mucous membrane can snag germs trapped in the nose and throat so the child can breathe, cough, or sneeze them back out. The mucus around the tonsils and adenoids can trap these germs, where they are then destroyed by the immune system.

If a child is not so healthy, the mucous membranes in the nose will either be too thick (causing a stuffy nose and congested throat) or too thin (causing a runny nose). The germs then will not be cleared away. Once the viruses enter the nose, they attach themselves to the cells found there. In response, the body's immune system swings into action. Injured cells in the nose and throat release chemicals called prostaglandins, which trigger inflammation and attract infection-fighting white blood cells. The throat will begin to feel scratchy and swollen.

Tiny blood vessels stretch, which allows spaces to open up and specialized white cells to enter. Body temperature rises, and histamine is released. This steps up the production of mucus in the nose, trapping and removing viral particles. The nose starts to run. As the nose and throat stimulate the extra mucus production, it irritates the throat and triggers a cough. Cold viruses are also responsible for congestion in the sinuses.

All of this activity is the underlying cause of the cold symptoms. By the time a child starts feeling sick, the body has already been fighting the invader for a day or two. When children are in the process of catching a cold, they probably feel fine. It is not until they are actually getting better that they feel sick.

In order to break through the body's defenses to cause a cold, viruses must attack in huge numbers. Most of the time, a brief encounter with a sick stranger will not cause disease, even if a child sits in a doctor's office filled with sick patients for 10 or 20 minutes.

On the other hand, going to school all day in a building filled with children who have colds could carry a risk. Traveling on a plane carrying sick passengers is an even bigger risk, since the recirculated air in a pressurized cabin evenly distributes viruses to everyone while drying out mucous membranes that would normally trap viruses.

Symptoms

A stuffy congested nose, sneezing, sore scratchy throat, cough, headache, runny eyes, and sometimes a low fever. Viruses that attack the lower respiratory tract (the windpipe, bronchial tubes, and lungs) are more serious, but less common; these viruses are responsible for PNEUMONIA and BRONCHITIS.

Because the symptoms are actually caused by the body's attempt at healing itself, there are times when it may be best to let the body handle itself. For example, it may be best to let a fever below 101.5°F burn itself out, since this type of fever will also help the body burn up viruses and toxins. However, if the child with a low fever is uncomfortable, it makes sense to try to lower the body's temperature.

Treatment

There is no treatment that will cure a cold. Symptoms may be treated by a wide variety of over-the-counter medications and many different types of home remedies. While the use of vitamin C to treat colds is still controversial, several well-controlled studies demonstrate that it can lessen the severity of a cold's symptoms and duration. In any case, vitamin C is not toxic and there is no harm in giving a child an extra dose, although megadoses should be avoided. Other studies have shown that zinc lozenges can shorten the duration of symptoms.

When to Call the Doctor

Parents should call a doctor if the child shows the following warning signs:

- fever of 102°F or above
- fever over 101°F that stays up after fever medication has been given
- any fever that lasts more than three days
- difficulty breathing, very rapid breathing, shortness of breath, or wheezing, noisy breathing
- blue or dusky color around mouth, nail beds, or skin
- extremely painful headache, throat, sinuses, or teeth
- skin rash
- white or yellow spots on tonsils or throat
- coughing episode lasting longer than the interval between coughs
- cough that produces yellow-green, gray, or bloody sputum, or that lasts longer than 10 days
- shaking chills
- delirium
- extreme difficulty swallowing

- headache and stiff neck (could be a sign of MENINGITIS)
- headache and sore throat (could be a sign of STREP THROAT)

Complications

A cold usually lasts for about 10 days, although it can range from three days to several weeks. A doctor should be consulted if the child still feels sick after 10 days, or if the child's face starts to swell or the teeth become extremely sensitive. These symptoms can signal a bacterial infection in the sinuses or middle ear.

When the sinuses become clogged with nasal secretions, they may become infected with bacteria. While antibiotics will not touch a cold, they will be effective in treating this type of secondary bacterial infection.

Colds also may trigger ASTHMA attacks in children with this condition, or they may lead to a middle EAR INFECTION. Pneumonia may also set in at the end of a cold. A child who suddenly develops a fever after the cold symptoms seem to be going away should see a doctor.

Colds vs. Flu and Allergies

A cold is not the same thing as influenza. The common cold is usually limited to the head, whereas the flu will affect the entire body. A cold usually begins slowly, with slight sore throat, mild chills or aches, and mild fever not usually over 100°F. The common cold causes a scratchy throat, runny nose, and itchy eyes.

The flu, on the other hand, strikes fast and hard, with much more severe symptoms, including nausea and vomiting, diarrhea, high fever (from 101°F to 104°F), body aches, severe chills, cough, eye pain, light sensitivity, and headache.

Allergies share a few symptoms with colds, but they have significant differences. A cold that seems to be hanging on for months is more likely an allergy. Winter allergies cause itchy eyes; itchy, runny, and stuffy nose; itchy throat; postnasal drip; coughing, sneezing, and season-long symptoms.

Prevention

A child remains infectious from 24 hours before symptoms appear until five days after symptoms begin, and is most infectious for the first three days. Young children are infectious for a longer period of time (up to three weeks), since it takes longer for their immature immune systems to fight off the virus.

While it may not seem practical, a child with a cold should stay home, especially to limit spreading of the virus. The most important factor in reducing the transmission of colds is effective hand washing. It's also important to avoid touching the nose and eyes. By scratching the nose or rubbing the eyes with a contaminated hand, the virus can easily be inhaled higher up into the nose. According to research, most children touch their nose or eyes about once every three hours.

Since most children find it hard not to touch their faces occasionally, washing hands often may help prevent colds. It is especially important for children who are already sick to wash hands, since they are even more likely to be wiping, blowing, scratching, or touching their faces. Washing the hands vigorously with soap and water for 20 seconds will remove the viruses.

Hands should be washed after sneezing or coughing; before eating; after wiping, blowing, or touching the nose; after using the toilet; and before touching another person.

Disposable tissues should be used instead of cloth handkerchiefs when coughing, sneezing, or blowing the nose and should be discarded immediately. A used tissue is filled with virus just waiting to be passed on to someone else.

In addition to not touching the face and washing hands, parents should disinfect areas likely to be contaminated with germs, such as door handles, telephones, light switches, and so on. The sick child should use a separate set of towels and washcloths, and parents should change their bedding more often. While it is not likely that rhinoviruses can cause illness by attaching themselves to a toothbrush, enteroviruses, which are found in the stomach and intestines, can occasionally cause a cold this way. Therefore, experts suggest replacing a toothbrush every three months. By being very careful, it is possible to stop the spread of colds even in a household where several children are sick.

cold sore A small skin blister also known as a "fever blister" that appears on the mouth during a cold. This is extremely common and is usually first transmitted during childhood. The term "fever blister" comes from the fact that such blisters often appeared during the high fevers of infectious illnesses before the invention of antibiotics.

Cold sores are harmless in healthy children and adults, although they are painful to the touch and can be unattractive. They are similar, but not identical, to "canker sores," which also appear on the mouth. Both usually cause small sores to develop in the mouth that heal within two weeks. However, canker sores are not usually preceded by a blister. Canker sores are usually larger than fever blisters, but they do not usually merge to form one large sore as fever blisters do. Finally, canker sores usually erupt on movable parts of the mouth (such as the tongue and the cheek or lip linings), whereas cold sores usually appear on the gums, roof of the mouth, lips, or nostrils.

People are most infectious when the sores first appear, but the cold virus is shed in the saliva for a long time (up to two months after the sores have healed). It can be spread to others during this entire time. Patients with an active cold sore should limit contact with newborns or anyone else with a weakened immune system.

Causes

Cold sores are caused by the contagious HERPES simplex virus. The viral strain usually responsible for cold sores is herpes simplex Type I (HSVI); up to 90 percent of all people around the world carry this virus. This strain usually appears on the mouth, lips, and face.

The virus is highly contagious when the blisters are present; it is often transmitted by kissing. The virus can also be spread by children who touch their blisters and then touch other children. About 10 percent of oral herpes cases in adults are acquired by oral-genital sex with a person with active genital herpes.

Most people have their first infection before age 10, although most will not have symptoms. About 15 percent will go on to develop many fluid-filled blisters inside and outside the mouth about five days after exposure, together with fever, swollen neck, and aches. This is followed by a yellow crust that forms over the blister, healing without scars in about two weeks. Once the infection occurs, the virus remains in a nerve located near the cheekbone. There it may remain, forever inactive, or it may travel down the nerve to the surface of the skin to cause a new blister.

Recurrent attacks tend to be less severe.

Cold sores tend to appear when the victim is stressed, exposed to sunlight, a cold wind, or another infection, or feels run down. Women tend to experience more cold sores around their menstrual periods, but some people are afflicted at regular intervals throughout the year. People with compromised immune systems may experience prolonged attacks.

One study suggests that the tendency for relapses might be inherited.

Symptoms

The first attack may not even be noticed; the first infection in childhood usually causes no symptoms. However, about 10 percent of newly infected children experience a mild to fairly severe illness with fever, tiredness, and several painful cold sores in the mouth and throat.

Subsequent outbreaks are often signaled by a tingling in the lips, followed by a small water-filled blister on a red base that soon grows, causing itching and soreness. Within a few days the blisters burst, encrust, and then disappear within a week. The virus then retreats back along the nerve where it lies dormant in the nerve cell; in some patients, however, the virus is constantly reactivated.

Treatment

There is no cure for recurrent fever blisters. For mild symptoms, the sore should be kept clean and dry and it will heal itself. For particularly virulent outbreaks, the antiviral drug ACYCLOVIR or idoxuridine paint may relieve symptoms. Otherwise, there are a range of nonprescription drugs available containing some numbing agent (such as camphor or phenol) that also contain an emollient to reduce cracking.

Some studies have suggested that zinc may help prevent outbreaks because the zinc interferes with herpes viral replication. Studies found that both zinc gluconate and zinc sulfate helped speed up healing time, but zinc gluconate was less irritating to the skin. Both zinc products are available at health food stores.

Sores can be protected with a dab of petroleum jelly (applied with a clean cotton swab); do not dip the swab that touched the affected area back into the jar. Patients should avoid drinks with a high acid content (such as orange juice).

Complications

Anyone with an impaired immune system is at risk of complications; the virus may spread throughout the body, causing a severe illness.

Prevention

While there is no effective preventive treatment, some patients find that using a lip salve before going out in the sun prevents outbreaks. Research has shown that the virus can live up to seven days on a toothbrush, causing a reinfection after the sore heals. Once a sore develops, an infected toothbrush can also lead to multiple sores, so a new toothbrush should be used during the outbreak. Once the sore has healed completely, a new toothbrush should be used. It is also better to use small tubes of toothpaste, since the paste can transmit germs, too. Using small tubes of paste will mean that you throw the tubes away more quickly.

An infected individual should not touch sores, which could spread the virus to new sites (such as the eyes or the genitals). Kissing should be avoided during an outbreak.

colitis See INFLAMMATORY BOWEL DISEASE.

communicable/contagious disease Any disease that is transmitted from one person or animal to another, either directly—by contact with feces or urine or other bodily discharges—or indirectly, via objects or substances such as contaminated glasses, toys, or water. It may also be transmitted via fleas, flies, mosquitoes, ticks, or other insects.

Control of a communicable disease rests on properly identifying the organism that transmits it, preventing its spread to the environment, protecting others, and treating the infected patients.

By law, many communicable diseases must be reported to the local health department. Communicable diseases include those caused by organisms such as fungi, CHLAMYDIA, parasites, rickettsiae, and viruses.

communication disorder A problem in being understood or in understanding. Students with communication disorders can quickly fall behind in class and have problems in vocabulary, memory, and problem solving. Many also encounter difficulty in social situations. While experts are not sure how many children have communication disorders, estimates suggest it may affect about 5 percent of the school age population. Early identification of a communication disorder is essential. Communication disorders can be grouped into two main categories—hearing disorders, or speech and language disorders.

A hearing disorder affects the ability to hear sounds clearly. Such disorders may range from hearing speech sounds faintly, or in a distorted way, to profound DEAFNESS. Speech and language disorders affect the way people talk and understand and may range from simple sound substitutions to the inability to use speech and language at all.

Hearing Disorders

Hearing disorders may be caused by a wide variety of problems either at birth or any time thereafter. Profound hearing loss from birth or an early age makes the acquisition of spoken language very difficult. However, deaf infants and children all go through the same developmental speech stages in acquiring gestural language such as American Sign Language.

Hearing loss acquired through disease, injury, or noise may be more subtle, but if not treated it may interfere with a child's ability to acquire spoken language.

Speech and Language Disorder

Evidence of a speech and language disorder may be seen when a person's speech or language significantly differs from that of others of the same age or background, or when there is a marked impairment in a person's ability to express himself.

Speech and language disorders may be caused by a broad range of factors, such as hearing loss, cerebral palsy, severe head injury, stroke, or heredity. Often, the cause is unknown.

Compassionate Friends, Inc. A national non-profit, self-help support organization that offers friendship and understanding to bereaved parents, grandparents, and siblings. There is no religious affiliation and there are no membership dues or fees. The mission of the Compassionate Friends is to help families toward the positive resolution of grief following the death of a child of any age and to provide information to help others be supportive. As seasoned grievers reach out to the newly bereaved, energy that has been directed inward begins to flow outward and both are helped to heal.

The Compassionate Friends was founded in Coventry, England, in 1969, following the deaths of two young boys, Billy Henderson and Kenneth Lawley, who had died just three days apart in the same hospital. The Compassionate Friends was incorporated in the United States as a nonprofit organization in 1978.

There are now Compassionate Friends chapters in every state in the United States—almost 600 altogether—and hundreds of chapters in Canada, Great Britain, and other countries throughout the world. In the United States, chapters are open to all bereaved parents, siblings, grandparents, and other family members who are grieving the death of a child of any age, from any cause. (For contact information, see Appendix I.)

Concerta An extended release form of methylphenidate (RITALIN) for ATTENTION DEFICIT HYPERACTIVITY DISORDER. Approved to be taken only once a day, this version of the drug eliminates the ups and downs that often come with traditional medications. Concerta is designed to give a very smooth sustained release and then to shut off after 10 to 12 hours, so that the child's appetite and sleep are fine at the end of the day.

Concerta is the first slow-release medication to be created for ADHD.

Concerta is approved for the treatment of ADHD in children over age six. It is designed to be taken just once a day in the morning, before a child leaves for school. The drug overcoat dissolves within an hour, providing an initial dose of methylphenidate, which is then released gradually in a smooth pattern, improving attention and behavior throughout the day. The advanced system was designed to help a child maintain focus without in-school and after-school dosing. Due to

its controlled release, Concerta minimizes the fluctuating levels of medicine in the blood associated with other medications when they are taken more than once per day.

Contraindications

Concerta should not be taken by patients who have significant anxiety, tension, or agitation, since the drug may make these conditions worse. It should not be used by anyone who:

- is allergic to Ritalin or any of the other ingredients
- has glaucoma
- has tics
- has TOURETTE'S SYNDROME or a family history of Tourette's syndrome
- takes a prescription monoamine oxidase inhibitor (MAOI).

Ordinarily, Concerta should not be given to patients with preexisting severe gastrointestinal narrowing, and it should be used with caution by anyone with a history of drug dependence or alcoholism. Chronic abuse can lead to psychological dependence.

conduct disorder A form of antisocial behavior characterized by extremely disobedient behavior in children, including vandalism, theft, lying, and drug use. Typically diagnosed in young boys, conduct disorders are characterized by antisocial behavior and patterns of "acting out" at home or at school. The child may have difficulty learning how to solve problems or establish peer relationships. As many as one in 10 children and adolescents may have a conduct disorder.

Individuals with conduct disorder are more likely to attract attention from teachers and parents, to be referred for services, and to receive some treatment at an early age for their misbehavior.

There is a high correlation between conduct disorder and ATTENTION DEFICIT HYPERACTIVITY DISORDER (ADHD). Individuals with both disorders are particularly at risk for continuing social and emotional difficulties into adulthood.

Cause

Research suggests that the most severe cases of conduct disorder begin in early childhood, especially in the presence of inconsistent rules and harsh discipline, lack of enough supervision or guidance, frequent change in caregivers, poverty, neglect or abuse, and a delinquent peer group.

Treatment

Because antisocial behavior in children and adolescents is very hard to change after it has become ingrained, the earlier the problem is identified and treated the better. Some recent studies have focused on promising ways to prevent conduct disorder among children and adolescents who are at risk for developing the disorder, since most children with conduct disorder are probably reacting to events and situations in their lives.

conjunctivitis The medical name for "pinkeye," an inflammation of the transparent membrane covering the white of the eye. This common infection of childhood, also referred to as a "cold in the eye," causes redness, discomfort, and a discharge from the eye.

Cause

Most conjunctivitis is caused by bacteria (staphylococci) spread by hand-to-eye contact, or by viruses associated with a cold, sore throat, or illness such as measles. Viral conjunctivitis can spread like wildfire through schools and other group settings.

Newborns sometimes contract a type of conjunctivitis called neonatal ophthalmia, caused by infection in the mother's cervix during birth from either GONORRHEA, genital HERPES, or CHLAMYDIA. The infection may spread to the entire eye and cause blindness.

Symptoms

All types of conjunctivitis lead to redness, itchy, scratchy feelings, discharge, and photophobia (dislike of bright lights). There may be so much discharge that the eyelids stick together in the morning.

Treatment

Antibiotic eye drops or ointments are given if a bacterial infection is suspected; however, this will not cure a viral infection. Warm water may wash away the discharge and remove crusts; in babies, the eye may be washed with sterile saline. In addition to eye drops, the discharge must be cleaned from the eyes, on an hourly basis for the first day.

Complications

A doctor should be called immediately if any of these symptoms appear: swollen red eyelids, blurry vision, severe headache, fever higher than 101°F, or a very painful eye. A doctor should be seen within 24 hours for any of the following symptoms: no improvement after drops or ointment, ear pain, or eyes that get more red or itchy *after* drops or ointment (which may be an allergic reaction).

Prevention

Hand washing may prevent conjunctivitis, since the disease is spread from hand to eye very easily. Anyone with the disease should have separate washcloths and towels. It is also important that swimming pools and hot tubs be properly chlorinated. Children with conjunctivitis should be kept at home until 24 hours after antibiotics have been taken. Newborns are treated with erthromycin opthalmic solution to prevent the infection.

consciousness, loss of See FAINTING.

convulsion See SEIZURES.

coxsackievirus Any of 30 different enteroviruses associated with a variety of symptoms, primarily affecting children during warm weather. The virus resembles the germ responsible for POLIO (especially in size). Among the diseases associated with these viruses are herpangina; HAND, FOOT, AND MOUTH DISEASE; myocarditis; and MENINGITIS.

Coxsackieviruses are separated into group A and group B viruses, with group B causing more serious infections. These viruses infect a child primarily via the gastrointestinal tract, although they may also enter the body through the respiratory tract via mucous droplets, especially when the droplets come from people with TONSILLITIS, PHARYNGITIS, or PNEUMONIA.

There are many viral types or strains identified by antibody testing or viral cultures, neither of which are often performed. These different strains may cause different symptoms. Some types of coxsackievirus are associated with specific clinical diseases:

• Coxsackievirus A16 and enterovirus 71 are linked with HAND, FOOT, AND MOUTH DISEASE

- Coxsackievirus A24 and enterovirus 70 with acute hemorrhagic conjunctivitis (pinkeye)
- Coxsackieviruses B1-B5 with myocarditis (inflammatory heart disease)

Treatment

Treatment is usually aimed at easing symptoms.

Prevention

Because these viruses spread chiefly by contact with fecal excretions, scrupulous hand washing is always the best defense against spread of these infections. Otherwise, there is no known way to prevent infection with these viruses other than isolating the affected patient.

cradle cap   A harmless, common skin condition in infants in which thick yellow greasy scales form in patches over the scalp. It is a form of seborrheic dermatitis, which may also occur on the face, neck, behind the ears, and in the diaper area. Without treatment, it may persist for months, but when properly cared for, the condition usually fades away within a few weeks. A doctor should be consulted if the skin looks inflamed, or if the condition worsens.

Treatment

The baby's hair should be washed with baby shampoo or a mild anti-dandruff shampoo once a day; after lathering, the scaly scalp should be massaged with a soft toothbrush for a few minutes. For very crusty conditions, olive or mineral oil should be rubbed into the baby's scalp an hour before a shampoo. The oil loosens and softens the scales, which can then be washed off. All the oil must be washed out, because if this is left in the hair it could aggravate the problem.

This treatment may need to be repeated for several days until the scales are all washed away. Baby's hair should be brushed daily with a soft bristle brush to help loosen scales that can then be removed with a fine-tooth comb.

A mild corticosteroid solution or cream may be prescribed in severe cases until the condition clears.

craniofacial conditions   A group of conditions which children may either be born with or develop later, in which the bones of the head and face grow inappropriately.

Craniosynostosis

This condition, which means "fused bones of the skull," occurs when the skull fuses too early. A child's skull is made up of a group of different bones that fit together like a jigsaw puzzle; the areas where the bones meet are called sutures. As a baby grows, the brain rapidly increases in size and causes the skull bones to expand. In craniosynostosis, the fused part of the skull cannot enlarge, which may lead to overgrowth and abnormalities in the shaped skull.

In "multi-suture craniosynostosis," more than one suture of the skull is prematurely closed. Multi-suture craniosynostosis includes the Apert, Crouzon, Pfeiffer, and Saethre-Chotzen syndromes.

The main treatment for craniosynostosis during infancy is surgery, which will relieve intracranial pressure, assure that the skull has the capacity to accommodate the brain's growth, and cosmetically improve the appearance of the child's head.

Apert syndrome   In this condition, the skull and the face grow abnormally, producing bulging eyes that are usually wide-set and tilted down at the sides. Children with this condition usually have problems with teeth alignment due to the underdevelopment of the upper jaw, and some have cleft palate, or webbed fingers and toes.

After the child is evaluated by a multispeciality craniofacial surgery team at a children's medical center, the condition can be surgically treated to correct the skull, mid-face, and palate. Hearing problems can be treated by a hearing specialist.

Crouzon syndrome   In this condition, the sutures in the head are prematurely fused so that the skull and face grow abnormally, producing bulging eyes, receding upper jaw, and protruding lower jaw. There also may be problems with teeth due to abnormal jaw growth.

There is no cure for Crouzon syndrome, but many of the symptoms can be treated with complex surgery best provided by comprehensive craniofacial teams at major centers. Surgeries used to treat the symptoms of Crouzon syndrome include the removal and replacement of portions of the cranial bone (craniectomy) as early as possible after birth. This can help prevent pressure and damage to the brain and can maintain a skull shape that is as normal as possible. Surgery to treat protruding eyeballs is done directly on the eye sockets or on the bones surrounding the eye sockets. Removing a portion of the jawbone can help treat a protruding lower jaw, which is often very successful in normalizing the appearance of the jaw. Finally, surgeons also can repair a cleft palate, and braces and other orthodontic treatments are usually necessary to help correct misalignment of teeth. An ophthalmologist and otolaryngologist (ear, nose, and throat specialist) should monitor infants and children with Crouzon syndrome. These specialists can check for problems and provide corrective treatment as necessary.

Pfeiffer syndrome In this condition, sutures that fuse too soon produce a high forehead and pointed top of the head. The middle face appears flattened, the nose is small and has a flattened appearance, eyes are widely spaced, and the upper jaw is underdeveloped, which causes the lower jaw to appear prominent. The thumbs and big toes are very broad, and teeth are often crowded.

Multiple staged surgery is usually recommended for patients with Pfeiffer syndrome. In the first year of life, doctors can release the sutures of the skull to allow for brain growth and expansion. Skull remodeling may need to be repeated as the child grows. If necessary, mid-facial advancement and jaw surgery can be done to provide adequate room for the eyes and to correct the occlusion. Although there is a significant malformation of the fingers and toes, usually these function adequately and do not require the surgical attention of a plastic surgeon and specialist.

Saethre-Chotzen syndrome In this condition, irregular head growth is caused when more than one suture is fused prematurely. Eyelids are droopy and eyes are widespread, bulging, and possibly crossed. The upper jaw may be underdeveloped, the nose may look "beaked," and the area between the nostrils is off center. Fingers are short and certain fingers may be fused. The hairline may be low.

Multiple staged surgery is also the general treatment plan for patients with Saethre-Chotzen syndrome, and is similar to the procedures for Pfeiffer

syndrome. In the first year of life the surgeon will release the synostotic sutures of the skull to allow adequate brain growth and expansion. This procedure may need to be repeated in the life of the child. Depending on the severity of the skull deformity, this procedure may be done in one stage or two stages.

If necessary, mid-facial advancement and jaw surgery can be done to provide adequate room for the eyes and to correct the occlusion to an appropriate functional position. Eye muscle surgery often needs to be performed by a pediatric ophthalmologist to correct the imbalance in the muscular structures of the eye as well as the drooping of the eyelids.

Cleft Lip and/or Palate

This type of craniofacial condition may lead to a separation of the parts or segments of the lip or roof of the mouth that are usually joined together during the early weeks in fetal development. A cleft lip is a separation of the two sides of the lip and often includes the bones of the maxilla and/or the upper gum. A cleft palate is an opening in the roof of the mouth that occurs when the two sides of the palate do not fuse as the unborn baby develops.

For a full discussion of this condition, its cause and treatment, see the separate entry for CLEFT LIP AND PALATE.

Facial Palsy

This condition may either be present at birth or acquired afterward, causing a complete or partial paralysis of the face, interfering with smiling, blinking, and frowning. The nerve impulses for facial movements begin in the brain and travel through the facial nerves to the muscles in the face. Diseases or injuries affecting the brain, the facial nerve, or the muscles of the face can cause facial palsy. In many cases, no treatment is necessary.

Frontonasal Dysplasia

Also known as median cleft face syndrome, this condition results in a flat, wide nose and wide-set eyes. There is a groove down the middle of the face, and in some cases, the tip of the nose is missing. A gap with extra folds of skin covering it may appear on the front of the head.

Treatment of this disorder depends on the severity of the child's physical characteristics. Surgery may correct the divided nose, cleft lip, and other facial deformities. In some cases, more surgery may be needed as the child gets older.

A team approach for infants and children with this disorder may help, including special social, educational, and medical services.

Hemifacial Microsomia/Goldenhar Syndrome

In this condition, the lower half of one side of the face does not grow normally, leading to a missing or partially formed ear. In Goldenhar syndrome (a variant of hemifacial microsomia) benign growths of the eye may be accompanied by neck problems, which are most commonly caused by a fusion of bony bridges between the bones of the neck.

Due to the delayed growth and development of the lower half of the face, the effects of this syndrome will be more evident as the child grows. The lack of the development of the upper and lower jaws can cause breathing problems as well as a dental malocclusion, which will need to be addressed surgically and orthodontically. Treatment generally requires the expertise of both a craniofacial surgeon and an orthodontist.

The jaw deformity may be reconstructed as early as age three if the problem is severe enough to cause airway problems. The best approach to reconstructing the jaw is determined by the surgeon and is specific for each patient. If it is needed, ear reconstruction is performed in four stages, usually at age six. Throughout life, these patients must maintain adequate dental occlusion through ongoing orthodontic treatment.

Microtia/Atresia

Microtia is the medical term for an incompletely formed ear that may range from an ear that is smaller than normal to just a bit of tissue at the location where the ear would normally be. Atresia is the absence of an ear canal in the middle ear. Microtia and atresia can occur alone or together, and they can also be associated with hemifacial microsomia. If both ears are affected, Treacher Collins syndrome may be involved.

There are several treatment options for a child with this condition, depending in part on how severely the ear is affected. In some cases, no treat-ment is necessary. For more severe cases, a new ear can be crafted from the child's rib cartilage in two separate operations. Because the cartilage must be mature, this technique is not offered until a child is at least 10 years old. After the cartilage is removed, surgeons carve it into an ear shape and slip it into a pocket of skin on the side of the child's head. At this stage it looks like an ear, but it lies flat against the side of the head where it will gradually stick. Six months later, a second operation is carried out to release the ear and create a groove behind it. The new ear is usually stiff but looks like an ear, feels warm, and will eventually have sensation. It will not grow, but by age 10, most children's ears are already adult size.

However, if a child had previous surgery to the ear or other scars, it might not be possible to use this technique to form a new ear. In this case, surgeons can insert a prosthetic ear anchored to fixtures embedded into the bone at the side of the child's head. The prosthesis is made of a soft silicone material and looks quite lifelike. The two required operations can be carried out when a child is about seven or eight years old. Any skin tags and vestiges in this area need to be removed prior to fitting the implants. During the first operation, surgeons place three titanium implants into the bone on the side of the small ear. In the second operation three months later, doctors will attach two screws to the implants.

A few months after the second operation, a bar will be fitted, and the new ear will be made to the same size, shape, and color of the child's other ear, which will clip onto the bar.

A good prosthesis of this kind will last about two years and can be worn even while swimming. The prosthesis can be worn at any time, but is generally taken off at night. The area around the screws that keep the ear attached to the skin must be cleaned every day.

Moebius Syndrome

In this very rare condition, the sixth and seventh cranial nerves are paralyzed, causing a lack of facial expression, lack of lateral eye movement, and lack of blinking. Children with this syndrome cannot smile.

Other symptoms may include deformed tongue and jaw, hand or foot deformities (such as clubfoot or missing fingers), poor muscle tone, and swallowing or breathing problems. Although a child with Moebius syndrome may crawl or walk later than other children, he or she eventually catches up.

Moebius syndrome does not get worse over time. Hand, foot, or jaw deformities, and crossed eyes, can be surgically treated. It is sometimes possible through surgery to counteract the facial paralysis by transferring nerves and muscles to the corners of the mouth.

A special feeding device or feeding tube may help the child get nourishment. Physical therapy can ease muscle problems, and occupational therapy can help the child learn how to wash and dress (especially for those with hand deformities). Speech therapy may help as well. A tracheotomy can ease severe breathing problems.

Miller Syndrome

This very rare condition is characterized by downward slanting eyelids, cleft palate, recessed lower jaw, small cup-shaped ears, and a broad nasal ridge. There are also shortened bowed forearms, incompletely developed bones in the arms, missing or webbed fingers and toes, and abnormal growth of the bones in the lower legs. Occasional problems include heart defects, lung disease, extra nipples, stomach or kidney reflux, undescended testicles, or dislocated hips.

The child should be treated by a qualified craniofacial medical team at a craniofacial center. Several surgeries may be necessary, depending on the severity of the child's condition. Some treatments may include a tracheostomy to help with breathing, a gastrostomy tube to assure proper nutrition, and craniofacial surgery to the jaw, ears, and eyes.

Nager Syndrome

This condition features downward slanting eyelids, absent or underdeveloped cheekbones, a severely underdeveloped lower jaw, malformed outer and middle ears, cleft palate, absence of lower eyelashes, scalp hair growing onto the cheeks, and underdeveloped or missing thumbs.

Several surgeries may be necessary, depending on the severity of the child's condition, including tracheostomy to help with breathing, a gastrostomy tube to assure proper nutrition, and craniofacial surgery to the jaw and ears.

Pierre Robin Syndrome

In this condition, the lower jaw is abnormally small and the tongue falls backward toward the throat; cleft lip and a cleft palate are also possible.

Infants must be kept face down, which allows gravity to pull the tongue forward and keep the airway open. These problems abate over the first few years as the lower jaw grows and assumes a more normal size. In moderate cases, the patient needs a tube placed through the nose and into the airway to avoid airway blockage. In severe cases, surgery is indicated for recurrent upper airway obstruction. Tracheostomy is sometimes required. Feeding must be done very carefully to avoid choking and inhaling liquids into the airways.

Treacher-Collins Syndrome

In this condition, the cheekbones and jawbones are underdeveloped, with notches in or stretching of the lower eyelids. The ears are frequently abnormal, part of the outer ear is usually missing, and hearing problems are common.

Treatment consists of testing for and treating any hearing loss so as to enable a child to perform at normal level in school. Plastic surgery can improve the receding chin and other physical defects.

crib death   See SUDDEN INFANT DEATH SYNDROME.

cri du chat syndrome   Also known as "cry of the cat syndrome" or "5p-syndrome," this is a rare congenital condition characterized by a kitten-like mewing cry caused by a small larynx. The cry usually disappears after the first few weeks of life, but the syndrome is usually linked with MENTAL RETARDATION, heart problems, unusual facial characteristics (such as widely spaced eyes), small head, and short stature.

Cause

The condition is the result of a chromosome abnormality in which a portion of chromosome 5 is missing in each of the child's cells.

Treatment

There is no treatment. The outlook is not good; the child may not survive infancy. (See also 5P-SOCIETY.)

Crohn's disease See INFLAMMATORY BOWEL DISEASE.

croup Inflammation and narrowing of the air passages in young children that causes a hoarse, barking cough and a wheezing on inhaling. Once very common in children from 6 months to 36 months of age, croup is a frightening but not terribly serious illness. In older children and adults, the air passages are too wide and the cartilage in the air passages too stiff for swelling or inflammation to cause the walls to collapse. Croup is known medically as laryngotracheobronchitis (LTB).

One bout of croup does not confer immunity, and some children get several attacks. However, most cases are mild and children recover uneventfully.

Cause

Croup is caused by one of several different types of viral infection (often a cold) that affects the larynx, windpipe, and airways into the lungs. The most common is parainfluenza virus (which usually occurs in late fall). RESPIRATORY SYNCYTIAL VIRUS (RSV) and INFLUENZA may appear in winter and early spring. ADENOVIRUS, rhinovirus, and sometimes MEASLES may lead to croup. While croup cannot be passed on to anyone else, it is possible to catch a virus that can cause croup.

Some babies appear to be more likely to get croup than others, possibly because of a sensitive larynx. Premature infants may also be prone to croup. Twice as many boys get croup as girls; some infants never get it, and others get it every time they have a cold.

Children outgrow the tendency toward croup, but there is no immunity.

Symptoms

Croup begins like a cold. About one to seven days later, fever, cough, and breathing problems appear, often at night. The child may awake with the characteristic barking cough, with shallow fast and noisy breathing. The high-pitched sounds occur during inhaling, not exhaling.

The child may feel better during the day but suffer the barking cough during the night for three or four nights.

Diagnosis

A doctor can diagnose croup from the symptoms; tests are not needed, although a neck X ray may be used to rule out foreign bodies or obstructions.

Treatment

Cool mist vaporizers or cool night air help a child to breathe; the child should be kept upright while breathing in the cool air. Steam from a shower will work if no vaporizer is available. If the swelling does not ease, the child may be taken outside for 20 minutes; the shock of the cold air usually eases the swelling.

A doctor should be called if the illness is severe (fever over 101°F and severe breathing problems). For serious cases, doctors may check oxygen levels in the blood and provide oxygen together with dexamethasone (Decadron). A tube may be inserted down or through the throat (tracheostomy). The infant may be placed in a croup or mist tent, but such a tent should not be constructed at home.

Complications

Croup that enters the windpipe and the small airways leading into the lungs is called acute laryngotracheobronchitis, a more serious condition that can interfere with breathing and may require hospitalization.

Epiglottitis is a rare but dangerous condition which may be confused with croup. However, today it is almost never seen since all American infants are given the Hib vaccine. Epiglottitis is caused by a sudden bacterial infection that causes so much swelling in the upper throat that the child's airway is almost blocked. A doctor should be called if there are any of these warning signs of epiglottitis:

- fever higher than 103°F
- drooling with open mouth
- agitation, restlessness, flaring nostrils
- bluish lips, skin, or nail beds
- muffled speech
- rapid, difficult breathing
- noisy breathing in and out
- movement in and out in the areas between the ribs during breathing
- severe sore throat
- refusal to swallow

Prevention

If the child has a tendency toward developing croup, there are some ways to prevent the disease from occurring:

- keep a cool-mist vaporizer in the room during sleep
- do not smoke in the house
- give clear fluids to a baby with a cold
- help calm an overexcited baby with a cold until sleep

cryptosporidiosis One of the more recently discovered types of food poisoning caused by a protozoan *Cryptosporidium,* which means "hidden spore" in Greek. The tiny invisible microbe infects cells lining the intestinal tract and was identified as a cause of human disease in 1976.

In the United States, many outbreaks in childcare centers are never identified. The number of cases that occur each year are not well documented.

Some immunity follows infection, but the degree to which this immunity occurs is not clear.

Cause

This parasite lives its entire life within the intestinal cells; it produces worms (oocysts) that are excreted in feces. These infectious oocysts can survive outside the human body for long periods of time, passing into food and drinking water, onto objects, and spread from hand to mouth. Unfortunately, chlorine does not kill the protozoan; instead, drinking water must be filtered to eliminate it. Many municipal water supplies do not have the technology to provide this filter.

Because the bacteria is transmitted by the fecal-oral route, the greatest risk occurs in those infected people who have diarrhea, those with poor personal hygiene, and diapered children.

Symptoms

Between one to 12 days after infection, the most common symptom is a watery diarrhea together with stomach cramps, nausea and vomiting, fever, headache, and loss of appetite. Some people with the infection do not experience any symptoms at all.

Healthy patients usually exhibit symptoms for about two weeks, but those with impaired immune systems may have a severe and lasting illness.

Diagnosis

The infection is diagnosed by identifying the parasite during examination of the stool. If cryptosporidiosis is suspected, a specific lab test should be requested, since most labs do not yet routinely perform the necessary tests.

Treatment

There is no standard treatment, but some patients may respond to some antiparasitic drugs. Intravenous fluids may be necessary, and antidiarrheal drugs may help.

***Cyclospora cayetanensis* infection** Infestation with a parasitic microbe that causes intense diarrhea, weight loss, and fatigue. It was identified as a cause of human disease only recently. The United States is currently battling its fourth epidemic of cyclospora, which began in the spring of 1996. Contaminated raspberries have sickened more than 1,000 people in 11 states east of the Rocky Mountains. In the most recent outbreak, scientists have found it hard to track the source of the problem because it takes a week between ingestion and onset of symptoms. While health officials did not find cyclospora in any raw fruit, they suspect it only takes a few microbes to infect a person.

The first outbreak in the United States was probably in 1979, although it was never properly identified; it came to the attention of officials in Chicago in 1989. This was followed by reports of outbreaks in Morocco, Peru, and New Guinea. The first full description of the disease was reported in the *American Journal of Tropical Medicine and Hygiene* in 1991.

Cause

Little is known about the parasite's life cycle, the way it spreads and whether birds or animals that feed on berries are involved. The organism is a distant cousin of cryptosporidium, the protozoan that infiltrated a Milwaukee water supply in 1993 and caused an epidemic of CRYPTOSPORIDIOSIS and 40 deaths. But this new organism is twice as large. Because the organism is a parasite of the small bowel, patients continue to lose weight even after the diarrhea stops because they cannot absorb nutrients.

The organism does not appear to be halted by iodine or chlorine and can even elude filtration systems. The only thing that kills it is boiling the water in which it lives.

Symptoms

About a week after ingestion, the disease begins with severe diarrhea, stomach cramps, nausea, and vomiting. It then progresses to weeks of mild fever, debilitating fatigue, and loss of appetite; patients can lose 15 to 20 pounds. While the disease is not normally fatal, some patients have been hospitalized because of dehydration.

Treatment

The antibiotic Bactrim, once used routinely to treat diarrhea, can shorten the term of the illness, although most other diarrhea-causing organisms are now resistant to the drug. Alternately, a combination of trimethoprim and sulfamethoxazole has been established as effective therapy. Those with impaired immune systems require higher doses and longer therapy.

Prevention

Scientists advise those in epidemic areas not to eat strawberries or raspberries, especially if they have impaired immune systems. In other locations, officials suggest all fruit and vegetables should be thoroughly washed before eating.

Cylert (pemoline) A stimulant medication sometimes used to treat ATTENTION DEFICIT HYPERACTIVITY DISORDER (ADHD). Because of its association with life-threatening liver failure, Cylert is not ordinarily considered as first-line drug therapy for ADHD, and it was withdrawn from sale in Canada in September 1999 because of complications.

Since Cylert's debut in 1975, 13 cases of acute hepatic failure have been reported to the Federal Drug Administration (FDA). While the number of reported cases is not large, the rate of reporting ranges from four to 17 times the rate expected in the general population. This estimate may be conservative because of underreporting and because of the long latency between the beginning of Cylert treatment and the occurrence of signs of liver failure. Of the 13 cases, 11 ended in death or liver transplantation, usually within four weeks of the onset of signs and symptoms of liver failure.

Unlike Ritalin and Dexedrine, which can take effect within an hour, Cylert takes from two to four weeks to become effective. It is used by children and adults and is usually prescribed as part of a treatment plan that includes behavioral or educational interventions. Stimulant medications like Cylert are generally taken for as long a period of time as is helpful.

Although experts are not sure how Cylert works, they believe it boosts the production of a neurotransmitter called dopamine.

Side Effects

In addition to the serious liver problems, common side effects include sleep problems and loss of appetite. It may decrease growth rate in children, so its use should be monitored carefully by a physician.

cystic fibrosis (CF) A chronic, progressive, and usually fatal genetic disease of the body's mucous glands that primarily affects the respiratory and digestive systems in children and young adults. The sweat glands and the reproductive system are also usually involved. Typically, children with CF have a lifespan of about 30 years. However, some milder cases of CF may not be diagnosed until young adulthood; patients with these milder cases may live into their 40s with excellent supportive care.

While the condition has existed for hundreds of years, the name "cystic fibrosis of the pancreas" was first applied to the disease in 1938. About 30,000 Americans have CF—mostly whites whose ancestors came from northern Europe, although it affects all races and ethnic groups. It is less common in African Americans, Native Americans, and Asian Americans. About 2,500 babies are born with CF each year in the United States, and about one in every 20 Americans is an unaffected carrier of an abnormal CF gene. These 12 million people are usually unaware that they are carriers.

Symptoms

Symptoms vary from child to child, but a baby born with the affected genes usually has symptoms within the first year of life, although signs of the disease may not show up until adolescence or young adulthood. Infants or young children should be tested for CF if they have persistent diarrhea, bulky foul-smelling and greasy stools, frequent wheezing or pneumonia, a chronic cough with thick mucus, salty-tasting skin, or poor growth. Babies born with an intestinal blockage (meconium ileus) also may have CF and should be tested.

Symptoms

CF affects different children in different ways and to varying degrees, although the underlying problem is the same—abnormal glands responsible for controlling sweat and mucus. Sweat is responsible for cooling the body, while mucus lubricates the respiratory, digestive, and reproductive systems, and prevents tissues from drying out, protecting them from infection.

Children with CF lose a great deal of salt when they sweat, which can disrupt the balance of minerals in the blood, triggering abnormal heart rhythms. In addition, CF patients have very thick mucus that builds up in the intestines and lungs, leading to malnutrition, poor growth, frequent respiratory infections, breathing problems, and permanent lung damage.

Death in most patients results from lung disease and infections, although CF can cause various other medical problems. These include sinusitis, nasal polyps, rounding and enlargement of fingers and toes, pneumothorax (rupture of lung tissue and trapping of air between the lung and the chest wall), coughing of blood, enlargement of the right side of the heart, abdominal pain and discomfort, gassiness, and protrusion of the rectum through the anus. Liver disease, diabetes, inflammation of the pancreas, and gallstones also are common in some people with CF.

Diagnosis

The sweat test, which measures the saltiness of sweat, is the most common test for CF, since excess levels of sodium and chloride suggest that the child has CF. However, this test may not work well in newborns because they do not produce enough sweat. In that case, an immunoreactive trypsinogen blood test (IRT) may be performed to search for a specific protein called trypsinogen. Also, a small percentage of people with CF have normal sweat chloride levels. They can only be diagnosed by chemical tests for the presence of the mutated gene.

Other tests that can help diagnose CF are chest X rays, lung function tests, sputum cultures, and stool examinations.

Cause

Genes are the basic units of heredity, which are found on structures called chromosomes within the heart of the cell. Most genes instruct cells to make particular proteins. Each child has 46 chromosomes, 23 inherited from each parent, and each of the 23 pairs of chromosomes contains a complete set of genes. Every child has two sets of genes, one from each parent. If a part of a gene is flawed, it can cause a biological malfunction that can cause disease.

In order for a child to have CF, each normal parent must carry one abnormal CF gene and one normal CF gene. The parent with an abnormal CF gene does not have the disease, because the normal CF gene is strong enough ("dominant") to suppress the action of the abnormal CF gene. But if both parents have one abnormal CF gene each, their child has a 25 percent chance of inheriting two copies of the abnormal CF genes—one from each parent. A child born to two parents who both have the disease (very unlikely) would have a 100 percent risk of developing CF.

The CF gene was identified in 1989. The biochemical abnormality in CF is caused by a mutation in a gene that produces a protein responsible for the movement of chloride ions through cell membranes. The protein is called CFTR—cystic fibrosis transmembrane regulator. However, this protein accounts for only 70 to 80 percent of all CF cases. This means that other mutations (there are at least 400) seem to be responsible for the remaining CF cases.

Differences in disease patterns are probably caused by the combined effects of a particular mutation and other unknown factors in the CF patient and the environment.

Prevention

Since CF is a genetic disease, the only way to prevent or cure it would be with gene therapy at an early age, which could repair or replace the defective gene. Another option for treatment would be to give a person with CF the active form of the protein product that is scarce or missing. At present, neither gene therapy nor any other kind of treatment exists for the underlying causes of CF, although several drug-based approaches are being studied.

Treatment

There is no cure for CF. Doctors can ease the symptoms of CF or slow the progress of the disease for better quality of life by antibiotic therapy combined with treatments to clear the thick mucus from the lungs. The therapy is tailored to the needs of each patient. Patients with advanced disease might consider a lung transplant.

Although CF was once always fatal in childhood, better treatment methods in the past 20 years have increased the average lifespan of CF patients.

Lung problems   The major focus of treatment aims to ease the obstructed breathing that triggers frequent lung infections, through physical therapy, exercise, and medications. Postural drainage allows drainage of the mucus from the lungs as the chest or back is clapped and vibrated to dislodge the mucus and help it move out of the airways. This process is repeated over different parts of the chest and back to loosen the mucus in different areas of each lung. Family members must perform this treatment for children, but as they grow older children can learn to do it by themselves. Mechanical aids that help chest physical therapy also are available.

Exercise also helps to loosen the mucus, stimulate coughing to clear the mucus, and improve overall physical condition.

Inhaled medications can help breathing; these include bronchodilators to widen the breathing tubes, mucolytics to thin the mucus, and decongestants to reduce swelling. Recently, an inhaled aerosolized enzyme that thins the mucus by digesting the cellular material trapped in it has been approved by the U.S. Food and Drug Administration. Antibiotics to fight lung infections may be taken orally, in aerosols, or by injection.

Digestive problems   The digestive problems in CF are less serious and more easily managed, with a well-balanced, high-calorie diet that is low in fat and high in protein. Pancreatic enzymes to help digestion also are often prescribed, and vitamin supplements of A, D, E, and K ensure good nutrition. Enemas and mucolytic agents can treat intestinal obstructions.

Gene therapy for CF is not yet possible, but scientists are trying to develop ways of treating the CF gene abnormality.

Prenatal Diagnosis

It is possible to find out if a baby has CF, but tests cannot detect all of the CF gene mutations. Because these tests are very expensive and carry certain risks to the mother, they are not used for all pregnant women. If a family already has one child with CF in the family, the expectant mother may request an amniocentesis or chorionic villus biopsy to see if the fetus has CF genes from both parents, is a carrier for one gene, or has no affected CF genes.

However, scientists cannot prevent CF. Babies with two abnormal CF genes already have the disease at birth in some organs, such as the pancreas and liver; problems in the lungs, however, develops only after birth. Someday, gene therapy may be used to prevent the lung disease from developing, or CF itself might be prevented in the future.

cystitis   See URINARY TRACT INFECTION.

cytomegalovirus (CMV)   One of the HERPES family of viruses, this strain is the largest, most complex virus that infects humans. First discovered in 1956, this extremely common infection has affected almost all adults in childhood, yet rarely produces symptoms. By adulthood, almost 85 percent of Americans may be infected.

However, those with impaired immunity may have more serious symptoms. It may also cause significant problems during pregnancy if a woman has a first infection, which would be transmitted to her unborn child. This can cause minor impairments affecting hearing, vision, or mental capacity. A few of these babies are born with severe brain damage, including mental retardation or severe hearing loss.

Once a person has been infected, the cyto-megalovirus (CMV) remains latent in the body like other herpes viruses and can be reactivated later on during periods of stress or weakened immunity.

Cause

CMV is present in almost all body fluids, including urine, saliva, semen, breast milk, and blood. Although it can be sexually transmitted, most children do not get it this way. It is commonly found in day care centers, where it is passed around in children's saliva or urine-soaked diapers and transmitted from unwashed hands or shared toys.

CMV transmission happens often in day care institutions. While young children rarely have symptoms, they excrete the virus in their urine and saliva for months to years. It is also possible to acquire CMV from transfused blood or transplanted organs, since so many individuals have the infection without having symptoms.

A child having an organ transplant or chemotherapy for cancer takes drugs that suppress the immune system; if a patient had been infected with CMV earlier in life, the dormant virus can reactivate, resulting in life-threatening illness. If a patient taking these drugs has a first exposure to the virus, the new infection can cause a serious illness. In AIDS patients, reactivation of a CMV infection can lead to PNEUMONIA, HEPATITIS, ENCEPHALITIS, colitis, or serious eye infections called retinitis.

Symptoms

Young children may experience a mild cold or flu-like illness with fever. Almost all babies infected before birth are normal; about 10 percent are sick. Of these 10 percent, 20 to 30 percent have serious symptoms and may die. Symptoms include problems with major organs including the liver, brain, eyes, and lungs; other symptoms include convulsions, lethargy, tiny pinpoint rash, and breathing problems. If the infant survives, there may be permanent damage (MENTAL RETARDATION, water on the brain, small brain, hearing loss, eye inflammation, poor coordination, and liver disease).

Some studies suggest a few apparently normal babies who were infected at birth may encounter health problems later in life. Babies infected before birth excrete the virus intermittently for years and are infectious when shedding virus.

While CMV does not usually use a problem for healthy people, it can sometimes lead to an acute form of MONONUCLEOSIS, including a fever of two to three weeks, hepatitis, and sometimes a rash. Healthy people with CMV mononucleosis have an excellent prognosis.

Diagnosis

Test results for CMV can be misleading. Blood can be tested for the CMV antibody, but all the presence of antibody indicates is that there was an earlier infection. The test will not reveal whether the virus is presently active in blood, urine, or saliva. If a patient has symptoms that imply a recently acquired infection, sequential tests may reveal changes in antibody levels that indicate an active infection. However, since these changes can be hard to distinguish from normal fluctuations, researchers are trying to develop tests that are more specific.

The test for virus in these fluids is available in most large hospital and commercial labs, but results may take between two and six weeks.

Newborns with possible congenital CMV infection must have virus cultured from their urine, nose, eyes, or spinal fluid to confirm CMV, which can be helpful in diagnosing potential problems such as hearing loss. Researchers are now refining tests that would measure CMV in saliva.

In patients with impaired immunity, tests can be helpful to measure the effectiveness of therapy.

Treatment

There is no cure for congenital CMV; babies with the disease need to be hospitalized. In AIDS patients, treatment includes two intravenous antiviral drugs, ganciclovir and foscarnet. These drugs are not recommended for those with healthy immune systems because the side effects from the drugs are more severe than the risks of the illness.

Prevention

Good hygiene can reduce the risk of transmission at day care centers, but intensive infection control is not practical when dealing with a virus as common as CMV. Scientists are presently researching a preventive vaccine.

Children who need organ transplants are tested for antibodies to CMV; those who do not have the antibodies will be matched to donors without antibodies as well. Because a match is not always possible, the recipient faces a risk of serious CMV infection from the transplanted organ later. To prevent this complication, a patient will receive an injection of CMV antibody.

CMV-negative organ recipients who need blood transfusions will be given special CMV-negative blood, which is rare and saved for special cases. Otherwise, the blood can be filtered to remove the CMV antibodies.

dacryocystitis   Inflammation of the lacrimal sac at the corner of the eye, caused by obstruction of the duct that causes tearing and discharge from the eye.

Symptoms
In the acute phase, the sac becomes inflamed and painful. The disorder almost always occurs only on one side and is usually seen in infants.

Treatment
Systemic treatment of antibiotics will usually cure the problem.

deafness and hearing disorders   Federal government projections have estimated that there are about 50,000 deaf and 325,000 hard-of-hearing children in the school-age population. Estimates suggest that one person in every 1,000 is born deaf, or is deafened before age three, and that one in 500 is hard of hearing or develops hearing problems by age 19. These figures vary, because it is especially hard to estimate the incidence of deafness among children since the condition so often goes unrecognized or misdiagnosed in the very young.

More than 90 percent of deaf children and 20 percent of hard-of-hearing children receive special education services, and in general, deaf children receive more intensive and comprehensive services than do children with a milder hearing loss.

The lack of early detection of hearing problems in children is a major public health problem. The average age at which moderate to severe hearing problems are detected in children is two to three years of age, but these problems can and should be identified and treated much sooner. If undetected and untreated, hearing loss in children leads to delayed speech and language development and can contribute to emotional, social, and academic problems later. Ideally, doctors should identify infants with hearing loss before three months of age, so that intervention can begin by six months.

Parents are usually the first to suspect a hearing loss. Any child should have a hearing test who experiences any of the following conditions:

- a history of frequent EAR INFECTIONS
- children at risk for hearing problems, such as those with abnormalities of the skull or face; prematurity; intrauterine infection; MENINGITIS; genetic conditions relating to deafness; family history of hearing loss
- a child who does not follow directions
- speech or language delay (such as no babbling in a six-month-old, no words by 18 months, or no word combinations by age two)
- behavioral problems
- any child whose parent is concerned about hearing

If a parent or doctor suspects a hearing problem, the child's primary care provider may choose to conduct a hearing screening for a preschooler, but infants and young toddlers will need a referral for special tests. A pediatrician should conduct ongoing exams when a child has middle ear fluid, until it has cleared. If the fluid is present for several months without clearing, consultation with an otolaryngologist should be considered.

If a parent has any doubt about slower-than-normal sound and speech/language development, these concerns should be discussed with the child's doctor and hearing tests should be seriously considered.

There are several ways to test hearing in children, including behavioral testing, brainstem evoked response testing, otoacoustic emissions, and central auditory processing testing.

Behavioral Testing

A behavioral test is a better measure of hearing and usually should be used first in most children, even older infants. In sound field audiometry, the child is placed in a soundproof booth and exposed to sound (even an infant of one or two months will startle after a loud noise). An infant who does not show a startle reaction may have a hearing problem. However, relying on startling alone may not identify infants with smaller but still significant losses.

In a type of test called visual response audiometry, older infants will turn their head toward noise that gets their attention. Eventually they can learn that a stuffed animal will light up when there is noise, and they will look for the animal when they hear the noise. If they do not look, they did not hear it.

Conditioned play audiometry is a type of test that teaches toddlers up to age three or four to put a toy in a box when they hear the noise. Failure to put a toy in the box is an indication that they did not hear the noise.

In an *air conduction audiometry* test, children with a developmental age of four or above wear earphones and raise their hands when they hear a sound.

Older children can respond to a bone vibration, which helps to determine whether a hearing problem is in the middle ear or inner ear, in cases where both ears do not hear equally well. This is called *bone conduction audiometry.*

Brainstem Evoked Response Testing (BER, ABR, BSER)

This testing method is not a direct measure of hearing but a measure of nerve activity. It is used with children who cannot respond in the soundproof booth because in this type of test, no responses are required from the child. As the child sleeps (with or without sedation), earphones and electrodes record activity from the hearing nerve. The test, which measures high-pitched sounds better than low-pitched sounds, is often used by hospitals to test newborns.

Otoacoustic Emissions

This is a very new method of rapid testing that can be used for screening in the newborn nursery and also with a child who cannot respond to behavioral testing. It is based on the fact that the ear not only hears noise but also makes noises. By measuring the very faint noises made by the ear, the test estimates how well the ear hears. An ear that does not hear will not make the expected noises. These noises are much too faint to be heard by human ears, but there are machines that can measure the sounds.

Central Auditory Processing Testing

A child must be able to speak in full sentences and have reasonably advanced language to take the central auditory processing test, so they must be at least age five. The test assesses the ability to process the sounds children hear. Some children hear very well but have trouble deciding what to do with the sound once they hear it. These children are typically intelligent but have trouble following directions in school, especially in noisy environments. They may have had many ear infections when they were younger and developed difficulty dealing with sound as a method of communication.

DEET (N1N-diethyl-m-toluamide) The most effective of all bug repellants, this product may be safely used on children—but not on infants. DEET should be kept out of the eyes. New preparations combine sunscreen with DEET in one cream.

Every year about a third of the U.S. population is expected to use DEET in a variety of liquids, lotions, sprays, and impregnated materials (such as wrist bands). DEET is available in formulations registered for direct application to human skin containing from 4 percent to 100 percent DEET. Except for a few veterinary uses, DEET is registered for use by consumers and should not be used on food. Consumers who use a repellent with DEET on children should use it only when outdoors and wash the child's skin after coming indoors. Children should be sure not to breathe in or swallow DEET or get it into the eyes. It should never be applied to wounds or broken skin.

DEET is designed for direct application to human skin to repel insects rather than kill them.

After it was developed by the United States Army in 1946, DEET was registered for use by the general public in 1957. More than 230 products containing DEET are currently registered with the Environmental Protection Agency (EPA).

The EPA recently issued a Reregistration Eligibility Decision (RED) for the chemical DEET, concluding that as long as consumers follow label directions and take proper precautions, insect repellents containing the substance do not present a health concern. Based on extensive toxicity testing, the EPA believes that the normal use of DEET does not present a health concern to the general population.

However, the EPA is no longer allowing child safety claims on product labels that had appeared on certain products with a DEET concentration of 15 percent or less. The scientific data on DEET do not support product label claims of child safety based on the percentage of active ingredient.

dehydration   A serious lack of fluids in the body that occurs when a child is not drinking enough to replace fluids lost through sweating. It is a serious medical condition that in extreme cases can be fatal.

Under normal conditions, children lose some body water every day in sweat, tears, urine, and stools. This fluid is usually replaced throughout the day from the water and salt content of what children eat and drink. Sometimes, however, children lose too much water and salts as a result of fever, diarrhea, vomiting, or heavy exercise. For example, a child can lose up to a quart of sweat during a two-hour sports game.

In the most severe cases, they may not be able to replace this water simply by drinking normally. This is especially true if an illness prevents a child from taking fluids by mouth, or if fluid loss is so extreme (as with severe diarrhea) that the child cannot replace it by simply drinking more often.

Symptoms

If a child is exercising heavily, or is suffering from fever, diarrhea, or vomiting, a parent or coach should watch for the following signs of dehydration:

- headaches
- fatigue

- thirst
- irritability
- dizziness and weakness
- muscle cramps
- nausea and vomiting
- decreased performance
- heat sensations
- general discomfort
- sunken soft spot (fontanel) on top of head (in infant)
- excessive sleepiness or disorientation
- muscle cramps
- deep, rapid breathing
- no urination for several hours (more than six to eight hours in infants; more than eight to 10 hours in children)
- fast or weakened pulse
- very dry mouth
- dry, wrinkled, or doughy skin (especially on abdomen, upper arms, and legs)
- inactivity or decreased alertness

Treatment

Treatment of dehydration should take place immediately. Depending on the severity of the situation, medical attention should be sought from a certified athletic trainer or emergency medical services via 911.

Prevention

Children who drink fluids regularly can prevent dehydration and a trip to the emergency room, but they need to drink at regular intervals and not wait until they are thirsty to start drinking. If they are thirsty, they are already dehydrated. They should always drink before, during, and after activity:

- Children should drink 12 ounces of fluid about 30 minutes before activity begins.
- During an activity, children weighing less than 90 pounds should drink five ounces every 20 minutes; children over 90 pounds should drink nine ounces every 20 minutes.

- After the activity is over, children should drink every 20 minutes during the first hour to make up for fluid loss.

What to drink Some drinks are better than others when it comes to replacing fluids. Although water is easily accessible, active children do not always drink enough water to stay fully hydrated. Studies show that when drinking water, children will only drink about half of the amount they need; a lightly flavored sports drink encourages them to drink 90 percent more than water, so they stay better hydrated. Research shows that a scientifically formulated sports drink helps children stay better hydrated because it will replace electrolytes that active children lose through sweat. In addition, flavored Pedialyte is also effective. (See also HEAT ILLNESSES.)

dental care Good tooth care begins at birth, when parents should begin wiping a child's gums with a wet cloth or gauze after feeding. It is important to take care of baby teeth, because they help a child chew and speak properly and guide the proper eruption of the permanent teeth.

Dentists recommend that parents establish a tooth-care routine from the beginning, brushing after breakfast, lunch, and before bedtime. By age one, when the front teeth erupt, they should be wiped with gauze after meals. By the time a child reaches 12 to 18 months, parents should begin brushing their child's teeth with a soft brush and water. By age two and three, a pea-sized bit of fluoridated toothpaste may be added to the brush. Any basic fluoride paste with the seal of the American Dental Association is a good choice. (Children should spit out and not swallow excess toothpaste after brushing.) Sometime between ages four through six, a child can begin to brush with parental supervision.

Parents might want to avoid whitening or bleaching toothpastes, since some children find these products cause some discomfort. If a child objects to the taste of toothpaste, a plain wet brush alone is just as effective in cleaning the teeth as toothpaste. Some children enjoy inexpensive electric children's toothbrushes, which do a very good job and can help kids want to brush.

Children can either visit the family's regular dentist, or choose a pediatric dentist. Pediatric dentists, who limit their practice to treating only children, receive two to three years of special training in pediatric dentistry after dental school. In just the way that pediatricians specialize in children's health, pediatric dentists specialize in caring for children's teeth. A pediatric dentist can provide both primary and specialty dental care for infants and children through adolescence. Pediatric dentists may be a particularly good choice for children with emotional, physical, or mental problems because these dentists are trained and qualified to treat special young patients.

Flossing

Many pediatric dentists also recommend flossing as soon as the first teeth touch—as early as age one or two. The parent should stand behind the child to floss teeth. Children old enough to floss independently might enjoy using colorful plastic floss holders in child-friendly shapes.

Fluoride

Fluoride prevents tooth decay, according to the American Academy for Pediatric Dentistry (AAPD). Most children drink fluoridated water from municipal supplies, but if water isn't fluoridated, the child needs a supplement. Fluoridated toothpaste alone does not provide enough fluoride.

Most dentists agree that mouthwash or a fluoride rinse is not really necessary for children, especially because of the risk that they may swallow the product. This is a concern especially if the mouthwash contains alcohol.

Cavities in Baby Teeth

Most dentists agree that cavities in baby teeth should be filled. Primary teeth can be infected and destroyed, and bacteria in one little cavity can grow and spread to other teeth, seeding the mouth with bacteria that may spread to permanent teeth as they erupt.

Sealants

Sealants protect the grooved and pitted surfaces of the teeth, especially the chewing surfaces of six- and 12-year molars, where most cavities in children are found. Made of clear or shaded plastic, sealants are applied to the teeth to help keep them cavity-free. A child with particularly deep grooves in the teeth may be ready for a sealant as young as age two and one-half to three years. Sealants are a good way to protect primary molars that are prone to decay.

Problem Foods

Many dentists say that plain chocolate is fine as a special treat, since the child's saliva washes away much of the chocolate afterward. It is much less likely to cause decay than a cookie or a cracker that gets chewed into the teeth, where it can remain for a long time.

depression   A mood disorder characterized by sadness, hopelessness, low self-esteem, fatigue, or agitation. As many as one in every 33 children (and one in five adolescents) may have clinical depression. Recent studies have shown that more than 20 percent of adolescents in the general population have emotional problems, and a third of teens attending mental health clinics suffer from depression.

A child who has experienced an episode of depression is at an increased risk for developing another episode of depression within the next five years. In addition, children who experience a depressive episode are five times more likely to become depressed as an adult. Indeed, depression in childhood may predict a more severe depressive illness in adulthood.

Clinical depression can have a devastating impact on children's school performance, friendships, and family relationships. Because children who are depressed are likely to experience depression in adulthood, treatment of this childhood disorder is critical.

Symptoms

Children who suffer from clinical depression lose interest in activities and have low energy, poor concentration, and sleeping problems. Some even fairly young children may feel so hopeless that they want to kill themselves. Major depression is almost always characterized by feelings of general sadness and total loss of pleasure for at least two weeks. There are a wide range of typical symptoms

related to a clinical depression, including at least three of the following:

- deep sadness or crying jags
- gain or loss of weight
- chronic insomnia or excessive sleepiness
- outbursts of shouting and anger
- loss of interest in hobbies and interests
- feelings of worthlessness, unattractiveness, guilt
- problems with concentration
- muddy, foggy thoughts
- anxiety, phobias, delusions, or fears
- restlessness
- slowed body movements
- suicidal thoughts

Depression in Adolescence

Teenage depression is increasing at an alarming rate and calls for prompt, appropriate treatment. Depression can take several forms, including BI-POLAR DISORDER (formally called manic depression), which is a condition that alternates between periods of euphoria (mania) and depression.

Depression can be difficult to diagnose in teens because adults may expect teens to act moody. Also, adolescents do not always understand or express their feelings very well. They may not be aware of the symptoms of depression and may not seek help; therefore, they may need encouragement from their friends and support from concerned adults to seek help and follow treatment recommendations.

Sometimes teens feel so depressed that they consider suicide. Each year, almost 5,000 young Americans aged 15 to 24 kill themselves—a rate of suicide in this age group that has nearly tripled since 1960, making it the third leading cause of death in adolescents and the second leading cause of death among college-age youth. Studies show that suicide attempts among young people may be based on long-standing problems triggered by a specific event; suicidal teens may look at a temporary situation as a permanent condition. Feelings of anger and resentment combined with exaggerated guilt can lead to impulsive, self-destructive acts.

Four out of five teens who attempt suicide have given clear warnings. Warning signs that should always be taken seriously include:

- suicide threats (direct and indirect)
- obsession with death
- poems, essays, and drawings that refer to death
- dramatic change in personality or appearance
- irrational, bizarre behavior
- overwhelming sense of guilt, shame, or rejection
- different eating or sleeping patterns
- severe drop in school performance
- giving away belongings

Cause

Experts believe there are many causes of depression. It is likely that a combination of biological, environmental, and psychological factors contribute to the onset of the disorder. Moreover, children who develop depression are likely to have a family history of the disorder. At even greater risk are those children who have a chronic illness or who experience abuse, neglect, or other trauma.

Depression in children often occurs together with other mental disorders such as anxiety disorders or disruptive behavior disorders. Adolescents who are depressed are also at risk for substance abuse.

Treatment

It is extremely important that depressed children and teens receive prompt, professional treatment. Depression is serious and, if left untreated, can worsen to the point of becoming life-threatening. If depressed children and teens refuse treatment, it may be necessary for family members or other concerned adults to seek professional advice.

Clinical depression is a serious disorder that responds well to a combination of medication and therapy. Some of the most common and effective ways to treat depression in children and adolescents are:

Psychotherapy   This provides children and teens an opportunity to explore events and feelings that are painful or troubling to them. Psychotherapy also teaches coping skills.

Cognitive-behavioral therapy   This type of counseling helps children and teens change negative patterns of thinking and behaving.

Interpersonal therapy   This type of treatment helps children and teens focus on how to develop healthier relationships at home and at school.

Medication   Antidepressants can be very effective in easing symptoms of depression and is often prescribed along with therapy. Currently only Prozac is officially approved for use in children and adolescents, but doctors can still legally prescribe other antidepressants to children on an "off-label" basis. Even very young children are taking many of the newest antidepressants.

So far, studies of citalopram (Celexa), Prozac, and Zoloft suggest that these newer antidepressants may help to relieve the suffering of children with depression. While only Prozac has been specifically approved for use in children, doctors can still prescribe antidepressants for children. It may be necessary to try several antidepressants before finding one that is effective.

dermatitis   The general term used to refer to a group of inflammatory conditions of the skin. While people often use the terms ECZEMA and dermatitis interchangeably, eczema is actually dermatitis in its advanced stages, with blisters, fissures, oozing, crusting, scabbing, thickening, peeling, and discoloration. While there are a wide variety of dermatitis conditions, there are three main categories: atopic dermatitis, contact dermatitis, and seborrheic dermatitis. (See also DERMATITIS, ATOPIC; DERMATITIS, CONTACT; DERMATITIS, SEBORRHEIC.)

dermatitis, atopic   Also known as atopic ECZEMA, this is a common condition in infants, often appearing between two and 18 months of age. It tends to occur in those with an inherited tendency to develop allergy and is found in 10 percent of the population. The condition is usually associated with ASTHMA, HAY FEVER, or ALLERGIC RHINITIS, and it may affect as many as seven to 24 of every 1,000 people. It is most common in children.

Typically, the condition begins in the first year of life, fading away about 40 percent of the time by age 15. However, children with very severe disease are more likely to have persistent problems as they get older. Although there is no cure, the long-term prognosis is good.

Symptoms

In acute cases, this form of eczema is characterized by a mild, very itchy rash on the face, inner elbow creases, and behind the knees, with red, scaling skin and pimples. If scratched, the pimples leak a clear liquid, forming large weeping areas; infection may occur if the condition appears in the diaper area.

Atopic dermatitis tends to wax and wane. In chronic cases there are scaling and skin color changes. Most children improve during the summer and worsen during the winter, which is probably related to humidity and temperature.

Treatment

Keeping adequate hydration of the skin and avoiding irritants may be all that is required of children with mild cases. Irritants include wool clothing, strong detergents, and water. Irritants can be avoided by using a mild detergent (such as Ivory Snow flakes or Dreft), by avoiding wool, and by adding bath oil to bath water. Emollients such as white petrolatum should be applied immediately after bathing, and topical corticosteroids and tar preparations are useful. Oatmeal (Aveeno) baths are helpful, as is daily moisturizing with emollients such as Eucerin cream.

In acute cases, a medium-potency topical corticosteroid lotion or cream should be applied after bathing or after applying aluminum acetate or saline compresses. For chronic cases, potent topical corticosteroids should be applied right after bathing; soaking or using compresses of water-soluble tar preparations may decrease the need for topical steroids. However, the risks of these drugs limit their use in long-term treatment.

Adequate doses of antihistamines can control itching and prevent scratching, which could lead to secondary infection; oral antibiotics are helpful if infection develops, which is a frequent complication in itchy children.

dermatitis, contact   An inflammation of the skin caused by an allergic reaction to direct contact with a substance to which a child is sensitive. Usually an itchy or scaly rash erupts at the point of contact, which can be anywhere on the body.

While the immune system normally protects against bacteria and viruses, an allergic response causes the immune system to overreact to usually harmless substances such as dyes or metals.

Causes

Substances that are often implicated in contact dermatitis in children include metals (especially nickel), dyes and chemicals, cleaning products or detergents, latex, POISON IVY, and insecticides. Latex is one of the most common irritating substances in children and may be found along the waist and legbands of underwear.

Contact dermatitis may also be caused by topical medications; about a third of all dermatology patients will test positive for a contact allergy to some type of ingredient in a topical drug or cosmetic. The most common are lanolin, local anesthetics, and preservatives such as parabens.

Symptoms

Contact dermatitis usually starts as an itchy red rash, evolving into blisters with cracking and peeling skin. The severity of this type of dermatitis depends on the particular substance, and how sensitive a person is. Symptoms should subside within a few days or weeks if the offending substance is avoided.

Diagnosis

Allergy patch tests may help determine the substances that are provoking the reaction. In the test, a doctor exposes small areas of skin to a variety of known allergens, observing the skin for a reaction.

Treatment

Mild cases do not require treatment, but frequent or severe outbreaks should be referred to a physician. Topical medications such as calamine lotion, ANTIHISTAMINES, or over-the-counter cortisone creams usually ease symptoms. Hydrocortisone cream (in the 0.5 percent strength) is available without a prescription; stronger creams, which are necessary for cases of significant outbreaks, can have serious side effects.

Regular bathing is a good way to reduce inflammation and soothe irritated skin. Water should not be too hot or cold. Two cups of colloidal oatmeal or AVEENO BATH or baking soda can be added to the water.

In severe cases of weeping sores, cold milk compresses or baking soda baths may help soothe the itch.

dermatitis, seborrheic An extremely common form of ECZEMA that causes scaling around the nose, ears, scalp, mid-chest, and along the eyebrows. There may be PSORIASIS-like plaques and secondary infection as a result of scratching. It is often misdiagnosed by non-physicians as simply dry skin. However, the flaking caused by this type of dermatitis is not caused by dryness.

Cause

This condition is believed to have a genetic link, although how the condition is inherited is not clear. It is most common in boys after puberty, and its incidence increases with age. Untreated dandruff also may lead to seborrheic dermatitis.

Treatment

Treatment is similar to other types of eczema, with shampoos containing tar, sulfur, SALICYLIC ACID, or selenium daily. Hydrocortisone 1 percent cream will control the skin condition on the face and chest. If shampoos do not work, a steroid solution such as fluocinolone may be applied to the scalp one or two times daily for very short periods.

developmental disability Technically, this term refers to any significant disability acquired before the age of 22. In actuality, however, "developmental disability" is used instead of the term MENTAL RETARDATION to describe the condition of individuals with severely impaired intellectual functioning from birth. The term brings the description of this particular spectrum of disability more into line with the general language used to define various types of difficulties, and its focus on development rather than retardation provides a more accurate way of describing the actual nature of these difficulties.

However, the term also has a legal definition as it appears in the Developmental Disabilities Assistance and Bill of Rights Act of 1990, Public Law 101-496, Section 102. In this law, the term "developmental disabilities" means severe, chronic disabilities of a person five years of age or older which

- is caused by a mental or physical impairment
- occurs before age 22
- is likely to continue indefinitely
- results in substantial functional limitations in at least three of the following areas: self-care, language, learning, mobility, self-direction, ability to live independently, and economic self-sufficiency
- reflects the person's need for special long-term services

Developmental Speech and Language Disorders

Children with developmental speech and language disorders have trouble producing speech sounds, using spoken language to communicate, or understanding what other people say. Speech and language problems are often the earliest indicators of a LEARNING DISABILITY. These speech and language disorders include developmental articulation disorder, developmental expressive language disorder, and developmental receptive language disorder.

With a *developmental articulation disorder*, children may have trouble controlling their rate of speech, or they may lag behind their friends in learning to make speech sounds. These disorders are common, appearing in at least 10 percent of children younger than age eight. Fortunately, articulation disorders can often be outgrown or successfully treated with speech therapy.

Some children with *developmental expressive language disorder* have problems expressing themselves in speech, such as calling objects by the wrong names, speaking only in two-word phrases, or not being able to answer simple questions.

Some people have trouble understanding certain aspects of speech; this is *developmental receptive language disorder*. This explains the toddler who does not respond to his name or a first grader who consistently cannot follow simple directions. While hearing is normal, these individuals cannot make sense of certain sounds, words, or sentences. They may seem as if they are not paying attention, but in fact they simply cannot understand certain types of speech. Because using and understanding speech are strongly related, many people with receptive language disorders also have an EXPRESSIVE LANGUAGE DISORDER.

Of course, some misuse of sounds, words, or grammar is a normal part of learning to speak. It is only when these problems persist that there is any cause for concern.

Dexedrine See DEXTROAMPHETAMINE.

dextroamphetamine (Dexedrine) A STIMULANT MEDICATION used to treat ATTENTION DEFICIT HYPERACTIVITY DISORDER (ADHD) in children and adults as a part of a treatment program that includes behavioral and psychosocial interventions.

It takes about three to four weeks to feel the full effects, and the drug works better for some people than others, depending on dosage and individual differences. The short-acting form of this medication reaches maximum effect in about two hours; the extended release form reaches peak effectiveness in about 10 hours.

Side Effects

Typical side effects may include nervousness, insomnia, and loss of appetite. Prolonged or excessive use can lead to dependence. Physicians may recommend periods of time when the medication is stopped temporarily so behavior can be evaluated.

Drug Interactions

Dexedrine and monoamine oxidase (MAO) inhibitors together can cause serious or fatal interactions; at least 14 days must pass after taking one of these before taking the other. Acidifying agents such as guanethidine, reserpine, and fruit juices can lower the absorption of Dexedrine, and drugs such as Diamox (acetazolamide) increase absorption of amphetamines. The effects of tricyclic antidepressants and norepinephrine may become more concentrated when taken with Dexedrine. Thorazine (chlorpromazine), lithium, and Haldol (haloperidol) can blunt the effects of Dexedrine (dextroamphetamine).

diabetes, juvenile A disorder of metabolism (also known as type I diabetes) that affects the way a child's body uses digested food for growth and energy. Type 1 diabetes accounts for about 5 to 10 percent of diagnosed diabetes in the United States.

Most food is broken down into glucose, the main source of fuel for the body. After digestion, glucose passes into the blood, where cells use it for growth and energy. Insulin must be present for the cells to be able to absorb glucose. Insulin is a hormone produced by the pancreas, a gland that is supposed to automatically produce the right amount of insulin to move glucose from blood into our cells. In children with diabetes, the pancreas either produces little or no insulin, or the cells do not respond correctly to the insulin that is produced.

As a result, glucose builds up in the blood, spills into the urine, and is excreted, robbing the body of its main source of fuel—even though the blood contains large amounts of glucose.

Type 1 diabetes is an autoimmune disease—a disease that occurs when a child's immune system attacks the child's own body. In diabetes, the immune system attacks and destroys the insulin-producing beta cells in the pancreas, which stops the pancreas from producing insulin. A child with type 1 diabetes needs to take insulin daily to live.

Cause

Scientists do not know exactly why the body's immune system attacks the beta cells, but they think that autoimmune, genetic, and environmental factors (and, perhaps, viruses) are involved.

Type 1 diabetes develops most often in children and young adults, although it can appear at any age. Symptoms of type 1 diabetes usually develop over a short period, although beta cell destruction can begin years earlier.

Symptoms

A doctor may suspect juvenile diabetes if the child complains of increased thirst and urination, constant hunger, weight loss, blurred vision, and extreme fatigue. If not diagnosed and treated with insulin, a child can fall into a life-threatening diabetic coma (diabetic ketoacidosis).

Diagnosis

A fasting plasma glucose test performed in the morning is the preferred test for diagnosing type 1 diabetes. However, diabetes can be diagnosed by any one of three positive tests, with a second positive test on a different day. The other tests include:

- A random plasma glucose value (taken any time of day) of 200 mg/dL or more, along with the presence of diabetes symptoms.
- A plasma glucose value of 126 mg/dL or more, after a child has fasted for 8 hours.
- An oral glucose tolerance test (OGTT) plasma glucose value of 200 mg/dL or more in the blood sample, taken two hours after a child drinks a drink containing 75 grams of glucose dissolved in water. This test, taken in a lab or the doctor's office, measures plasma glucose at timed intervals over a three-hour period.

Diabetes is widely recognized as one of the leading causes of death and disability in the United States and is associated with long-term complications that affect almost every part of the body. It often can lead to blindness, heart and blood vessel disease, strokes, kidney failure, amputations, and nerve damage.

Type 1 diabetes occurs equally among boys and girls, but it is more common in whites than in nonwhites. Data from the World Health Organization's Multinational Project for Childhood Diabetes indicate that type 1 diabetes is rare in most African, American Indian, and Asian populations. However, some northern European countries, such as Finland and Sweden, have high rates of type 1 diabetes. The reasons for these differences are not known.

Treatment

Children with type 1 diabetes are treated with a healthful diet, physical activity, and insulin via injection or an insulin pump. The amount of insulin must be balanced with food intake and daily activities. Blood glucose levels must be closely monitored through frequent blood glucose checking. Before the discovery of insulin in 1921, everyone with type 1 diabetes died within a few years after diagnosis. Although insulin is not a cure, it allows a person to live normally by replacing the vital insulin the diabetic no longer produces.

Children with diabetes must take responsibility for their day-to-day care, which primarily includes keeping blood sugar levels from getting too low or too high. When blood sugar levels drop too low (hypoglycemia), the child can become nervous, shaky, and confused, and even faint. A child also can get sick if blood sugar levels get too high (hyperglycemia).

Children with diabetes should see an endocrinologist, who can help them learn to manage their diabetes. In addition, children with diabetes often see ophthalmologists for eye examinations, podiatrists for routine foot care, and dietitians and diabetes educators to help teach the skills of day-to-day diabetes management. The goal of diabetes management is to keep blood glucose levels as close to the normal range as safely possible.

Keeping blood glucose levels as close to normal as safely possible reduces the risk of developing major complications of type 1 diabetes, according to one major government study. The 10-year study, completed in 1993, included 1,441 people with type 1 diabetes. The study compared the effect of intensive management and standard management on the development and progression of eye, kidney, and nerve complications of diabetes. Intensive treatment aims to keep hemoglobin A1C as close to normal (6 percent) as possible. Hemoglobin A1C reflects average blood sugar over a two- to three-month period. Researchers found that study participants who maintained lower levels of blood glucose through intensive management had significantly lower rates of these complications. More recently, a follow-up study showed that the ability of intensive control to lower the complications of diabetes has persisted eight years after the trial ended.

In recent years, advances in diabetes research have led to better ways to manage diabetes and treat its complications. Major advances include the development of quick-acting and long-acting types of insulin, better ways to monitor blood glucose, research advances in noninvasive blood glucose monitoring, development of external insulin pumps (replacing daily injections), laser treatment for diabetic eye disease, and successful transplantation of kidneys and pancreas in people whose own kidneys fail because of diabetes.

Scientists also have demonstrated that two types of high-blood-pressure drugs, ACE (angiotensin-converting enzyme) inhibitors and ARBs (angiotensin receptor blockers), are more effective in slowing a decline in kidney function than other high-blood-pressure drugs in people with diabetes. Promising results with islet transplantation for type 1 diabetes also was recently reported by the University of Alberta in Canada.

Prevention

Researchers continue to search for the cause of diabetes and ways to prevent or cure it. Since some genetic markers for type 1 diabetes have been identified, it is now possible to screen relatives of people with type 1 diabetes to see if they are at risk.

Researchers are working on a way to help people with type 1 diabetes live without daily injections of insulin. In an experimental procedure called islet transplantation, islets are taken from a donor pancreas and transferred into another person. Once implanted, the beta cells in these islets begin to make and release insulin. Scientists have made many advances in islet transplantation in recent years. According to reports, as of June 2003 about half of the patients who had a transplant have remained healthy and insulin-free for up to a year after receiving a transplant. The goal of islet transplantation is to infuse enough islets to control the blood glucose level without having to resort to insulin injections.

diaper rash   A common condition of infancy caused by skin irritation from substances in feces or urine. It is probably worsened by friction from rough diapers and prolonged wetting of the skin.

While babies vary in their susceptibility to diaper rash, skin inflammation in some infants can be severe. In general, breast-fed babies have a lower incidence of diaper rash than bottle-fed babies, and the resistance continues long after the baby has been weaned. In some infants, diaper rash is the first indication of sensitive skin heralding a long series of later skin problems, such as ECZEMA.

About half of all cases of diaper rash go away by themselves within a day. The other half may last up to 10 days or more.

Symptoms

The skin appears reddened at first and, as the rash becomes chronic, the skin becomes dry and scaly.

In chronic severe cases, the skin is covered with papules, blisters, and erosions that can be mistaken for bacterial infections or even burns. A long-term rash that will not clear up may be caused by a fungal infection or PSORIASIS.

Treatment

Some of the oldest advice is still the best for diaper rash: expose the rash to air—take off the diaper and lay the baby face down (with face turned to one side) on a towel over a waterproof sheet. Protective ointment will help prevent and clear the problem. In severe cases, a mild corticosteroid drug is necessary to control inflammation, often given in combination with an antifungal drug to kill any organisms that might cause THRUSH.

Prevention

Prevention of this skin condition is always better than trying to cure it once it appears. The aim in a preventive diaper rash program is to keep the baby's skin as dry as possible for as long as possible. Since a newborn breast-fed baby urinates about 20 times a day, and has a bowel movement after each feeding, this can be a major undertaking. Still, diapers should be changed as often as possible followed by a water repellant emollient with each change. If possible, the diaper should be left off at least an hour a day.

Critics still disagree on the relative merits of cloth vs. disposable diapers and diaper rash, with each contingent asserting that only one type of diaper prevents diaper rash. Recent research has indicated that diapers containing absorbent gelling material significantly reduce skin wetness, leaving skin closer to the normal pH than either conventional disposable diapers or cloth. Proponents of cloth diapers insist that the cloth allows for more air circulation to the skin and, because the cloth diapers do not hold as much water, this type of diaper tends to get changed more often than do disposables.

While it is important to keep the diaper area clean, drying sensitive baby bottoms with a towel can be irritating to some infants. Experts suggest drying irritated bottoms with a hair dryer set on low; afterward, zinc oxide ointment should be applied. Since a baby's urine is sterile and clean, the infant's bottom need not be cleaned after urination; only patted or air dried.

If cloth diapers are used, one ounce of vinegar should be added to one gallon of water during the final rinse water to help match the cloth's pH to the baby's skin. The cloth diapers should then be well rinsed. Diaper rash enzymes are most active in an environment with high pH, often found in cloth diapers after washing. Cloth diapers provided by diaper services are usually very close to a baby's pH level and are usually tested at regular intervals to ensure the products' pH level.

diarrhea Frequent passage of loose, watery stools that also may contain pus, mucus, blood, or fat. In addition to frequent trips to the bathroom, a child with diarrhea may complain of abdominal cramps and weakness, nausea, and vomiting. This is a common problem in childhood that usually lasts a day or two and goes away on its own without any special treatment. However, prolonged diarrhea can be a sign of other problems.

Infection with the ROTAVIRUS is the most common cause of acute childhood diarrhea. Rotavirus diarrhea usually resolves in three to nine days. Other cases of acute diarrhea are usually caused by eating contaminated food or drinking contaminated water, or from an infectious disease.

Diarrhea is not a disease in itself, but simply a symptom of an underlying condition. While it may seem to be more of a nuisance than a serious health problem, untreated severe diarrhea can lead to dehydration and electrolyte imbalance. This means the body lacks enough fluid to function properly. It is particularly serious in infants and young children, and in any child with an impaired immune system.

Diarrhea usually starts suddenly and lasts between a few hours and two to three days. It may be caused by a temporary problem, such as an infection, or a chronic problem, such as an intestinal disease. A few of the more common causes of diarrhea are:

- *Bacterial or viral infections* Diarrhea can be caused by several types of bacteria in contaminated food or water, including *Campylobacter, Salmonella, Shigella,* and *Escherichia coli.* Viruses

causing diarrhea include rotavirus, NORWALK VIRUS, HERPES SIMPLEX, CYTOMEGALOVIRUS, and viral HEPATITIS. Diarrhea beginning within six hours of eating usually indicates that the food has been contaminated by toxins such as *Staphylococcus,* clostridium, or *E. coli* bacteria. If it takes longer (between 12 to 24 hours after eating), the diarrhea is probably from contamination of food or water by bacteria such as *Campylobacter* or *Salmonella,* or by a virus such as rotavirus or Norwalk virus. Infective gastroenteritis may be caused by inhaling droplets filled with ADENOVIRUS or ECHOVIRUS. Less often, diarrhea may be related to SHIGELLOSIS or GIARDIASIS.

- *Food intolerance* Some children cannot digest some component of food, such as lactose, the sugar found in milk.

- *Food allergy* Some FOOD ALLERGIES (such as some fruits, poultry, nuts, and so on) cause nausea and vomiting, among other symptoms.

- *Parasites* Those that can cause diarrhea include *Giardia, Entamoeba histolytica,* and *Cryptosporidium.*

- *Drug reactions* Some children may react to certain medicines, such as antibiotics or antacids containing magnesium.

- *Intestinal diseases* Some conditions, including inflammatory bowel disease or celiac disease, may cause diarrhea.

- *Functional bowel disorders* Irritable bowel syndrome, characterized by intestines that do not work normally, can cause diarrhea.

When to Visit the Doctor

Parents should take a child to the doctor if any of the following symptoms appear:

- black stools
- stools containing blood or pus
- temperature above 101.4°F.
- no improvement in diarrhea after 24 hours
- signs of dehydration (thirst; less frequent urination; dry skin; fatigue; light-headedness; dark colored urine; dry mouth and tongue; no tears when crying or no wet diapers for at least three

hours; sunken abdomen, eyes, or cheeks; irritability; skin that does not flatten when pinched and released)

Treatment

Medications to treat diarrhea in adults can be dangerous to children and should be given only under a doctor's guidance. Diarrhea can be dangerous in newborns and infants. In small children, severe diarrhea lasting just a day or two can lead to dehydration. Because a child can die from dehydration within a few days, the main treatment for diarrhea in children is rehydration using water and electrolytes. Doctors often recommend a special rehydration solution for children containing the nutrients they need. Available without a prescription, examples include Pedialyte, Ceralyte, and Infalyte.

diphtheria A preventable bacterial disease that affects the tonsils, throat, nose, or skin that was once widespread and greatly feared. Through the 1920s diphtheria killed 13,000 babies and children in the United States each year and made another 150,000 sick. It is most common in low socioeconomic groups where people live in crowded conditions. Unimmunized children under age 15 are likely to contract the disease.

Today the conquest of diphtheria is one of the greatest success stories of modern vaccination. In 1992 only four people in the United States were reported to have diphtheria, and by 1993 and 1994 no cases were reported. This does not mean that the disease has been eliminated.

Many Russian children did not get vaccines, so a serious outbreak began in Moscow in 1990; by 1992 there were 4,000 cases in the Russian federation and 24 deaths in Moscow. The problem has gotten worse since then, spreading throughout Russia with 1,100 deaths in 1994. Most of the victims are adults, but the outbreak has spread because many children had not been receiving their vaccines and adults who had been vaccinated were no longer immune.

Travelers to these areas must have completed a series of the vaccine and must have had a booster within the previous five years. There is no risk if the traveler is fully immunized.

In this country, confirmed cases of diphtheria must be reported to and investigated by the local and state health departments.

Cause

Diphtheria is caused by a bacterium *(Corynebacterium diphtheriae)* found in the mouth, throat, and nose of an infected individual; it is easily transmitted to others during coughing or sneezing, or through close contact with discharge from nose, throat, skin, eyes, and lesions. However, the bacteria do not travel very far through the air, and they infect only humans. The infection can also be spread by carriers, those who have the bacteria but have no symptoms.

Untreated patients who are infected can be contagious for up to two weeks, but not usually more than a month. Recovery from the disease does not always confer immunity.

Symptoms

Symptoms usually appear within two to five days of being exposed. There are two types of diphtheria; one type involves the nose and throat, and the other involves the skin.

Diphtheria usually develops in the throat, causing fever, red sore throat, weakness, and headache. There may be swelling and a gray membrane that completely covers the throat. This membrane can interfere with swallowing and talking and causes an unpleasant, distinct odor; if the membrane covers the windpipe, it can block breathing and suffocate the patient. Other symptoms include slight fever and chills. In the skin variety, skin lesions may be painful, swollen, and red.

Diagnosis

A sample of the nose or throat discharge is cultured; results are provided within eight hours.

Treatment

Diphtheria is a preventable and treatable disease, but if treatment is inadequate or not begun in time, a powerful toxin may be produced by the bacteria and spread throughout the body. This poison may cause serious complications.

Intensive hospital care and prompt treatment with diphtheria antitoxin offer the best hope for cure. The antitoxin neutralizes the toxin if it has not yet invaded cells but is still circulating in the blood. Antibiotics (penicillin or erythromycin) can help destroy the bacteria and decrease infectiousness in the respiratory secretions. Patients are kept isolated and in bed for 10 days to two weeks and are fed a liquid or soft diet. Secretions in nose and throat must be suctioned; tube feeding may be necessary if swallowing is impossible. A tracheotomy may be necessary if the breathing muscles are paralyzed.

A person is infectious from two to four weeks, or until after two to four days of antibiotic treatment. Anyone with a confirmed case must be isolated until negative results are obtained from two cultures from the nose and throat taken 24 hours apart, after completion of antibiotic treatment.

Complications

If the bacteria has time to produce the toxin, its complications can include bronchopneumonia, heart failure, or paralysis in the throat, eye, and breathing muscles. Severe paralysis of the breathing muscles or diaphragm can be fatal. The toxin will inflame the heart muscle (myocarditis), which can lead to heart failure and death. About one out of every 10 patients with diphtheria will die.

Prevention

Diphtheria vaccine is almost always given to infants in a combination with acellular pertussis and TETANUS (DTaP), given as a shot at ages two, four, six, and 15 months and once more as a booster before entering school at ages four to six.

All infants should be immunized; boosters throughout life will prevent resurgence. The vaccine is made of a toxoid (weakened form of the toxin) that stimulates the immune system to make antibodies against the toxin. However, this immunity wanes; a booster is required every 10 years.

The toxoid comes in two strengths; children under age seven need a higher concentration to develop immunity. Older patients should get the lower concentration, since it has fewer side effects yet will still boost immunity.

Anyone exposed to diphtheria must receive a vaccine booster (DTP, DT, or Td) if one has not been given within five years. Exposed people must have a throat culture and be under observa-

tion for one week; anyone with a positive culture (even without symptoms) needs seven days of antibiotics.

Anyone with a high fever or serious illness should not get a vaccination until recovered, but children with mild colds and low fevers should be vaccinated.

Common side effects of the vaccine and booster include slight fever and irritability in the first 24 hours with redness, swelling, or pain at the injection spot. Giving acetaminophen at the time of the shot may prevent a fever. A fever more than one day after the shot requires a call to the physician. (See also DIPHTHERIA, SKIN; DIPTHERIA TOXOID.)

diphtheria, skin A bacterial infection common in the tropics but also found in Canada and the southern United States that causes a rash similar to IMPETIGO. It is found in any area of crowded conditions and poor hygiene.

Cause

Skin DIPHTHERIA is caused by the same organism that causes diphtheria *(Corynebacterium diphtheriae)*, found in the mucous membranes of the nose and throat and probably on human skin. Rarely it is caused by food contaminated with the bacteria. A person can catch skin diphtheria by touching the open sores of a patient.

Symptoms

Superficial ulcers on the skin with a gray-yellow or brown-gray membrane in the early stages that can be peeled off; later, a black or brown-black scab appears, surrounded by a tender inflammatory area. Nasal discharge also may be present.

Treatment

Antibiotics and specific antitoxin; oral penicillin V potassium is effective in mild cases. While the antibiotics will inhibit the bacteria, diphtheria antitoxin is required to inactivate the toxin.

diphtheria toxoid A vaccine against DIPHTHERIA that is often combined with tetanus toxoid and acellular pertussis vaccine (DTaP) and given as a series of injections during infancy and childhood.

The toxoid is prepared by mixing formaldehyde with the poisonous toxin produced by *Corynebacterium diphtheriae,* rendering the toxin harmless.

Alternatively, diphtheria toxoid may be combined with tetanus toxoid alone (DT) and given to children, or combined with tetanus toxoid (Td) in an adult vaccine. The Td version only contains about 15 to 20 percent of the diphtheria toxoid found in the DTaP vaccine and is used for older children and adults.

The vaccine, which was introduced more than 50 years ago, led to a dramatic reduction of the incidence of diphtheria throughout the world. Primary preventive programs aimed at immunizing all infants and children in the community have almost eliminated the disease.

Yet while the reported incidence of diphtheria has been almost the same since the 1960s, it still occurs in isolated epidemics, primarily because some countries have taken a complacent attitude toward vaccination. The disease continues to represent a serious public health problem because it is possible for even fully immunized people to carry the *C. diphtheriae* bacteria in nose and throat, transmitting it to non-immunized individuals.

disinfection The elimination of most germs on surfaces. Low-level disinfection is used in most hospitals for items that will only come in contact with intact skin; this is usually all that is required in the home. Alcohol, chlorine bleach, and other chemical disinfectant products are used for low-level disinfection.

Household detergents or cleaners are not disinfectants nor germicides; they usually contain phosphates and are good for general cleaning.

Most disinfectants should not be used on human skin. Any household product that is called a disinfectant contains either ethyl alcohol (ethanol) isopropyl alcohol (isopropanol), hydrogen peroxide, chlorine, ammonia, phosphoric acid, or pine oil.

- *Alcohol* Sold at drug stores or supermarkets; can be used to wipe off thermometers. It is also an antiseptic.

- *Ammonium* Found in many household disinfectants; quaternary ammonium compounds are used in hospitals to wipe down floors, walls, and furniture.

- *Chlorine* The ingredient in household bleach that kills germs, usually found as sodium hypochlorite. It will kill bacteria and viruses and can be used to wipe down bathrooms, diaper changing tables, diaper pails, toys, and cutting boards. Chlorine can be used in solution: 1/4 cup (4 tbs.) bleach in 1 gallon water, or 1 tbs. bleach to 1 quart water. NEVER USE CHLORINE WITH ANY ACID PRODUCT OR AMMONIA; the resultant chlorine gas will react with water to form hydrochloric acid, which can cause serious symptoms ranging from eye irritation to lung damage and pneumonia.

- *Hydrogen peroxide* Three percent hydrogen peroxide can be found in drugstores and can be useful in cleaning small surface areas and as an antiseptic.

divorce and children One out of every two marriages today ends in divorce, and many divorcing families include children. However parents may feel about the divorce—and many may be relieved—children are almost always frightened and confused by the perceived threat to their security.

Divorce can be misinterpreted by children unless parents tell them what is happening, how they are involved and not involved, and what will happen to them. If possible, both parents should be present when telling the children about divorce. They should not feel they have to take sides or worry about losing the love of either parent. Parents should answer questions such as where they will live and with whom, when they will see each parent, where the other parent will be, how they can contact either parent, school arrangements, involvement in activities, and so on. If one parent chooses not to be involved in a child's life, it is best not to be dishonest with your child or misrepresent the truth.

Children often believe they have caused the conflict between their mother and father; they need to understand the decision to divorce had nothing to do with them or their behavior. At the same time, many children assume the responsibility for bringing their parents back together, sometimes by sacrificing themselves.

Some parents feel so hurt or overwhelmed by the divorce that they may turn to the child for comfort or direction.

Vulnerability to both physical and mental illnesses can originate in the traumatic loss of one or both parents through divorce. With care and attention, children can be helped to deal constructively with the resolution of parental conflict.

Parents should be alert to signs of distress in their children. Young children may react by becoming more aggressive and uncooperative or withdrawn. Older children may feel deep sadness and loss, and their schoolwork may suffer. Behavior problems are common.

Children will do best if they know that their mother and father will still remain involved with them. Long custody disputes or pressure on a child to "choose sides" can be particularly harmful for the youngster and can add to the damage of the divorce. Research shows that children do best when parents can cooperate on behalf of the child.

Parents' ongoing commitment to the child's well-being is vital. If a child shows signs of distress, the family doctor or pediatrician can refer the parents to a child and adolescent psychiatrist for evaluation and treatment. In addition, the child and adolescent psychiatrist can meet with the parents to help them learn how to make the strain of the divorce easier on the entire family. Psychotherapy for the children of a divorce, and the divorcing parents, can be helpful.

Down syndrome A congenital form of MENTAL RETARDATION caused by an extra chromosome, characterized by distinct physical features as well as developmental disabilities. Down syndrome affects people of all ages, races, and economic levels, occurring once in about every 800 to 1,000 live births. More than 350,000 people in the United States alone have Down syndrome. The condition was first described in 1959 by French physician Jerome Lejeune, who discovered that instead of the usual 46 chromosomes present in each cell, there were 47 in the cells of individuals with Down syndrome. Because 95 percent of all cases of Down syndrome occur because there are three copies of the 21st chromosome, it is also referred to as "trisomy 21."

While Down syndrome is usually caused by an error in cell division, two other types of chromosomal abnormalities (mosaicism and translocation) are also implicated. Regardless of the type of Down syndrome a person may have, all people with Down syndrome have an extra portion of the number 21 chromosome present in some of their cells. This additional genetic material alters the course of development and causes the characteristics associated with the syndrome.

Women age 35 and older have a significantly increased risk of having a child with Down syndrome: A 35-year-old woman has a one in 400 chance of conceiving a child with Down syndrome, and this chance increases gradually to one in 110 by age 40. At age 45 the incidence is about one in 35. Since many couples are postponing parenting until later in life, the incidence of Down syndrome conceptions is expected to increase. Therefore, genetic counseling for parents is important.

Maternal Diagnosis

Pregnant women have access to both screening and diagnostic tests to find out if an unborn child has Down syndrome. Screening tests estimate the risk of the fetus having Down syndrome, whereas diagnostic tests tell whether or not the fetus actually has the condition.

Screening tests are typically offered between 8 and 20 weeks of gestation, but they can accurately detect about 60 percent of cases. Many women who undergo these tests will be given false-positive readings, and some women will be given false-negative readings. Prenatal diagnosis of Down syndrome is by chorionic villus sampling (CVS), amniocentesis, and percutaneous umbilical blood sampling (PUBS).

Each of these procedures carries a small risk of miscarriage as tissue is extracted from the placenta or the umbilical cord to examine the fetus's chromosomes, but the procedures are about 98 to 99 percent accurate in the detection of Down syndrome. Amniocentesis is usually performed between 12 and 20 weeks of gestation, CVS between eight and 12 weeks, and PUBS after 20 weeks.

Diagnosis of Child

The diagnosis of Down syndrome is usually suspected after birth as a result of the baby's appearance. Among the most common traits are low muscle tone, a flat facial profile, an upward slant to the eyes, an abnormal ear shape, a single deep crease across the center of the palm, and an excessive ability to extend the joints. Other common symptoms include an extra finger with one furrow instead of two, small skin folds on the inner corner of the eyes, too much space between the large and second toe, and an enlarged tongue compared to the size of the mouth.

Most people with Down syndrome have some level of mental retardation ranging from mild to moderate range, but most children with Down syndrome learn to sit, walk, talk, play, toilet train, and do most other activities. Because speech is often delayed, careful attention should be paid to the child's hearing, as retention of fluid in the inner ear is a very common cause of hearing and speech difficulties.

Treatment

Early intervention services should begin shortly after birth to help children with Down syndrome develop to their full potential. These programs offer parents special instruction in teaching their child language, cognitive, self-help, and social skills, and specific exercises for gross and fine motor development. Research has shown that stimulation during early developmental stages improves the child's chances of developing to his or her fullest potential. Continuing education, positive public attitudes, and a stimulating home environment have also been found to promote the child's overall development.

Because children with Down syndrome respond well to their environment, those who receive good medical care and who are included in community activities can attend school, make friends, find work, participate in decisions that affect them, and make a positive contribution to society. Just as in the normal population, there is a wide variation in mental abilities, behavior, and developmental progress in these children. Their level of retardation may range from mild to severe, but most function in the mild to moderate range. Due to these individual differences, it is impossible to predict future achievements of children with Down syndrome.

Because of the range of ability in children with Down syndrome, it is important for families and all members of the school's education team to place few limitations on potential capabilities. It may be effective to emphasize concrete concepts rather than abstract ideas.

Teaching tasks in a step-by-step manner with frequent reinforcement and consistent feedback has been successful. Improved public acceptance of children with disabilities, along with better opportunities for adults with disabilities to live and work independently in the community, has expanded goals for individuals with Down syndrome.

drowning Drowning is the second leading cause of injury-related death for children aged one through 15 years, accounting for 1,003 deaths in 1998. Boys are more likely than girls to drown, and blacks are more likely to drown than whites. In 1998 black children aged five through 19 years drowned at two-and-a-half times the rate of whites. However, black children aged one through four years had a lower drowning rate than white children, largely because drownings in that age group typically occur in residential swimming pools, which are not as accessible to minority children in the United States.

Children most often drown in swimming pools. According to the U.S. Consumer Product Safety Commission, among children younger than five years old, about 320 fatal drownings in 1991 and nearly 2,300 nonfatal near-drownings in 1993 occurred in residential swimming pools. Between 60 percent and 90 percent of drownings among children under age four occur in residential pools; more than half of these occur at the child's own home. Sixty percent fewer drownings occur in inground pools with four-sided isolation fencing than in inground pools without four-sided fencing.

Alcohol use also is involved in between a quarter and half of all adolescent deaths associated with water recreation; it is a major contributing factor in up to half of drownings among adolescent boys.

Prevention

Following some simple safety tips can greatly reduce the chance of accidental drowning among children. They include:

- *Supervision* Whenever young children are swimming, playing, or bathing in water, an adult should constantly watch them. This means that the supervising adult should not read, play cards, talk on the phone, mow the lawn, or do any other distracting activity while watching children.

- *Buddy up* Children should never swim alone or in unsupervised places but should always swim with a buddy.

- *Beware of buckets* Small children can easily drown in a bucket containing liquid; five-gallon industrial containers are a particular danger. Buckets always should be emptied when household chores are finished.

- *No alcohol* No one should drink alcohol during or just before swimming, boating, or water skiing, and no adults should drink alcohol while supervising children. Teenagers should be taught about the danger of drinking alcohol and swimming, boating, or water skiing.

- *Prevent choking* To prevent choking, children should never chew gum or eat while swimming, diving, or playing in water.

- *Learn to swim* Every child over age four should learn to swim, but swimming classes are not recommended for children under age four.

- *Learn cardiopulmonary resuscitation (CPR)* A sound knowledge of CPR is particularly important for pool owners and individuals who regularly participate in water recreation.

- *Beware swimming aids* Parents should not use air-filled swimming aids such as water wings in place of life jackets or life preservers with children, because this can give parents and children a false sense of security and increase the risk of drowning.

- *Check water depth* The American Red Cross recommends nine feet of water as a minimum depth for diving or jumping.

Swimming Pool Safety

Homeowners should be familiar with a number of safety tips to ensure swimming pool safety. They include:

- *Fence it in* A four-sided, isolation pool fence with self-closing and self-latching gates should be installed around the pool. The fence should be at least four feet tall and completely separate the pool from the house and play area of the yard.

- *Phone* A telephone should be available near the pool, and homeowners should know how to contact local emergency medical services. The emergency number (911) should be posted in an easy-to-see place.

- *CPR* All pool owners should know CPR.

- *Safety equipment* Pool owners should keep a long pole and life preserver rings handy for emergencies.

Open Water Safety

Adult swimmers should know the local weather conditions and forecast before swimming or boating, because sudden thunderstorms and strong winds can be extremely dangerous to swimmers and boaters. Water activities should be restricted to designated swimming areas, which are usually marked by buoys. When boating, everyone should use U.S. Coast Guard–approved personal flotation devices (life jackets), regardless of distance to be traveled, size of boat, or swimming ability of boaters.

Open water usually has limited visibility, and conditions can sometimes change from hour to hour. Currents may be unpredictable, moving quickly and changing direction rapidly. A strong water current can carry even expert swimmers far from shore.

Adults should watch for signs of rip currents—water that is discolored, unusually choppy, foamy, or filled with debris. Make sure everyone knows how to evade a rip current—swimming parallel to the shore, *not directly in to shore*. By swimming parallel to shore, the swimmer can move out of the current; at this point, the swimmer can head directly in toward the shore.

DTaP vaccine Abbreviation for DIPHTHERIA, TETANUS, and acellular pertussis (WHOOPING COUGH) vaccine that is now the recommended immunization for all children. This acellular vaccine contains only pieces of the pertussis bacterial cell, which causes fewer side effects than the original DTP shot, yet it is just as effective.

Diphtheria, tetanus, and whooping cough are all serious childhood diseases that can be fatal. Since the organisms that cause them are still widely present in the community, continued vaccinations and regular booster shots are highly recommended. The DTaP vaccine is recommended as a five-dose series: three doses given to infants at two, four, and six months of age, followed by two additional booster doses at 12 to 18 months and at four to six years. Tetanus and diphtheria toxoids (Td) is recommended at age 11 to 12 years if at least five years have elapsed since the last dose of tetanus and diphtheria toxoid-containing vaccine. Subsequent routine Td boosters are recommended every 10 years.

The original "whole-cell" form of the vaccine (DTP) was reported to cause side effects including high fever and seizures. However, researchers believe that, contrary to rumors, there is no link between the DTP vaccine and SUDDEN INFANT DEATH SYNDROME.

DTP vaccine   See DTaP VACCINE.

dwarfism   Unusually short stature that can be caused by a variety of genetic and other conditions. Between one in 14,000 and one in 27,000 babies are born each year with some form of dwarfism. Dwarfism is generally defined as adult height of four feet 10 inches or less.

Many types of dwarfism are conditions marked by abnormal bone growth that are divided into two types: short-trunk and short-limb dysplasias. Children with short-trunk dysplasia have a shortened trunk with relatively longer limbs, whereas those with short-limb dysplasia have a near-normal size trunk but small arms and legs. Both types result in parts of the body that are not in proportion to one another. In the past, the term *dwarfism* was only used to refer to these cases of disproportionate short stature, while *midget* was applied to conditions in which all parts of the body match in size. However, the word *midget* is today considered offensive by many people of short stature. Today the terms *little person, person of short stature*, or *person with dwarfism* are the preferred terms.

Cause

More than 200 conditions cause dwarfism, most of which result either from a spontaneous mutation or from defective genes inherited from one or both parents. It is possible for two average-size parents to have a child with short stature; 85 percent of children with the most common form of dwarfism (achondroplasia) have average-size parents.

In instances of spontaneous genetic change, for some unknown reason a single normal gene in a chromosome inherited by the child suddenly mutates, leading to dwarfism. Spontaneous mutation can occur in any pregnancy and is a more common cause of a child with dwarfism born to average-size parents.

Inherited dwarfism is caused by a genetic trait carried by one or both parents. If both parents carry a recessive gene for a particular condition that produces dwarfism (which means they do not have the condition themselves), and they each pass that gene to their child, the child would be born with dwarfism.

Skeletal Dysplasias

The most common causes of dwarfism are the skeletal dysplasias, including: achondroplasia, diastrophic dysplasia (diastrophic dwarfism), and spondyloepiphyseal dysplasias (SED).

Achondroplasia   This is a form of short-limb dwarfism caused by a single autosomal dominant gene, which means that a spontaneous mutation in the gene can produce the condition, or a child can inherit the gene from a parent with achondroplasia. Children with achondroplasia have a relatively long trunk and shorter upper arms and legs, together with a large head, prominent forehead, pronounced abdomen, bowed legs, short feet and fingers, and limited flexibility of the elbows and hips.

Diastrophic dysplasia   This is another form of short-limb dwarfism, which causes shortened forearms and calves of the arms and legs. Significant bowing of the legs further reduces the child's height. Other characteristics often include clubfoot, broad hands with low-set thumbs that turn out, cysts on the upper ear that progress to swelling and thickening of the ears. Although the size of the head appears normal at birth, the face usually develops a long, full appearance with a high, broad forehead and square jaw. Originally believed to be a variation of achondroplasia, researchers now recognize it as a distinct condition with its own characteristics.

Spondyloepiphyseal dysplasias This is a very large group of skeletal conditions causing short-trunk dwarfism characterized by abnormal growth in the spine and long bones of the body. In one form (spondyloepiphyseal dysplasia tarda), the lack of growth in the trunk may not become obvious until the child is between five and 10 years old. On the other hand, the characteristics of children with spondyloepiphyseal dysplasia congenita (short neck and trunk and a barrel-shaped chest) are apparent at birth.

Proportionate Types of Dwarfism

Unlike the skeletal dysplasias, which largely produce disproportionate forms of dwarfism, proportionate types of dwarfism are usually caused by metabolic or hormonal problems in infancy or childhood. Chromosomal abnormalities, pituitary gland disorders, absorptive problems, MALNUTRITION, FAILURE TO THRIVE, and kidney disease can all lead to short stature if the child fails to grow at a normal rate.

Symptoms

The symptoms of dwarfism vary depending on the specific underlying condition, but obviously short stature and short limbs are the most recognizable signs. In addition, some children have large heads or bulging foreheads and may experience HYDRO-CEPHALUS (fluid on the brain) in infancy. Other possible complications include APNEA (a temporary breathing interruption) caused by abnormally small airways or by a compressed brain or spinal cord.

As children get older, other symptoms may appear, including delayed motor development, susceptibility to ear infections, weight problems, curvature of the spine, BOWED LEGS, joint inflexibility, and teeth problems. The combination of limited joint flexibility and a curved spine often leads to joint and back problems and fatigue in later childhood and adolescence. Early ARTHRITIS is a common complication during early adulthood.

Diagnosis

Some types of dwarfism can be identified through prenatal testing, if a doctor suspects a particular condition, but most cases are not identified until after birth. In these cases, a doctor reaches a diagnosis based on the child's appearance, failure to grow, and X rays of the bones.

Treatment

There is no treatment for most of the conditions that lead to dwarfism. If dwarfism is caused by hormonal or metabolic problems, the child can be treated with hormone injections or special diets to trigger growth. Skeletal dysplasias, however, cannot be cured, although medical care can lessen some of the complications of their short stature. For example, surgery to replace joints can ease joint pain, and hip surgery can help line up the hips and ease the stress on joints. These children may also have hip-replacement surgery in adulthood. Some children with dwarfism may have operations to fuse part of the spine to strengthen the neck or back.

One controversial procedure for children with achondroplasia involves lengthening limbs by cutting the bones in the arms or legs and inserting pins into the bones to hold the ends apart. New bone growth gradually fills in the space, lengthening the limb. Critics of the surgery argue that short stature does not need to be "corrected." Limb lengthening is a prolonged, painful process that can take two or more years and may carry complications, such as infections around the inserted pins. And since limb lengthening has been done only since the 1980s, the long-term physical results of the process have not been thoroughly evaluated. There is some evidence that the surgery might help spinal alignment and decrease the incidence of neurological problems in the lower spine. If that proves to be true, the surgery could be recommended in some cases in the future.

Prognosis

Typically, most children with dwarfism have normal intelligence and can live a normal life, marry, have children, and have fulfilling careers. Although people with dwarfism are protected under the Americans with Disabilities Act, many people with dwarfism argue that they do not have a disability.

dyscalculia A significant learning disability involving mathematics that affects between 2 percent and 6 percent of elementary school aged children in the United States. Dyscalculia is a medical term associated with brain dysfunction that is presumably present at birth. Many students identified as having a specific LEARNING DISABILITY or attention disorder may have associated problems with learning or applying mathematical concepts, functions, and procedures.

It also may relate to a variety of more basic disorders such as confusion or deficits in perception, spatial skills, sequencing, and so on. It is sometimes referred to as acalculia, which is technically a total inability to do arithmetic.

However, because the cause of problems with arithmetic and mathematics may vary widely, it is important to understand the underlying sources of the learning difficulty in this area before deciding what educational remedies to choose.

Symptoms

There are a variety of symptoms with this condition, including normal or advanced language and other skills and often good visual memory for the printed word. This is accompanied by poor mental math ability, often with problems in using money (such as balancing a checkbook, making change, and tipping). This may develop into an actual fear of money and its transactions.

In addition, a person with dyscalculia has problems with math processes such as addition, subtraction, or multiplication, as well as with math concepts (such as sequencing numbers). The student may have trouble retaining and retrieving concepts or have problems grasping math rules.

This is combined with a poor sense of direction, as well as trouble reading maps, telling time, and grappling with mechanical processes. There is difficulty with abstract concepts of time and direction, schedules, keeping track of time, and the sequence of past and future events.

Common mistakes in working with numbers include number substitutions, reversals, and omissions. Students also may have trouble learning musical concepts, following directions in sports that demand sequencing or rules, and keeping track of scores and players during games such as cards and board games.

Treatment

Individuals with dyscalculia need help in organizing and processing information related to numbers and mathematical concepts. Since math is essentially a form of language using numbers instead of words as symbols, it is important to communicate frequently and clearly with a child as to what is needed to do a mathematical problem. While the condition is lifelong, performance can be improved with intensive intervention. The child should have real-life exposure to how math is a part of everyday life, counting ingredients in a cake, how to make change, and so on.

dyslexia   A specific learning difficulty, usually with spelling and writing, and sometimes with reading and numbers. It is characterized by problems in coping with written symbols, despite normal intelligence. Dyslexic children and adults may have problems putting things in order or following instructions and may confuse left and right. The word *dyslexia* comes from the Greek meaning "difficulty with words."

Experts estimate that dyslexia occurs in about 8 percent of the population. It is a permanent disability, which is often accompanied by strengths in areas such as creativity or physical coordination. Each dyslexic person's difficulties are different and vary from slight to very severe disruption of the learning process.

Its cause has not been fully established, but the effect creates neurological anomalies in the brain. These anomalies trigger varying degrees of difficulty in learning when using words and sometimes symbols. Children or students who are dyslexic have trouble sorting out the sounds within words, which is why they have problems with reading, writing, and spelling. Most children with dyslexia have difficulty with text, memory, and basic mathematics.

Children are either born with dyslexia or they acquire the difficulty during early childhood, but it is when they begin to learn using words and sometimes other symbols that it becomes a noticeable problem.

Symptoms

Dyslexia may include a variety of reading problems, such as:

- lack of understanding what is read
- lack of awareness of sounds that make up words, often including a difficulty with blending sounds to make words

- problems with spelling
- problems with the order of letters in words
- trouble rhyming words
- difficulty with pronouncing words
- delay in speaking
- delay in learning the alphabet, numbers, days of the week, months, colors, shapes, and other basic information
- difficulty understanding subtleties of language such as jokes or slang

Cause

Modern experts believe dyslexia may be caused by differences in brain structure and function present since birth, with a strong genetic component. A number of studies have indicated a strong heritability for dyslexia, predominantly among boys within a family. In general, the ratio of males to females identified with dyslexia is about four to one. Because of this, the role of the hormone testosterone before birth is being investigated as a possible cause of inherited dyslexia.

The reading difficulties associated with dyslexia are not related to intelligence or motivation; students often possess unusual talents, especially in areas that require visual, spatial, and motor skills. This disorder is not due to a physical disability, such as a visual problem. Instead, it is a problem in how the brain processes the information as the individual is reading.

Traditional definitions of dyslexia have relied on an unexpected gap between learning aptitude and achievement in school, particularly in the area of reading. However, contemporary research has indicated that difficulties or delays in developing awareness of sounds and processing abilities play a primary factor in the development of the reading problems associated with dyslexia. Word-finding difficulties are a second factor in the case of some individuals with severe reading difficulties.

Dyslexia is the most researched and most fully understood of all the learning disabilities. Some research links it to low levels of the brain chemical dopamine. Still a great many research questions remain unanswered.

Treatment

Although dyslexia is a lifelong condition, with appropriate instruction individuals with dyslexia may largely overcome their reading difficulties. Individuals with a reading disability most often benefit from a language program that provides direct instruction in understanding the letter-sound system. The earlier this instruction is given, the greater the chance the person will become a fluent reader.

Typically, the more senses that can be used when learning something, the better the person will learn. For individuals with reading disabilities, it is important to learn as much as possible by seeing, hearing, writing, and speaking. For example, a teacher of students with this disability can provide a written outline of the day's lecture in addition to giving the lecture itself. Books on tape can help someone access literature with all of its benefits, including vocabulary and ideas.

Parents of children with reading disabilities can encourage their children to read by providing reading materials on subjects in which they have an interest. Several decades of teacher-based and clinical research support the need for a multisensory, sequential, phonetic-based approach to reading instruction as the essential foundation for the development of reading skills. For example, a student learning the consonant blend *"bl"* might listen to the sound while looking at the letters, then say it aloud while tracing the two letters on a rough-board. This method of instruction increases the chance that the information will be stored and retained in long-term memory.

There is no total cure, but the effects can be eased by skilled specialized teaching of phonics, sequencing, and techniques to raise the person's self-esteem. Given proper support, dyslexic students are able to go on to college and pursue successful careers. (For contact information see LEARNING DISABILITY; Appendix I.)

dyspraxia A general term used to describe a range of different conditions involving difficulty with learned patterns of movement ("motor planning") without any muscle or nerve damage. In some cases dyspraxia is used to describe coordination problems, gross-motor, and fine-motor body movements. It causes an underdevelopment of the brain in which messages are not properly transmitted to the body, producing a number of problems in physical and thinking areas. It affects at least 2 percent of the population in varying degrees; 70 percent of those affected are male. Dyspraxia can be subtle or more pronounced, and often a person's disability is not readily apparent.

The term is also commonly used in the field of speech-language therapy to describe the condition of developmental verbal dyspraxia, in which a child has significant problems in producing speech sounds and sequencing sounds into words. This condition may also be accompanied by a difficulty in making and coordinating the physical movements required to produce speech, called oral dyspraxia. There are many other types of dyspraxia, including:

- *Ideomotor* Inability to perform single motor tasks, such as combing hair or waving good-bye
- *Ideational* Difficulty with multilevel tasks, such as taking the proper sequence of steps for brushing teeth
- *Dressing* Problems with dressing and putting clothes on in order
- *Constructional* Difficulty with spatial relations
- *Verbal* Problems and delay with expressive language

Symptoms

Dyspraxia causes a range of symptoms such as coordination problems (awkwardness, clumsiness, trouble with hopping, skipping, throwing and catching a ball, or riding a bike). There may be confusion about which hand to use for tasks, problems with holding a pen or pencil properly, and sensitivity to touch (the child may find some clothes uncomfortable; there may be an intolerance to having hair or teeth brushed, or nails and hair cut). In addition, there may be problems with short-term memory, trouble with reading and writing, poor sense of direction, speech problems, phobias, or obsessive behavior.

While older children may be verbally adept, they may not develop the social skills to get along with their peers. While children with dyspraxia can be of average or above average intelligence, they often have immature behavior. Logic and reasoning may be challenging.

Treatment

These is no cure for dyspraxia, but the earlier a child is treated, the greater the chance of improvement. Occupational therapists, physiotherapists, and accommodations at school can all help a child to cope with the condition. A child with dyspraxia wants to communicate but often cannot, so pressuring such a child will only lead to further inhibition. Repetitive verbal activities can help develop language skills, including songs, poems, nursery rhymes, and so on. A child who has trouble communicating can use sign language or a communication board to supplement speech temporarily.

To improve motor function, the child should practice tasks to learn the correct sequence of movements that must be followed. Physical activities should be encouraged to strengthen a child's overall performance and coordination, beginning with simple physical tasks and leading up to more complicated tasks involving multiple steps.

earache A severe, stabbing pain in the ear usually caused by an infection in the middle ear. This occurs most often in young children, when the stabbing pain is accompanied by a fever and a temporary loss of hearing. If the eardrum breaks, the pain and pressure are relieved immediately.

Another common cause of earache is SWIMMER'S EAR (otitis externa), which is an inflammation of the outer ear canal usually caused by an infection. This infection may affect the entire canal, or only parts of it, and may form an abscess or boil. There may be irritation or itching, discharge, and temporary mild deafness as well.

Much more rarely, an earache may be caused by HERPES zoster (shingles), which can cause blisters in the ear canal and can produce pain for weeks or months after the infection has ended.

Earaches that come and go could occur from many different problems, including tooth pain, TONSILLITIS, or pain in the lower jaw. In fact, almost any disorder that affects areas near the ear can cause an earache, since the same nerves that serve the ear also supply many nearby areas.

Earaches may be treated with painkillers, and antibiotics are often prescribed for infection. Pus in the outer ear may need to be removed or drained. (See also EAR CONDITIONS; EAR INFECTION.)

ear conditions There are a number of ear conditions that may plague a child's life, including SWIMMER'S EAR, EAR INFECTION, EARACHE, and MIDDLE EAR BAROTRAUMA.

Swimmer's Ear

Swimmer's ear is a painful infection in the delicate skin of the outer ear canal caused by frequent exposure to water that keeps the skin of the ear canal damp, providing an ideal environment for bacteria and fungi to grow. Swimmer's ear is also known as an external ear infection (otitis externa). The resulting irritation may first cause itching, followed by swelling of the skin of the ear canal and drainage. This may be accompanied by severe pain that is worsened when the ear lobe or other outside part of the ear is touched.

Ear Infection

A common childhood infection involving the middle ear (that cavity between the eardrum and the inner ear) known medically as otitis media. Symptoms of a middle ear infection include hearing loss and the presence of pus or fluid. The infection may be treated with antibiotics. An ear infection can cause a great deal of pain, but since it can be treated simply and effectively, there are rarely any serious, long-term complications.

Serious cases may occur in some children who experience recurring ear infections. This most commonly develops within two months of birth and is characterized by persistent fluid in the middle ear and temporary hearing loss. This condition may be hereditary, and sometimes must be treated with long-term use of antibiotics or surgery.

Children are very susceptible to ear infections. Nearly all children experience an ear infection before the age of six, and they are at their most vulnerable up to age two. Bacteria enter from the back of the throat via the eustachian tube, the passage that connects the back of the nose to the middle ear. The angle and shortness of the eustachian tube in children facilitates the bacterial transmission.

Middle Ear Barotrauma

Another kind of earache can occur when a child is in a descending airplane. Called middle ear barotrauma, it is related to abnormal pressure changes in the air space behind the eardrum. Even in a pressurized aircraft cabin, there is a drop in the cabin air pressure as the plane climbs. As the plane descends, air pressure rises. When a plane descends and the pressure in the cabin increases, the air pressure in the middle ear must be equalized. If it is not, the increased cabin air pressure pushes on the eardrum and causes pain. Normally the eustachian tube will open to equalize pressure (this is what happens when a child yawns or swallows), and the result is the "popping" sensation in the ear. However, children have a relatively small eustachian tube that may not function effectively. This can cause pain.

ear infection   The common name for otitis media, this is an infection involving the middle ear (that cavity between the eardrum and the inner ear). A middle ear infection can produce pus or fluid and cause hearing loss. While an ear infection is painful, it is not terribly serious; it is easily treated and there are not usually any long-term complications.

Ear infections are most common in children because of the shortness of their eustachian tubes (the passage that connects the back of the nose to the middle ear), which makes it easier for bacteria to enter from the back of the throat. Almost all children have had at least one infection by the time they are six years old. They are most susceptible to ear infections during the first two years of life.

Some children (especially babies with ear infections within two months of birth) have recurrent ear infections. They seem to run in families and are characterized by persistent fluid in the middle ear and short-term hearing loss. These conditions may require long-term antibiotics or surgery.

Cause

During a cold, the eustachian tube can swell and become blocked, allowing fluid to accumulate in the middle ear. The fluid produced by the inflammation cannot drain off through the tube and instead collects in the middle ear, where it can allow bacteria and viruses drawn in from the back of the throat to breed.

The usual cause of a middle ear infection is bacteria that are normally present in a child's throat, including *Streptococcus pneumoniae, Haemophilus influenzae,* and *Moraxella catarrhalis.*

Risk factors for the developing of an ear infection include being male, bottle-fed, Native American or Hispanic, and younger than two. Other risk factors include living in crowded conditions, going to day care, having allergies, and inhaling household cigarette smoke.

Symptoms

Acute middle ear infection causes sudden, severe earache, deafness, ringing of the ear (tinnitus), sense of fullness in the ear, and fever. Occasionally, the eardrum can burst, which causes a discharge of pus and relief of pain. Parents may notice a baby or young child suffering cold with thick discharge, irritability, pulling or tugging at the ear, crying in the middle of the night, shaking his head, and exhibiting poor appetite. There may be fluid draining from the ear, although this is not always the case. A low fever is common. The worst symptom is ear pain.

Chronic middle ear infection is usually caused by repeated attacks of acute otitis media, with pus seeping from a perforation in the eardrum together with some degree of deafness. Complications include otitis externa (inflammation of the outer ear), damage to the bones in the middle ear, or a matted ball of skin debris which can erode the bone and cause further damage (called a "cholesteatoma"). Rarely, infection can spread *inward* from an infected ear and cause a brain abscess.

Diagnosis

Middle ear infection can be detected by examining the ear with an instrument called an otoscope. A sample of discharge may be taken to identify the organism responsible for the infection, but it is not often done.

Treatment

Acute middle ear infection usually clears up completely with antibiotic drugs, although sometimes there may be continual production of a sticky fluid in the middle ear known as "persistent middle ear infection." A doctor may also remove pus and skin debris and prescribe antibiotic ear drops. Ephedrine nose drops can help establish draining of the ear in children.

Since the mid-1980s, some strains of bacteria have developed resistance to amoxicillin and other antibiotics. Some children may not improve after 10 days of antibiotics and may need three or four more weeks of drug treatment.

Acetaminophen may be given to relieve pain or to reduce fevers above 101°F. A warm towel or hot water bottle over the sore ear, or an ice pack wrapped in a towel, may ease pain. The child should lie with the infected ear down to help drain the fluid.

Complications

Rarely, a middle ear infection can lead to bacterial MENINGITIS and MASTOIDITIS (a serious infection of the air cells behind the middle ear). Warning signs of mastoiditis include: high fever, severe ear pain, pus-like drainage, and redness, swelling, and tenderness behind the ear.

Prevention

Breast-feeding prevents ear infections during the first six months. Bottle-fed babies should not drink with the bottle propped or while lying on the back. Adults should not smoke around an infant, since the smoke irritates the lining of the nose and throat. Early treatment prevents most problems.

early childhood assessment Testing that identifies early developmental and learning problems in preschool and primary grade children. Early childhood assessment practices allow for accurate and fair identification of the developmental needs of infants, preschoolers, and young children.

Sound early childhood assessment should involve a multidisciplinary team, including school psychologists with specialized training in the assessment of the young child, and those who view behavior and development from a longitudinal perspective.

Early assessment of potential problems is essential because of a child's broad and rapid development. Intervention services for any psychological and developmental problems are essential and cost-effective.

Standardized assessment procedures should be used with great caution in educational decision-making because such tools are inherently less accurate when used with young children. Multidisciplinary team assessments must include multiple sources of information, multiple approaches to assessment, and multiple settings in order to yield a comprehensive understanding of children's skills and needs. Therefore, assessments should center on the child in the family system and home environment, both substantial influences on the development of young children.

early intervention program A program designed to identify and provide intervention for infants and young children who are developmentally delayed and at high risk for school failure. The purpose of this type of program is to help prevent problems as the child matures.

These programs address the needs of young children from birth to the beginning of school with a collaborative effort from parents and medical personnel, social services, and educational professionals. The pre-academic skills that may need help include self-concept, fine and gross motor skills, awareness of sounds, visual discrimination, communication and language development, thinking skills, and social skills. Nationally recognized early intervention programs include Project Head Start and Reading Recovery.

eating disorders Complex conditions caused by a combination of long-standing behavioral, emotional, psychological, interpersonal, and social factors. Scientists and researchers are still learning about the underlying causes of these emotionally and physically damaging conditions. While eating disorders may start with a preoccupation with food and weight, they are usually triggered by many other factors besides food.

Children with eating disorders often use food and the control of food in an attempt to compensate for feelings and emotions that may otherwise seem overwhelming. For some, dieting, bingeing, and purging may begin as a way to cope with painful emotions and to feel in control, despite the fact that these behaviors will eventually damage the child's health, self-esteem, and sense of competence.

Scientists are still researching possible biochemical or biological causes of eating disorders. In some individuals with eating disorders, certain chemicals in the brain that control hunger, appetite, and digestion may be imbalanced. The exact meaning and implications of these imbalances are unclear. While eating disorders are complex conditions that can be triggered by a variety of potential causes, they can create a self-perpetuating cycle of physical and emotional destruction that can be hard to stop. All eating disorders require professional help.

Daughters born to mothers with past or present eating disorders may be at high risk of developing an eating disorder themselves. Studies have found that mothers with eating disorders interact differently with their daughters than other mothers when it comes to feeding and weight issues. This suggests that the risk factors for the later development of an eating disorder may begin very early in life.

In one recent California study, baby daughters of women with eating disorders sucked significantly faster, whether breast- or bottle-fed, and were weaned from the bottle an average of more than nine months later than offspring of women without eating disorders. When their children were age two or older, mothers with eating disorders fed their children on a less regular schedule, used food as a reward or to calm the child, and showed greater concern about their daughters' weight than did other mothers. Scientists believe that these differences may pose a serious risk for the later development of an eating disorder.

EBV See EPSTEIN-BARR VIRUS.

ECHOvirus A type of virus associated with many infections including MENINGITIS, upper respiratory tract infection, CONJUNCTIVITIS, and infantile diarrhea. ECHOvirus, which is an acronym for enteric cytopathogenic human orphan virus, includes more than 30 types. The virus is found throughout the world and peaks in summer and fall. Outbreaks are common in day care centers.

Most ECHOvirus infections are mild, but symptoms may vary from mild to lethal and acute to chronic. Other symptoms and infections with which the virus is associated include muscle weakness and paralysis, pericarditis, myocarditis, the common cold, and acute febrile respiratory illnesses.

E. coli **infection** See *ESCHERICHIA COLI* 0157:H7.

Ecstasy (MDMA) An illegal stimulant drug that can kill nerve cells in the brain, also known as 3,4 methylenedioxymethamphetamine (MDMA). The drug, related to the drugs mescaline and amphetamine, is also known as "Adam," "XTC," or just "E."

Ecstasy was first synthesized and patented in 1914 by the German drug company Merck as an appetite suppressant; in the 1970s it was given to therapy patients because it helped them talk about their feelings. This practice was stopped in 1986 when animal studies showed that Ecstasy caused brain damage.

Users say Ecstasy lowers their inhibitions and relaxes them, increases awareness and feelings of pleasure, and gives people energy. However, some people report side effects after taking MDMA, such as headaches, chills, eye twitching, jaw clenching, blurred vision, and nausea. Unlike the drug LSD, low doses of MDMA do not cause people to hallucinate.

Ecstasy gained national attention when it became the drug of choice at parties called "raves." In a survey taken in 2000, 8.2 percent of 12th graders, 5.4 percent of 10th graders, and 3.1 percent of 8th graders reported that they had used MDMA at least once within the year.

Ecstasy appears to have several effects on the brain, boosting the levels of certain neurotransmitters. Recent data suggest that MDMA may be toxic to the brain, according to the brain scans of people who have used the drug an average of 200 times over five years. Those who used the drug more often had more brain damage than less frequent users. Moreover, memory tests of people who have taken Ecstasy as compared to non-drug users have shown that Ecstasy users had lower scores. Brain scans also show that there is a 20 percent to 60 percent loss of healthy serotonin cells in the drug users, which could affect a person's ability to remember and to learn. Scientists do not yet know if this damage is permanent, if those damaged cells will replace themselves, or if this loss of cells affects behavior or the ability to think.

ecthyma A shallow ulcerative skin infection caused by bacteria that often results in scarring, similar to a deep form of IMPETIGO, usually found on legs and protected areas of the body. The condition commonly occurs during unfavorable conditions, such as poverty, war, or captivity.

Cause

The infection is caused by group A streptococci or *Staphylococcus aureus*.

Symptoms

The condition begins with one lesion, which enlarges and encrusts; beneath this crust is a pus-filled "punched ulcer." Children are more commonly affected with ecthyma, which is usually associated with poor hygiene and malnutrition and minor skin injuries from trauma, insect bites, or SCABIES.

Treatment

Erythromycin or dicloxacillin is administered. The lesions should also be soaked and crusts removed.

ectodermal dysplasia (ED) A group of genetic disorders that are identified by the absence or deficient function of at least two of these: teeth, hair, nails, or glands. At least 150 different EDs have been identified. Charles Darwin identified the first EDs in the 1860s, and today the number is believed to affect as many as seven out of every 10,000 births.

There is usually no reason to expect anything but normal intelligence with ectodermal dysplasia, though some of the extremely rare forms have been associated with mental retardation. As with the general population, some individuals affected by ED may be very bright, some may be average, and others may find challenges in learning.

Symptoms

Individuals affected by EDs have abnormalities of sweat glands, tooth buds, hair follicles, and nail development. Some types of EDs are mild while others are devastating. Many individuals affected by EDs cannot perspire. Air conditioning in the home, school, and workplace is a necessity. Other symptoms may include deficient tears and saliva, frequent respiratory infections, poor hearing or vision, missing fingers or toes, cleft lip and/or palate, poor immune system, sensitivity to light, and lack of breast development.

Life span can be affected in some rare types of EDs, but there are very few documented examples of a death because of an inability to perspire.

There are four different types of ectodermal dysplasia: anhidrotic, anhydrotic, hypohidrotic, and hypohydrotic.

- anhidrotic means "no sweating" and is derived from the Greek words *an* ("none") and *hidros* ("sweat"). A person who does not sweat at all could be said to be anhidrotic.

- anhydrotic means "no water" from the Greek *an* ("none") and *hydro* ("water"). Those who are totally devoid of water could be said to be anhydrotic.

- hypohidrotic means "deficient sweating" from the Greek *hypo* ("under/deficient") and *hidros* ("sweat"). Someone whose sweat function is diminished (sweats little in response to heat or in response to stress only) could be said to be hypohidrotic.

- hypohydrotic means "deficient water." Those who are partially or totally devoid of water could be said to be hypohydrotic.

Cause

As a baby is developing, three layers of tissue can be identified: an inner layer (the endoderm), a middle layer (the mesoderm), and an outer layer (the ectoderm). Defects in formation of the outer layer lead to ED. The reason that so many parts of the body are affected is because the ectoderm of the surface of the developing baby forms the skin, nails, hair, sweat glands, parts of the teeth, the lens of the eye, and the parts of the inner ear. Another portion of ectoderm forms the brain, spinal cord, nerves, the retina of the eye, and the pigment cells of the body.

Treatment

At this time, there is no cure. Because most people with EDs have missing or malformed teeth, dental treatment is necessary beginning with dentures as early as age two, multiple replacements as the child grows, and perhaps dental implants thereafter. Orthodontic treatment may also be necessary.

Precautions must be taken to limit upper respiratory infections, and care must be provided for the skin to prevent cracking, bleeding, and infection.

Professional care may minimize the effects of vision or hearing deficits, and surgical or cosmetic procedures may improve other deformities.

Prognosis

There is no evidence that the life span for a person diagnosed with one of the common ectodermal dysplasias is shorter than average, but a few rare syndromes may lead to a shortened life span.

eczema   An allergic skin disorder (also called atopic dermatitis) that usually appears in babies or very young children and may last until the child reaches adolescence or adulthood. Eczema causes the skin to itch, scale, and flake. Parents with eczema are more likely to have children with eczema. About 60 percent of children with eczema will develop signs in the first year of life; 85 percent will have symptoms within the first five years. Some children only have a few episodes of flare-ups, while other children will have atopic dermatitis all their lives. Eczema is very common; about 10 percent of infants and children have the condition.

Cause

Different triggers can make eczema worse, including stress, other allergies, scratching, and sweating.

Symptoms

As a child gets older, the location of symptoms tends to change. In infants and young children, the dry skin is usually located on the face, outside of the elbows, and on the knees. In older children and adults, eczema tends to be on the hands and feet, the front of the arms, and on the back of the knees.

Symptoms may include dry, scaly skin; small bumps; redness; and swelling. Chronic eczema may lead to thickened, hardened skin.

Treatment

There is no cure for eczema. The main goal of treatment is to remove any irritants and decrease the amount of dryness and irritation. Daily application of creams, lotions, and antihistamines may help stop itching.

Children with atopic eczema should be bathed quickly with a mild, neutral soap no more than three times a week. Bath oil may prevent excess skin drying, and fingernails should be clipped to decrease damage from scratching. Children should avoid contact with things that irritate the skin. The child should wear lightweight clothes, since sweating can make eczema worse.

Medications may be prescribed in severe cases. Most common drugs include antihistamines to help decrease the itch, such as diphenhydramine (Benadryl) or hydroxyzine (Atarax). These medications may cause drowsiness. Some new antihistamines are also available that do not cause drowsiness, such as loratadine (Claritin) or Clarinex.

Steroid creams such as hydrocortisone ointments, mometasone (Elocon), or triamcinolone (Kenalog) help decrease the inflammation in the skin, thus decreasing the itching and swelling. New nonsteroidal creams are also available.

educable mentally handicapped (EMH)   See MENTAL RETARDATION.

Ehrlichia   A genus of bacteria that includes several well-known species infecting domestic animals. Ehrlichiae are small, gram-negative bacteria that primarily invade white blood cells, the same cells that fight disease by destroying invading microorganisms. Ehrlichiae typically appear as minute, round bacteria ranging from 1 to 3 micrometers in diameter.

The genus is in the same family (Rickettsia) as the bacterium that causes another tick-borne human disease, ROCKY MOUNTAIN SPOTTED FEVER. The species were first reported in dogs in 1935 but were only documented as causes of human disease in 1986.

The genus Ehrlichia is currently classified as a member of the family Rickettsiaceae, in the order Rickettsiales. The genus includes seven recognized species: *E. canis, E. chaffeensis, E. equi, E. phagocytophila, E. risticii, E. ewingii,* and *E. sennetsu.* A number of other named ehrlichiae, such as *E. platys, E. bovis, E. ovina,* and *E. ondiri,* also cause disease in animals. The names of the latter organisms are enclosed in quotation marks because they have not been formally proposed and accepted according to the rules of the International Code of Nomenclature of Bacteria, Bacteriological Code.

E. ewingii is the most recently recognized human pathogen that causes EHRLICHIOSIS, a potentially fatal disease that has been limited to a few patients in Missouri, Oklahoma, and Tennessee, most of whom have had underlying suppressed immune systems.

Ehrlichia ewingii is transmitted by the lone star tick *(Amblyomma americanum),* which is also able to transmit the disease among dogs. Other potential carriers of the disease remain to be identified. Canine granulocytic ehrlichiosis caused by *E. ewingii* has been described in south central and southeastern states, including Arkansas, Georgia, Mississippi, Missouri, North Carolina, Oklahoma, Tennessee, and Virginia.

Scientists do not know whether *E. ewingii* infection in humans is a new phenomenon or merely a newly recognized one. Because *E. ewingii* is closely related to *E. chaffeensis* and both are found in Missouri, it is possible that previous cases of *E. ewingii* have been misdiagnosed as *E. chaffeensis.*

ehrlichiosis, human granulocytic   A disease (HGE) identified in 1990 that is spread by the type of ticks that carry LYME DISEASE. Although the disease can be treated with antibiotics, treatment is often delayed because it is confused with a summer flu. If it is treated early and properly, the disease is not associated with brain damage or arthritis.

The Centers for Disease Control and Prevention reported at least two deaths in 1990–93 due to the disease in Wisconsin and Minnesota. Some researchers believe this is not a new disease at all, but one of which doctors were simply unaware. New York and New England states are believed to have patients who have had the disease but who have instead been diagnosed with Lyme disease.

It is also possible that some patients are infected with both Lyme and HGE disease at the same time, making a proper diagnosis more difficult. For every 12 Lyme-infected ticks a child might find during an hour's walk in tick-infested areas of Nantucket, there would be four HGE-infected ticks and two ticks infected with both diseases, which raises the possibility of getting two infections from one bite.

Some Harvard University researchers believe that the HGE bacterium was discovered by Dr. Ernest Tyzzer of Harvard in 1938 in voles and mice from Martha's Vineyard, but that it was believed to be exclusively an infection of rodents.

Cause

Ehrlichiosis represents a group of clinically similar yet distinct diseases caused by *Ehrlichia chaffeensis,*

E. ewingii, and a bacterium extremely similar or identical to *E. phagocytophila.* Human ehrlichiosis caused by *E. chaffeensis* was first described in 1987 and is found primarily in the southeastern and south central parts of the country. It is primarily transmitted by the lone star tick *(Amblyomma americanum).* Human granulocytic ehrlichiosis (HGE) was first identified in 1994, the second recognized Ehrlichia infection of humans in the United States.

The name for the species that causes HGE has not been formally proposed, but this species is closely related or identical to the veterinary pathogens *E. equi* and *E. phagocytophila.* HGE is transmitted by the blacklegged tick *(Ixodes scapularis)* and the western blacklegged tick *(Ixodes pacificus)* in the United States. *E. ewingii* is the most recently recognized cause of ehrlichiosis, which has been limited to a few immunocompromised patients in Missouri, Oklahoma, and Tennessee.

Most patients are infected in the spring and summer when they are more commonly exposed to disease-carrying ticks. Up to 90 percent of all ehrlichiosis cases occur between April and September; about 55 percent to 70 percent of all cases occur during May through July. A history of tick bites or exposure to tick-infested habitats is reported in 50 percent to 90 percent of cases.

From 1986 to 1997 health departments and laboratories reported more than 1,200 cases of human ehrlichiosis to the CDC. Although ehrlichiosis is a nationally notifiable disease, not all state health departments have reported cases. Most of the recognized cases have originated from states that also have a high incidence of Lyme disease, such as Connecticut, Minnesota, New York, and Wisconsin. This distribution is consistent with the fact that the ticks that transmit ehrlichiosis *(Ixodes scapularis)* also transmit the bacteria that causes Lyme disease *(Borrelia burgdorferi).*

Symptoms

While Lyme disease often produces a telltale circular rash around the tick bite site, HGE does not usually cause visible symptoms. Instead, about 10 days after a person has been bitten, the bacteria multiplies inside white blood cells, and then suddenly causes fever, chills, headache, and muscle ache. Its flu-like symptoms are far more severe than those associated with Lyme disease.

Severe symptoms of the disease may include prolonged fever, kidney failure, meningoencephalitis, seizures, or coma. Between 2 percent and 3 percent of patients may die from the infection. While many of the symptoms overlap with Lyme, the HGE symptoms tend to peak very quickly, moving from health to severe debilitation in a few hours.

Preliminary evidence suggests that infection caused by the *E. chaffeensis* bacteria may become more severe than other ehrlichia infections. The severity of ehrlichiosis may also be related in part to the health of the child's immune system. Patients with compromised immunity caused by corticosteroids or cancer chemotherapy, HIV infection, or removal of the spleen appear to develop more severe disease.

Children who are not treated can develop serious liver and lung problems that can lead to organ failure. Untreated ehrlichiosis can be a severe illness; as many as half of all patients require hospitalization.

Diagnosis

Only four labs in the United States can test for HGE, which takes a week. Diagnosis is difficult and testing has not been standardized. If it is summer and a child develops sudden, flu-like symptoms without coughing or nasal congestion, HGE is a likely suspect—especially if the child remembers a recent tick bite. (Lyme disease symptoms usually appear more gradually.)

Treatment

Prompt treatment is essential; the longer a case is untreated, the worse the outcome. HGE responds to doxycyclines and other tetracycline antibiotics; it does not respond to amoxicillin and other antibiotics used to treat Lyme disease.

The antibiotic suppresses the growth of microbes but does not kill them, so the immune system must fight off the infection. Co-infection with another type of bacteria at the same time can suppress the immune system, increasing a patient's vulnerability to other infections. In these cases, treatment time may need to be longer.

Signs of the disease fade away within two months and the disease does not appear to cause

the chronic, arthritis-like symptoms that haunt Lyme disease patients for years.

Prevention

The same precautions that prevent Lyme disease should also be taken to prevent HGE. Avoiding tick habitat is the best way to prevent tick bites, but ticks may also be found in lawns, gardens, and on bushes adjacent to homes.

When walking in the woods, children should stay on trails and avoid brushing up against low bushes or tall grass. Ticks do not hop, jump, fly, or descend from trees—a child must come in direct contact with them. To prevent bites, children should wear protective clothing (light-colored, long-sleeve shirts and light-colored pants tucked into boots or socks). The light-colored clothing allows ticks to be more easily spotted.

Ticks and their hosts (mice, chipmunks, voles, and other small mammals) need moisture, a place hidden from direct sun, and a place to hide. The clearer the area around a house, the less chance there will be of getting a tick bite. All leaf litter and brush should be removed as far as possible away from the house. Low-lying bushes should be pruned to let in more sun. Leaves should be raked up every fall, since ticks prefer to overwinter in fallen leaves. Woodpiles are favorite hiding places for mammals carrying ticks, so woodpiles should be neat, off the ground, in a sunny place, and under cover.

Gardens should be cleaned up every fall, since foliage left on the ground over the winter can provide shelter for mammals that may harbor ticks. Stone walls on the property increase the potential for ticks.

ehrlichiosis, human monocytic   The first type of ehrlichiosis that was discovered in 1985, and which is transmitted by the lone star tick *(Amblyomma americanum)*. About 425 cases have been reported from 30 states, including 10 deaths. Since 1986 about 400 cases have been confirmed in 30 states, mostly in the southeastern and south central United States; nine people have died.

Cause

The disease is caused by *Ehrlichia chaffeensis* or *E. ewingii,* bacteria in the genus Ehrlichia that were only recently identified.

Symptoms

Symptoms are similar to human granulocytic ehrlichiosis (EHRLICHIOSIS, HUMAN GRANULOCYTIC), including fever, headache, chills, malaise, sweating, muscle aches, nausea, and vomiting. The infection may range from a mild illness to a severe, life-threatening disease. It may cause leukopenia (reduction of white blood cells), thrombocytopenia (reduction in blood platelets), anemia, or abnormal liver function.

Treatment

Antibiotics are effective if begun early enough in the disease.

emergency room information   When a child is taken to the emergency room for an injury or illness, there is some important information caregivers should always be prepared to provide. This includes a list of the child's allergies (especially to medications), drugs the child is currently taking, preexisting illnesses, height and weight, plus a record of immunizations.

Allergies

It is vital that emergency room doctors know of any drug allergies a child may have, but any allergies—including food or latex—are important to note. Knowing these details may help emergency personnel find a cause for problems such as seizures or breathing difficulties.

Current Medications

Because some medications should not be taken together, it is important to provide emergency doctors with a list of any drugs (and dosages) the child is currently taking. It is also important to know when the last dose was given.

Preexisting Illnesses

Any preexisting health problems, such as diabetes or asthma, could have a big impact on the kinds of tests or treatments a child might be given in an emergency room. This is so important that a child with a serious chronic condition should ideally wear a medical alert tag, bracelet, or necklace. This is especially important if a child suddenly gets sick at day care, school, or a friend's house. It is also important to keep a record of the dates and types of surgeries a child may have undergone.

Immunizations

Keeping an up-to-date record of a child's immunizations can help doctors rule out some kinds of problems in an emergency. Knowing a child has had a HEPATITIS B injection, or is protected against tetanus, could be very important.

Height, Weight, Blood Type

Knowing a child's accurate height and weight can be important in calculating drug dosages. One thing that is not crucial is knowing a child's blood type. In a true emergency, only the "universal donor" blood type—O negative—will be given in a transfusion.

Emergency Information for Caretakers

Caregivers should know not only how to get in touch with parents at all times but also the name and phone number of the child's doctor. This is vital in case of medical emergency, if the parents cannot be reached. Parents who are going to be separated from a child on a vacation or business trip should leave a medical release allowing the child's caregiver to authorize medical care. However, in a life threatening emergency a medical release would not be necessary, because medical personnel are authorized to do what they must to save the life of someone involved in an accident or other emergency.

encephalitis   Inflammation of the brain usually caused by a viral infection. Often, the meninges (membranes covering the brain) are affected. An attack may be very mild, but in most cases it is a serious condition.

The most common strains of encephalitis in North America include St. Louis encephalitis (SLE), eastern equine encephalitis (EEE), California encephalitis (CE), western equine encephalitis, La Crosse encephalitis, Venezuelan equine encephalitis, WEST NILE VIRUS encephalitis, and Powassan encephalitis (spread by ticks, not mosquitoes). Japanese encephalitis is not found in the United States, but it is very common throughout Asia and poses a risk to international travelers.

Cause

Most of the time, the virus responsible is the HERPES simplex virus type I, which also causes COLD SORES. In the United States it may also be caused by a virus transmitted to humans via mosquito bite, causing St. Louis encephalitis. More and more cases are related to infection with HIV, the organism responsible for AIDS. Occasionally, encephalitis is a complication of other viral infections such as MEASLES or MUMPS.

Symptoms

Usually, symptoms begin with headache, fever, and prostration, leading to hallucinations, confusion, paralysis of one side of the body, and disturbed behavior, speech memory, and eye movement. There is a gradual loss of consciousness and sometimes a coma; epileptic seizures may develop. If the meninges are affected, the neck is usually stiff and the eyes are unusually sensitive to light.

Central nervous system symptoms include some (not all) of these:

- abnormal reflexes
- changes in consciousness
- confusion
- disorientation
- dizziness
- inability to speak
- irritability
- listlessness
- loss of balance
- odor hallucinations
- seizure
- sleepiness
- spasticity
- tremor
- weakness

Diagnosis

Symptoms, signs, and the results of CT scans, EEG, and a spinal tap will help diagnose the disease.

Treatment

The antiviral drug ACYCLOVIR administered intravenously is an effective treatment for encephalitis caused by the herpes virus. If the disease is related to other viral infections, there is no known effective treatment. Depending on the virus causing the problem, some patients will die and some who recover will have brain damage, with mental impairment, behavioral disturbances, and epilepsy. Supportive care is the treatment of choice in these cases.

encephalitis, California   The most common form of a group of viruses that cause encephalitis. First discovered in Central Valley, California, in 1943, this variety is the most common type of encephalitis and infects more boys than girls under age 15 in both rural and suburban areas. La Crosse encephalitis (a widespread encephalitis common in young children) belongs to this group.

The California virus belongs to a group of viruses called bunyavirus. It is a zoonosis (disease passed from animals to humans) and is carried by many different types of mosquitoes, which catch the virus from and give it to both squirrels and chipmunks in wooded areas. La Crosse encephalitis is carried by the *Aedes triseriatus* mosquito.

The infected mosquitoes remain infected for life; because the virus does not remain present in human blood, it is not possible to transmit the virus between humans.

Most adults who live in areas where the mosquitoes live are immune because they have antibodies produced when they were bitten as children. Elderly people may be susceptible, because the immunity appears to wear off with age.

Since the original virus was isolated, other viruses have been isolated that are closely related to California encephalitis. This group of related viruses is now classified as the California serogroup. Several other human pathogens (such as the La Crosse virus) also belong to the California serogroup. Although little human disease was associated with these viruses until 1960, now the California serogroup virus infections are the most commonly reported cause of mosquito-transmitted encephalitis in the United States. From 1996 to 1998 approximately three times as many reported human cases of mosquito-borne encephalitis were caused by the California serogroup viruses as were reported for western equine encephalomyelitis virus, St. Louis encephalitis, and eastern equine encephalitis viruses combined.

Cause

When an infected mosquito bites a child, the virus passes into the blood and then travels to the brain and spinal cord. It multiplies in the central nervous system, inflaming and damaging nerve cells, interfering with signals sent from the brain to other parts of the body.

Symptoms

Only a small percentage of children with the disease exhibit any symptoms, beginning with fever, irritability, drowsiness, headache, and nausea/vomiting. This can lead to convulsions or seizures. Most people recover completely.

Diagnosis

Spinal tap (lumbar puncture) will reveal antibodies to the specific encephalitis virus in cerebrospinal fluid (CSF). The actual virus may be found in brain tissue from those who have died from the disease. Only the antibodies will appear in blood or CSF, not the virus itself; the patients are not infectious and cannot pass the disease on to others; it is spread to humans only by infected mosquitoes.

Complications

Less than 1 percent of children who contract the disease will die. Some may experience occasional seizures or behavioral changes (such as reduced attention span).

Treatment

There is no cure for viral encephalitis. When a child's immune system produces enough antibodies to destroy the virus, the person recovers. Generally, a child with the symptoms of encephalitis is admitted to the hospital for treatment in a darkened room and given medication to reduce fever and treat the severe headache.

Prevention

There are no drugs that prevent California encephalitis.

encephalitis, eastern equine (EEE) The least common of all the arboviral infections, but the most deadly, since one-third of patients will die. This type of encephalitis primarily affects horses, donkeys, and mules along the eastern seaboard; it only affects about five to 10 humans each year in the United States. The viral disease is characterized by inflammation of the brain and spinal cord, often causing serious or fatal nerve damage.

Outbreaks of the disease in horses have occurred along the east coast since 1831. The first human to die of the disease was a Massachusetts baby in 1938. EEE is related to a similar virus that infects horses and humans in the western states called western equine encephalitis.

Most recently a 1996 outbreak in Rhode Island sent oceanside residents into panic, as experts discovered that one out of every 100 mosquitoes in the area were carrying the disease. High school football and outdoor games were moved out of town, and children were urged to stay away from woods and swamps. A state of emergency was declared as tests showed a tenfold increase in infected mosquitoes, and the state sprayed an entire town with an insecticide called resmithrin. Only four people in Rhode Island have ever been recorded as having the virus, however; one of them, a teenager, died in 1993.

In 1991 five older people in northern Florida contracted EEE; two died and three partially recovered. Other cases cropped up in Georgia, Michigan, Louisiana, and South Carolina; at the same time, an epidemic in horses swept along the southeastern states, killing many animals. Two years later, only 88 cases of EEE were reported in horses and only five humans contracted the disease.

Three types of encephalomyelitis occur in horses in the United States: eastern equine encephalomyelitis, western equine encephalomyelitis, and Venezuelan equine encephalomyelitis. Eastern equine encephalomyelitis is a severe form of equine encephalitis; it lasts longer and causes more deaths and problems than either the western or Venezuelan versions. Venezuelan equine encephalomyelitis occurs in Central and South America, as well as Florida and Texas.

Cause

Four different types of mosquitoes carry the virus responsible for EEE. The virus enters the bloodstream through the mosquito bite, traveling directly to the spinal cord and brain. As the virus multiplies in the central nervous system, it damages the nerve cells, interfering with the signals the brain sends to the body.

Despite its name, the primary natural hosts of the viruses of both eastern and western encephalomyelitis are birds, not horses.

Because the virus is not present in the blood of humans, it is not transmitted between people. Since the disease is transmitted primarily by mosquitoes, it occurs most often during the insect season, especially in low, marshy areas. Most people who live in areas where the mosquito carries the virus are immune, since they were bitten as children and developed antibodies without ever becoming sick.

Symptoms

Unlike St. Louis encephalitis in which only a few patients have symptoms, most people with EEE get symptoms, which begin five to 15 days after a mosquito bite. Symptoms begin with headache, fever, chills, muscle aches, and nausea, followed by paralysis, convulsions, and coma. Infants and young children are most at risk for serious cases, but those who are sick for a few days before the paralysis and convulsions appear will probably recover completely.

Diagnosis

Rapid tests to identify antibodies to the EEE virus in blood and cerebrospinal fluid are now available.

Treatment

There is no cure for encephalitis. Pain medication for fever and headache will be given in the hospital.

Complications

Long-term damage may include facial palsy, weakness, seizures, or mental problems. Children younger than five have a poor outlook for recovery.

Prevention

A vaccine can prevent the disease in horses, and should be given in areas where EEE is prevalent. All foals must be vaccinated, and older horses must be revaccinated during the EEE season. An experimental vaccine is available for those who work in labs with the virus.

encephalitis, La Crosse A major type of ENCEPHALITIS in the eastern United States, this disease is caused by the La Crosse virus in the family Bunyaviridae. The encephalitis caused by this virus is most common in children and young adults under the age of 19. The 30 to 180 annual cases of La Crosse encephalitis represent between 8 percent and 30 percent of all cases of encephalitis.

Symptoms

Patients may have all or some of the following symptoms: fever, vomiting, stiff neck, headache, lethargy, seizure, and coma.

Treatment

There is no specific therapy, but most patients recover. The disease is fatal in fewer than 1 percent of cases.

Prevention

There is no vaccine available.

encephalitis, tick-borne A viral infection of the central nervous system caused by a tick bite, usually in children who visit forested areas. Tick-borne ENCEPHALITIS occurs from April through August when the ticks are alive.

Cause

In addition to the bite of ticks, this type of encephalitis can be transmitted by consuming unpasteurized dairy products from infected animals.

Symptoms

Symptoms appear between one to two weeks after the bite of an infected tick or ingesting infected dairy products and resemble symptoms of mosquitoborne encephalitis.

Treatment

Treatment is symptomatic. (See also ENCEPHALITIS, EASTERN EQUINE; ENCEPHALITIS, CALIFORNIA.)

encephalitis, western equine Like eastern equine ENCEPHALITIS, this virus affects horses and humans; this version affects humans primarily in the central and western plains of the United States. It is much rarer than its eastern cousin, with more than 639 confirmed cases since 1964. Human infections are usually first detected in June or July.

Symptoms

Symptoms, which appear between five and 10 days after being bitten, range from mild flu-like illness to full-blown encephalitis, coma, and death. While western equine encephalitis is less often fatal than its eastern cousin, it is still serious and can lead to brain damage and other major complications in about 13 percent of people infected with the disease. About 3 percent of those who develop severe symptoms will die.

Cause

The disease is caused by the western equine encephalitis virus, which is closely related to the eastern and Venezuelan equine encephalitis viruses. The virus flourishes in birds that live near irrigated fields and farming areas.

Treatment

Treatment is supportive.

encephalitis, West Nile   See WEST NILE VIRUS ENCEPHALITIS.

encephalomyelitis   See ENCEPHALITIS, EASTERN EQUINE; ENCEPHALITIS, WESTERN EQUINE.

encephalomyelitis, acute disseminated   (ADE)
A neurological disorder characterized by inflammation of the brain and spinal cord caused by damage to the myelin sheath covering the nerves. The myelin sheath is the fatty covering that acts as an insulator on nerve fibers in the brain.

ADE appears more often in children and typically follows vaccination or infection. A variety of terminologies is used to describe it, including post infectious, parainfectious, or post-vaccinial encephalomyelitis. ADE predominantly affects the white matter of the brain; under a microscope, an invasion of white blood cells around small veins can be seen. Where these cells accumulate, myelin is destroyed. The association of the disease with a prior infection or immunization suggests an immune system problem. Research of ADE patients found that their bodies mount an allergic response against their own brain constituents.

The viral agents most often linked to ADE infections are the viruses that cause St. Louis encephalitis, western equine encephalomyelitis, California encephalitis (see ENCEPHALITIS, CALIFORNIA,) and the MUMPS virus, ECHOVIRUSes, and COXSACKIEVRUS.

ADE was first described 250 years ago by an English physician, who noted that it occurred occasionally in patients who had smallpox.

Diagnosis

A spinal tap will often reveal abnormal cerebrospinal fluid and an increase in white cells and protein. An electroencephalogram usually abnormal shows diffuse slowing. An MRI typically shows multiple areas of abnormality in the white matter of the brain.

Symptoms

Symptoms appear suddenly, with fever, headache, stiff neck, vomiting, and appetite loss quickly followed by confusion, stupor, delirium, and occasionally coma. Neurological examination usually reveals inflammation of the optic nerve, clumsiness, paralysis on one side, and seizures. Some symptoms may last a month; fatal cases may progress in a matter of days. Typically, once the disease ends, further attacks are rare. Recent long-term studies of patients with ADE have shown that a small number later develop multiple sclerosis.

Treatment and Prognosis

There is no specific treatment for viral encephalomyelitis, although high doses of corticosteroids can often quickly improve symptoms, with an excellent prognosis. Overall, the outlook is good where the diagnosis is made early and the appropriate therapy is instituted without delay, but the prognosis for children with ADE varies. Some youngsters experience a complete or nearly complete recovery, but permanent complications are common in infants and children who survive the initial infection.

encopresis   Incontinence with feces. Encopresis is a problem that children can develop due to chronic constipation. Once children become constipated, they may avoid using the bathroom to avoid discomfort. As stools become impacted and unable to move forward, the rectum and intestine become enlarged due to the hard, impacted stool. Eventually, the rectum and intestine have problems sensing the presence of stool, and the muscle at the end of the digestive tract that helps retain the stool loses its strength. At this point, liquid stool can start to leak around the hard, dry, impacted stool, soiling a child's clothing.

Cause

Any child with chronic constipation may develop encopresis. Constipation can be caused by a junk-food diet, drinking too many sodas and sugared drinks, not drinking enough water and fruit juices, lack of exercise, and stress.

Boys are six times more likely to develop encopresis. Even though family stress can be linked to constipation, there does not seem to be any link between developing encopresis and number of siblings, birth order, age, or the family's income

Complications

Encopresis can cause both physical and emotional problems. Impacted stool in the intestine can cause abdominal pain, appetite loss, and bladder infections. In addition, affected children may feel ashamed or embarrassed and may avoid going to school, playing with friends, or spending the night away from home. Parents may feel guilt, shame, anger, or distaste, which can further upset the child.

Symptoms

Symptoms may include loose, watery stools; needing to have a bowel movement with little or no warning so that a child cannot get to the bathroom in time; scratching or rubbing of the anal area due to irritation by watery stools; withdrawal from friends, school, and/or family.

Diagnosis

A physician may order a number of tests, including an abdominal X ray to evaluate the amount of stool in the large intestine; a barium enema to check the intestine for blockage, narrow areas, and other problems.

Treatment

Treatment for encopresis may include removing the impacted stool, keeping bowel movements soft so the stool will pass easily, retraining the intestine and rectum to gain control over bowel movements. An enema may be prescribed to help remove the impacted stool. In addition, medications may be prescribed to help keep the child's bowel movements soft for several months. This will help prevent stool impaction from occurring again. Often, boosting the amount of fiber in the child's diet will help, including adding more fruits and vegetables, more whole grain cereals and breads, with fruit juice and water. Children should not eat too much junk food or drink too many caffeinated beverages. Whole milk should be limited to 16 ounces a day for children over two but should not be eliminated altogether. Since eating a meal will often stimulate a bowel movement within 30 minutes to an hour, meals should be served on a regular basis. Increasing the amount of exercise a child gets can also help with constipation. Exercise aids digestion by helping the normal movements the intestines make to push food forward as it is digested, and children who do not move around much are often constipated.

Until the intestine and rectum regain their muscle tone, children may still have "accidents" and soil their underwear on occasion. Preschool children may wear disposable training pants until they regain bowel control. Taking a change of underwear to school can help lessen a child's embarrassment and improve self-esteem as bowel control improves.

endotoxin shock   See SEPTIC SHOCK.

enterovirus   A virus that multiplies primarily in the intestinal tract. This type of virus includes COXSACKIEVIRUS, ECHOVIRUS, and poliovirus.

enuresis   See BED-WETTING.

ependymoma   A common slow-growing childhood brain tumor that may be either benign or malignant. This type of tumor may alter the flow of cerebrospinal fluid, causing buildup of fluid in the brain (HYDROCEPHALUS). The third most common brain tumor in children, up to 30 percent of ependymomas occur in children younger than three. Half of all ependymomas occur in the first two decades of life.

Ependymomas do not usually grow rapidly, they are not invasive and usually do not spread. In unusual cases, the risk of sudden death from a large ependymoma results from increased intracranial pressure of the tumor and excess fluid pressing on the brain.

Symptoms

Nausea and vomiting occur in about 80 percent of patients, together with a headache caused by pressure that is usually worst in the morning. There may be behavior changes such as lethargy, irritability, diminished social interaction, and loss of appetite, and problems with balance.

Treatment

An ependymoma usually cannot be completely removed because of its location, either on the brain floor or deep in the cerebral hemisphere. The best treatment depends on the tumor's location and whether it has spread. However, in general, the preferred treatment of an intracranial ependymoma is aggressive surgical removal of as much as possible.

If complete removal is impossible, treatment with radiation therapy and/or chemotherapy is considered.

Recurrence of an ependymoma depends upon how much of the tumor was removed, as well as the success of radiation or chemotherapy. Most recurrent ependymomas reappear close to their original location. An ependymoma can, however, spread within the central nervous system. Treatment options for a child with a recurrent ependymoma may include another surgery, chemotherapy, and further radiation.

epiglottitis Inflammation of the epiglottis, a thin flap of cartilage lying behind the root of the tongue that covers the entrance to the larynx during swallowing. Acute epiglottitis is a severe form of the condition that usually affects children. The condition is also called epiglottiditis.

Cause

Epiglottitis is caused by *Haemophilus influenzae* type B, an aggressive bacterium that at one time caused many serious infections in children under age five. The vaccine against this bacteria has essentially wiped out all cases of *H. influenzae* epiglottitis, MENINGITIS, CELLULITIS, and PNEUMONIA, diseases that used to kill or cripple several thousand chil-

dren a year. Rare cases of epiglottitis still occur, now caused by other bacteria such as *Staphylococcus aureus* and *Streptococcus pneumoniae.*

Symptoms

The severe form is characterized by sore throat, fever, noisy breathing, croupy cough, and a swollen epiglottis. The patient may turn blue and require an emergency tracheostomy to maintain breathing.

Treatment

Antibiotics, rest, oxygen, and supportive care.

epilepsy A chronic condition of the nervous system marked primarily by recurrent seizures. Epilepsy may express itself in major *(grand mal)* seizures causing unconsciousness, or in minor *(petit mal)* seizures. It is sometimes associated with other conditions including specific LEARNING DISABILITIES or attention disorders.

About 1 percent of all children will develop epilepsy, which means that about 690,000 children and young adults in the United States have some type of epilepsy. About 55,000 new cases of epilepsy are diagnosed each year in children under age 18.

Cause

In 70 percent of cases there is no known cause for the condition. Of the remaining cases of epilepsy, the cause may be linked to head injury, birth trauma, brain malformations, poisoning, infection, brain tumors, mother's illness during pregnancy, heredity, or degenerative brain disorders.

Symptoms

Seizures may include convulsions, brief stares, muscle spasms, odd sensations, or episodes of automatic behavior and altered consciousness.

Diagnosis

One of the most important clues in diagnosing epilepsy is usually found in the child's medical history, which includes as much information as possible about the actual seizures. Family members often will be asked to record details about the seizures to help the doctor determine the type of epilepsy.

A doctor can diagnose epilepsy from a number of different tests. Which tests are ordered may vary, depending on how much each test reveals, but they may include:

- a thorough physical examination, especially of the nervous system
- blood work (blood sugar, complete blood count, electrolytes, and liver and kidney function tests)
- electroencephalogram (EEG)
- brain scans (magnetic resonance imaging [MRI], computed tomography [CT] scans, or PET scans [positron emission tomography])

Treatment

Epilepsy is a lifelong condition that is usually controllable with some combination of medication, diet restriction, surgery, or a new type of therapy called vagus nerve stimulation. Unfortunately, about 20 percent of children with epilepsy are unable to gain complete control over their seizures.

Of all available treatments, medications known as antiepileptic drugs are the most often prescribed therapy for seizures. More than 20 medications are available to treat epilepsy. If medicines are not able to prevent seizures, other methods such as surgery or a special diet may be tried. The goal of all epilepsy treatment is to prevent further seizures, avoid side effects, and make it possible for the patient to lead a normal, active life.

Most epilepsy medicines are taken by mouth in the form of tablets, capsules, sprinkles, or syrup. They may include:

- carbamazepine (Tegretol, TegretolXR, Carbatrol)
- clonazepam (Klonopin)
- ethosuximide (Zarontin)
- phenobarbital
- phenytoin (Dilantin)
- primidone (Mysoline)
- valproic acid (Depakene)
- divalproex sodium (Depakote)

Newer drugs which are also prescribed for epilepsy include felbamate (Felbatol); gabapentin (Neurontin); lamotrigine (Lamictal); levetiracetam (Keppra); oxcarbazepine (Trileptal); tiagabine (Gabitril); topiramate (Topamax); and zonisamide (Zonagran). Other new drugs are in development.

A rectal gel form of diazepam (Diastat) may be prescribed to stop cluster seizures or prolonged seizures. Some doctors may prescribe pills of diazepam (Valium), lorazepam (Ativan), or clonazepam (Klonopin) for the same purpose.

A steroid drug (ACTH) may be injected to treat children with a type of epilepsy called infantile spasms, or for severe seizures that cannot be controlled with other drugs.

The particular drug that is prescribed depends on what kind of seizure a child is having, since different drugs control different types of seizures. People also react to these medicines in different ways. Some experience side effects, others may not. Some people's bodies break down medicines at a faster or slower rate than the average person. Once a medication is found to be successful, it can be closely monitored by blood tests to ensure that the correct amount of medication remains in the blood at all times.

Diet A special diet called a ketogenic diet may help treat seizures by changing the way the body derives energy. When the diet is first introduced, a child may need to be hospitalized so the physician can closely supervise the process. Although this diet was first introduced 80 years ago before the advent of most antiepileptic drugs, it has recently become more popular, especially with children whose seizures do not respond to medication. About 30 percent of children may control their epilepsy by the ketogenic diet alone.

Surgery Up to 30 percent of children who have epilepsy are candidates for surgery because they either do not respond to antiepileptic drugs or experience unpleasant side effects and may not succeed on the ketogenic diet. At least one-half of these children may be successfully treated through epilepsy surgery, if the seizures are confined to a small segment of the brain.

Surgery for epilepsy is a delicate, complicated operation that must be performed by an experienced surgical team. In addition to operations that remove a small part of the brain where seizures begin, other procedures may be done to interrupt the spread of electrical energy in the brain.

Vagus nerve stimulation This newer type of treatment may help children whose seizures are hard to control. With this treatment, a surgeon implants a small pacemaker under the skin below the collarbone that is attached to wires programmed to deliver a small burst of electrical energy to a nerve in the neck.

Epilepsy Foundation A national, charitable organization founded in 1968 and dedicated to the welfare of people with EPILEPSY. The foundation's mission is to work for children and adults affected by seizures through research, education, advocacy, and service. More than 60 affiliated Epilepsy Foundations serve people with seizures, and their families, in hundreds of communities nationwide.

The foundation is composed of volunteers committed to the prevention and cure of epilepsy and to a positive quality of life for everyone who lives with seizure disorders. Goals include broadening and strengthening research, providing easy access to reliable information, and assuring access to appropriate medical care for those affected by seizures.

On the local level, affiliate groups offer a variety of services including School Alert, camping, information and referral, education, and support groups. Respite care, assisted living, employment services, advocacy, and case management may also be offered. Nationally, the foundation offers research and research training grants and fellowships to scientists working to find the answers to epilepsy. The foundation supports national public education, legal and government advocacy, a national library, toll-free information services, media campaigns, and a broad array of educational materials. (For contact information, see Appendix I.)

Epstein-Barr virus (EBV) One of the most common human viruses that occurs around the world. A member of the HERPES family, EBV infects almost everyone at some point. In children, the virus causes no symptoms or only mild signs. In the United States and other developed countries, many children are not infected by the virus; if they become infected during adolescence, the virus causes infectious MONONUCLEOSIS.

Epstein-Barr virus (EBV) does not leave the body but establishes a lifelong dormant infection in some of the body's immune system cells. A very few carriers will go on to develop Burkitt's lymphoma and cancer of the nose and throat, two rare cancers that are not normally found in the United States. EBV appears to play a major role in the development of these cancers, but it is not considered to be the only cause.

Transmission of the EBV requires contact with saliva of an infected person, since the virus is not normally transmitted through air or blood.

erysipelas Contagious infection of the facial skin and subcutaneous tissue caused by *Streptococcus pyogenes* and marked by rapid-spreading redness and swelling, which is believed to enter the skin through a small lesion. While this disease is contagious, it does not produce huge epidemics like those of SCARLET FEVER.

Before the advent of antibiotics, this disease could be fatal, especially for infants and the elderly. Today it is quickly controlled with prompt treatment.

Symptoms
After a five- to seven-day incubation period, the patient experiences a sudden high fever with headache, malaise, and vomiting. The skin feels tight, uncomfortable, itchy and red, with patches appearing most often on the face, spreading across the cheeks and bridge of the nose. It also occurs on the scalp, genitals, hands, and legs. Within the inflammation, pimples appear, blister, burst, and crust over.

Treatment
Penicillin-class antibiotics will cure the infection within seven days. Bed rest, hot packs, and aspirin for pain and fever may also help.

erythema infectiosum See FIFTH DISEASE.

erythematous shellfish poisoning See SHELLFISH POISONING.

erythrasma A bacterial infection of the toe web, groin, and underarms that causes mild burning and itching. It is more common in warmer climates and among diabetics.

Cause

The infection is caused by *Corynebacterium minutissimum*. Recurrences are common.

Treatment

C. minutissimum is very sensitive to a wide variety of antimicrobial drugs; extensive cases may also require oral administration of erythromycin. Tolnaftate and Whitfield's ointment are also beneficial.

erythromycin (E-mycin, Erythro, Erythrocin, Robimycin, Ery-Tab, Erycette) An antibacterial antibiotic used to treat many bacterial and mycoplasmic infections, especially those that cannot be treated with penicillin. In children under age eight, it is the alternative to TETRACYCLINE, an antibiotic that can permanently stain developing teeth.

Because the drug is destroyed by acid in the stomach, the drug should be taken in coated forms, or as a compound. Patients with liver disease should not use this drug.

Side Effects

Possible side effects include nausea and vomiting, stomach pain, diarrhea, and an itchy rash. Certain brands of erythromycin may be taken with food to reduce the chance of irritating the stomach.

Escherichia A genus of gram-negative rodlike bacteria that are found in the intestines of humans and many animals. Named for the 19th century German physician Theodor Escherich who identified it, the genus is the most frequent cause of urinary tract infections and is commonly found in wounds.

Escherichia coli (E. coli). is a species of coliform bacteria normally found in the intestines, milk, water, and soil. Part of the reason it can be dangerous is that it comes in so many different strains that are capable of reproducing at extraordinary rates, doubling its population every two hours. If enough food were available, one *E. coli* cell could reproduce into a mass bigger than the earth in three days. Fortunately, most of the strains are harmless to the majority of children most of the time. However,

E. coli blood poisoning can be rapidly fatal as a result of shock caused by the action of the endotoxin it releases.

There are five groups of *E. coli* whose toxins can cause traveler's diarrhea. The worst is ESCHERICHIA COLI 0157:H7, which can cause a dysentery-type of fatal bloody diarrhea.

Escherichia coli 0157:H7 One of hundreds of strains of the bacterium *Escherichia coli*—a type that has emerged during the past 10 years as a cause of food-borne illness leading to HEMOLYTIC UREMIC SYNDROME (kidney failure and death). The combination of letters and numbers in the name of this bacterium refers to specific markers found on its surface and distinguishes it from other types of *E. coli*. The number of this type of *E. coli* food poisoning cases appears to be increasing, as has the frequency of complications from infection.

Although most strains of *E. coli* are harmless and live in the intestines of both humans and animals, the 0157:H7 strain produces a powerful toxin that can cause severe illness. An estimated 10,000 to 20,000 cases of infection occur in the United States each year. Most illness has been associated with eating undercooked, contaminated ground beef.

This particular *E. coli* mutation, which has 62 subtypes, was first recognized as a cause of illness in 1982 during an outbreak of bloody diarrhea which was traced to contaminated hamburgers. During this outbreak, scientists discovered that the *E. coli* 0157:H7 strain had somehow acquired the gene for Shiga toxin, caused by the organism *Shigella dysenteriae*. The strain of *E. coli* caused three outbreaks in 1982 among scores of patients who came down with an alarming type of diarrhea that appeared as if it were all fresh blood. The strain continued to appear sporadically, until in 1993 four children died and hundreds more fell ill after eating *E.-coli*-tainted hamburger in a fast-food restaurant in Washington. The incident set off a furor throughout the country, as consumer safety groups urged the government to beef up its meat inspection system.

The Washington outbreak was followed within months by more outbreaks of food-borne illness caused by *E. coli*, forcing the closing of two other restaurants and sickening 60 more consumers.

Annually the CDC estimates that *E. coli* alone is responsible for 20,000 cases of food poisoning, although these estimates may not be accurate since physicians are not required to report these poisonings.

A study by the Western States Meats Association found that *E. coli* was present in 1.5 percent of ground pork and also in poultry, and 3.7 percent in beef. In the past, people got *E. coli* food poisoning by drinking tap water in foreign countries. In the wake of the mass poisonings and deaths from *E. coli* poisoning, the government vowed to revamp the federal meat inspection system, which relied on visual inspections. In related action, the United States Dairy Association (USDA) decided to issue new labels for raw meat and poultry that discuss safe handling and cooking methods.

The Shiga gene has continued to spread and has now been found in other strains of *E. coli,* as well as other bacteria common to the human intestine, such as enterobacter.

Figures from the Centers for Disease Control suggest there may be 20,000 illnesses a year in this country, with 250 to 500 deaths from *E. coli* 0157:H7 alone. According to experts at the Food-borne Diseases Epidemiology Section of the federal centers, an additional 10,000 to 20,000 cases of food poisoning may be caused by Shiga toxin from other strains of bacteria for a total of perhaps 40,000 cases in the United States. This is part of an estimated total of about seven million cases of food-borne illness in general.

Recent epidemics have included the November 1996 cases involving a 15-month-old Colorado child who died after drinking tainted unpasteurized Odwalla apple juice; another 50 people became sick. In the summer of 1996 a similar epidemic swept Japan, killing seven people and infecting almost 9,000 Japanese. In the biggest outbreak, 6,500 people came down with *E. coli* infection in Sakai; the infection was traced to city-supplied school lunches.

Outbreaks have been traced to many different types of food. It has been found to survive in dry fermented meat despite production standards that meet federal and industry food processing requirements, scientists say. It has been found in salami, where the bacteria may have been present on raw meat that was brought into a plant and subsequently survived the fermentation and drying steps involved in salami production.

Primarily, the organism is found in a small number of cattle farms, living in the intestines of healthy cattle. Meat becomes contaminated during slaughter, and organisms can be mixed with beef when it is ground in huge vats. Alternatively, bacteria on a cow's udders or on milking equipment can find its way into raw milk.

Since contaminated meat looks and smells normal, it is possible to eat tainted meat unknowingly. Although the number of organisms needed to cause disease is not known, it is believed to be very small.

The problem is not with steak; a bit of bacterial contamination on the surface of a steak is not much of a threat, because it is quickly killed when the meat hits the pan. It is the practice of grinding the meat that gives bacteria its chance. When a contaminated steak is minced up and mixed with other beef from other animals, the bacteria become widely distributed—not just on the surface but throughout the meat. Contaminated and undercooked hamburger is suspected of causing more than half of all outbreaks of bloody diarrhea. Many outbreaks have begun in fast-food restaurants, but since the large chains have begun to sample their meat, the real problem today lies in grocery store hamburger, according to experts. The meat in grocery stores, the experts say, goes largely untested.

The toxin-making bacteria are killed only if the hamburger is cooked to an inside temperature of 155°F, hot enough to eliminate all meat pinkness.

Drinking unpasteurized milk, as well as swimming in or drinking sewage-contaminated water, also can cause infection.

The disease can also be transmitted from person to person through contact with contaminated stool, if hygiene or handwashing is not adequate. This is especially common in day care centers and among toddlers who are not yet toilet trained.

Symptoms

The *E. coli* 0157:H7 bacterium produces toxins that cause severe cramps and then watery or bloody diarrhea lasting for several days. Other symptoms include nausea and vomiting appearing within hours to a week after eating, but not usually any fever. Most people recover quickly and completely, but the complications are what make this a serious disease.

In certain people at risk (such as among the very young or old), the bacteria may cause hemolytic uremic syndrome (HUS), in which the red blood cells are destroyed and the kidneys fail. Between two and seven percent of infections lead to this complication. In the United States HUS is the main cause of kidney failure in children; most cases are caused by infection with this type of *E. coli*.

Patients are infectious for about six days while bacteria are being excreted in the stool. There is no solid evidence, but it appears that victims can get this infection more than once.

Diagnosis

The infection is diagnosed by identifying the bacterium in stool. Most labs that culture stool do not test for *E. coli* 0157:H7, so it is important to request that the stool be tested for this organism. Everyone with sudden diarrhea with blood should have the stool checked for this bacterium.

Treatment

Most patients recover within 10 days without need of specific treatment. There is no evidence that antibiotics help, and there is some evidence to suggest they may set off kidney problems. Antidiarrhea medicine should also be avoided.

HUS, on the other hand, is a life-threatening condition that is treated in a hospital intensive care unit, with blood transfusions and kidney dialysis. With intensive care, the death rate from this complication is between 3 and 5 percent. There is no cure for HUS.

Complications

Children who have had only mild infection, with diarrhea, usually recover completely. Of those who develop HUS, one-third have abnormal kidney function years later and a few need long-term dialysis. Another eight percent suffer with other complications, including high blood pressure, seizures, blindness, and paralysis, for the rest of their lives.

Prevention

To protect against this type of food poison, travelers should not use untreated water and ice, salads, raw fruits and vegetables that cannot be peeled, and uncooked milk products. Diners should always make sure hamburgers are well done.

Parents can prevent infection by thoroughly cooking ground beef, avoiding unpasteurized milk, and washing hands carefully. Undercooked beef should not be served to young children or anyone with an impaired immune system.

When caring for an infected patient, hand washing is crucial to avoid person-to-person spread of the disease.

About 38 states now ask doctors to report outbreaks of the disease but none regularly test for other strains of *E. coli* that produce the toxin.

exanthem subitem   See ROSEOLA.

expressive language disorders   Impairments in the ability to express ideas through language characterized by problems with vocabulary, grammatical structures, word order, and overall language development. Expressive language disorders may have a severe impact on an individual's ability to generate spoken language and may be associated with other language-based learning disorders, such as reading disability or written expression disorder. Three to 10 percent of all school-age children have an expressive language disorder.

There are a number of disorders relating to expressive language. *Dysnomia* refers to the inability to remember and express specific words. Individuals with dysnomia may "talk around" a word in order to express an idea without finding the appropriate words. For example, someone with dysnomia might say, "that thing you eat that is yellow and long" when attempting to say "banana."

Expressive language disorders also include those patients who can remember the word they want to say but cannot physically manipulate their speech muscles to produce the word. This disorder is called apraxia. Disorders in oral expressive language are called expressive aphasia. Students would be considered aphasic if they have problems expressing themselves orally but have no difficulty understanding language spoken to them and are successful with nonverbal tasks.

Cause

Although the cause of these disorders is unknown, brain damage and malnutrition have been associated as underlying factors. The condition can be present at birth or acquired at a later time, if brain damage or a medical condition affects otherwise normal development.

Diagnosis

Expressive language disorders are diagnosed by tests of discrepancy between verbal performance and nonverbal and receptive measures of potential performance. Because of a general cultural bias toward associating intelligence with communication, individuals with an expressive-language disorder may often be seen by others as less capable and intelligent than they actually are, even when nonverbal measures indicate extremely high intellectual potential.

Treatment

Expressive language disorders are treated by speech language pathologists.

eye infections The most common infection of the eye is CONJUNCTIVITIS, also known as pinkeye. Most of these infections are caused by bacteria such as staphylococci, or by viruses associated with a cold, sore throat, or illness such as MEASLES. Viral conjunctivitis is the version that often appears in schools, sweeping through classrooms in massive epidemics.

Newborns may contract a serious type of conjunctivitis from their mothers during birth caused by common bacteria, organisms responsible for gonorrhea or genital herpes, or by a chlamydial infection; this may cause blindness in the newborn unless promptly treated. Keratoconjunctivitis is an inflammation of both the conjunctiva and the cornea, often caused by a virus. Corneal infections are more serious and can lead to blurry vision or perforation if not treated.

Infection within the eye may make it necessary to remove the eyeball. This can occur after a penetrating injury to the eye, or as a result of infections that travel to the eye from elsewhere in the body.

failure to thrive A description applied to a child whose weight or rate of weight gain is significantly below others of similar age and sex. Failure to thrive can be caused by a wide variety of problems, such as genetic, physical, psychological, or social factors.

Although it is not unusual for newborns to lose a little weight in the first few days, some infants fail to pick up on expected weight gain and growth. Usually caused by inadequate nutrition or a feeding problem, failure to thrive is most common in children younger than age three. Failure to thrive also may be a symptom of a physical problem such as an infection. Child neglect or abuse also may be associated with failure to thrive.

During the first few years of life, most children gain weight and grow very quickly. Many children who lag behind these standards are perfectly normal—they simply fall at the lower end of the growth chart. Others, however, are considered to suffer from "failure to thrive."

Because this general diagnosis has many possible causes, it is important to identify any underlying problems for children who fail to thrive. Once the cause is understood, doctors and the family can work together to encourage the child to maintain a healthy growth pattern.

Although it has been recognized for more than a century, there is no one precise definition for "failure to thrive," primarily because it describes a condition rather than a specific disease. Children who fail to thrive do not receive, or are unable to take in or retain, adequate nutrition to gain weight and grow as expected. The condition is common in babies born prematurely, usually in conjunction with other medical problems linked to prematurity.

Symptoms

Typically, a child who is failing to thrive starts out growing well but over time begins to lag behind, first in weight and then in height. Symptoms of failure to thrive include height, weight, and head circumference in an infant or young child that do not progress normally according to standard growth charts (weight is lower than the third percentile, weight is 20 percent below ideal weight for height, or drops off from a previously established growth curve). Physical skills such as rolling over, sitting, standing, and walking are slow to develop, and mental and social skills are delayed.

If the condition is allowed to continue, the undernourished child may become apathetic and irritable and may begin to miss developmental milestones such as sitting up, walking, and talking at the usual age.

Cause

Some children fail to thrive because of a medical problem. There are multiple causes of failure to thrive that will disturb the body's metabolism enough to result in delayed growth. These include:

- chromosome problems such as DOWN SYNDROME and Turner's syndrome
- defects in major organ systems
- endocrine abnormalities, such as thyroid or growth hormone deficiency
- brain or central nervous system damage
- abnormalities in the cardiac and respiratory systems causing disturbed mechanisms to deliver oxygen and nutrients
- anemia or other blood disorders
- abnormalities in the gastrointestinal system, which may result in malabsorption or absence of digestive enzymes resulting in inadequate nutrition

Some conditions such as CEREBRAL PALSY, chronic GASTROENTERITIS, and gastroesophageal reflux (usually temporary) may contribute to this problem. Psychological and social causes may include emotional deprivation as a result of parental withdrawal, rejection, or hostility. Economic factors can affect nutrition, living conditions, and parental attitudes. Environmental factors may include exposure to infections, parasites, or toxins. Sometimes the cause is undetermined.

With reflux, the esophagus may become so irritated and painful that the child refuses to eat. Persistent diarrhea can interfere with the body's ability to use the calories from food. Problems with absorption such as CYSTIC FIBROSIS, chronic liver disease, and celiac disease all interfere with the body's ability to absorb nutrients, so that no matter how much the infant eats, the body does not retain enough of that food.

An intolerance of milk protein can lead to restrictions of the child's diet. Infections or parasites place great demands on the body, and can trigger short- or long-term failure to thrive. INBORN ERRORS OF METABOLISM can also limit a child's capacity to make the most of calories. Many other medical causes, such as neurologic, cardiac, endocrine, and respiratory problems can be suspects as well.

Sometimes doctors find that parents' attitudes or behaviors are causing the failure to thrive. Some parents restrict the amount of calories they give their infants out of fear that the child will get fat. Other children fail to thrive as a result of neglect—the parents simply do not feed them enough. Although in the past doctors tended to categorize cases of failure to thrive as either organic (caused by an underlying medical disorder) or inorganic (caused by caregiver actions), they are less likely to make such sharp distinctions today. This is because medical and behavioral causes often appear together. For example, a baby with a CLEFT PALATE who is reluctant to eat may cause stressful feeding times for a parent, who then becomes tense and frustrated, making it hard to sustain attempts to feed the child adequate amounts of food.

Risk Factors
Risk factors for failure to thrive are related to the causes and may include underlying undiagnosed diseases, poverty, negative emotional environments, and crowded or unsanitary living conditions.

Diagnosis
Most diagnoses of failure to thrive are made in infants and toddlers in the first few years of life. Because a child's brain grows as much in the first year as it will during the rest of the child's life, poor nutrition during this period can permanently harm mental development. It is perfectly normal for many babies to go through brief periods when their weight gain slows or they even lose a little weight. However, doctors usually get concerned if a baby does not gain weight for three consecutive months during the first year of life.

Doctors diagnose failure to thrive by plotting the child's weight, length, and head circumference on standard growth charts. Children who fall below a certain weight range for their age or who drop down two or more percentile curves on the weight chart over a short period of time will likely be evaluated further to determine if there is a problem.

The following laboratory tests may be performed:

- complete blood count (CBC) to detect anemia
- electrolytes (basic chemistries)
- urinalysis
- thyroid function tests
- other hormone studies
- hemoglobin electrophoresis to determine the presence of conditions such as sickle-cell disease
- X rays to determine bone age

If the doctor suspects a particular disease or disorder as a possible cause, specific tests to identify that condition can help. To determine whether the child is receiving enough food, the child's doctor can do a calorie count after asking the parents what the child eats every day. Talking to the parents can help a doctor identify any problems at home, such as neglect, poverty, household stress, or difficulty during feedings. A Denver Developmental Screening Test reveals delayed development.

Treatment
Treatment depends on the cause of delayed growth and development. Delayed growth due to nutri-

tional factors can be resolved by educating the parents and planning a well-balanced diet. Parental attitudes and behavior may contribute to a child's problems and need to be examined. In many cases, a child may need to be hospitalized to focus on implementing a comprehensive medical, behavioral, and psychosocial treatment plan.

If the period of failure to thrive has been short and the cause is determined and can be corrected, normal growth and development will resume. If failure to thrive is prolonged, however, the effects may be long lasting.

An entire medical team may be needed to help solve the problem, including a primary doctor, a nutritionist to evaluate the child's dietary needs, and an occupational or speech therapist to help the parent and child develop successful feeding behaviors and address any sucking or swallowing problems the child might have. For simple cases of poor nutrition, the doctor will recommend high-calorie foods and place the child on a high-density formula like Pediasure. The treatment can usually be carried out at home, with frequent visits to the doctor's office. More severe cases may require tube feedings at home. The tube runs from the nose into the stomach (or directly into the stomach) and the child is usually fed at night so as not to interfere with daytime activities or limit the desire to eat during the day. About half of a child's caloric needs can be delivered at night through a continuous drip. Once the child is better nourished and begins to feel better and eat more, the tube can be removed.

A child with extreme failure to thrive may need to be hospitalized for continuous feeding and monitoring. During this time, any possible underlying causes of the condition are treated. This also gives doctors the chance to watch the parents' feeding technique and to assess the interaction between parent and child.

Weight gain takes time, so several months may pass before a child is back in the normal range. Children who require hospitalization usually stay for 10 to 14 days or more, but it can be many months until the symptoms of severe malnutrition fade away.

Failure to thrive caused by a chronic illness or disorder may have to be monitored periodically and treated for a long time.

Prevention

The best way to prevent failure to thrive is by early detection at well-baby checkups, and periodic follow-up with school-age and adolescent children.

fainting Loss of consciousness caused by a temporary lack of oxygen to the brain. Known by the medical term *syncope,* fainting may be preceded by dizziness, nausea, or a feeling of extreme weakness. Fainting is extremely common in childhood—about one in five children faint at some point. In a small number of children it is a sign of heart disease, but that is really very rare. In most it occurs when they are ill, under physical or psychological stress, when they are hungry—or for no good reason at all.

An attack may be caused by extreme pain, fear, or stress resulting from an overstimulation of the vagus nerve, which helps control breathing and circulation. A child could faint from prolonged coughing or by straining to defecate or to blow a wind instrument. Another cause could be remaining in a stuffy environment without enough oxygen. In addition, standing still or standing erect for long periods of time can cause fainting due to blood that pools in the leg veins, cutting down on the blood available for the heart to pump to the brain.

Treatment

A fainting episode fades away as soon as normal blood flow to the brain is restored. This usually happens as soon as the child hits the ground, because the head is then placed at the same level as the heart. To head off an attack, a child should not stand for 10 to 15 minutes after regaining consciousness.

If a child does not regain consciousness after a minute or two, medical help should be obtained immediately. Repeated attacks should be checked out by a pediatrician.

Prevention

When a child senses an impending fainting attack, losing consciousness can be prevented by having the child sit with the head between the knees, or lying flat with the legs raised above the level of the heart.

Fainting should not be confused with a breath-holding spell, a type of temper tantrum in children usually under six years of age.

fears Fears are a normal part of growing up as youngsters explore the world around them, having new experiences and confronting new challenges. In fact, up to 43 percent of children between ages six and 12 have many fears and concerns.

Common Fears

One of the most common anxieties is a fear of darkness—especially being left alone in the dark—and a fear of animals, such as large barking dogs. Some children are afraid of fires, high places, or thunderstorms, while others worry about burglars, terrorists, kidnappers, or nuclear war. If there has been a recent serious illness or death in the family, children may worry about the health of remaining family members.

SEPARATION ANXIETY DISORDER is also common in young children. Sometimes this fear can intensify when the family moves to a new neighborhood or children are placed in a child-care setting where they feel uncomfortable. Youngsters might become afraid of going to summer camp or even attending school. Their phobias can cause physical symptoms like headaches or stomach pains and eventually lead the children to withdraw into their own world, becoming clinically depressed.

In middle childhood, fears come and go. While the concerns of most children this age are fairly mild, sometimes these fears can become so extreme that they develop into phobias. Phobias are strong and irrational fears that can become persistent and debilitating, significantly influencing and interfering with a child's usual daily activities.

For instance, a 10-year-old child might become so terrified about news reports on terrorism that he keeps a baseball bat under his bed or a Swiss army knife under his pillow. Some youngsters in this age group develop phobias about the people they meet in their everyday lives. This severe shyness can keep them from making friends at school and relating to most adults, especially strangers. They might consciously avoid social situations like school dances or birthday parties, and they often find it difficult to talk comfortably with anyone except their immediate family.

Phobias

It is normal for children to have fears, such as taking a test, facing a growling dog, or waiting out a thunderstorm. A phobia is more than fear, however—it is an extreme response, a kind of fear that does not go away. A child with a phobia will be afraid of something every time it is seen or experienced, not just afraid once or twice. Children with phobias often go out of their way to avoid the situation or object that frightens them. The fear can be so severe that facing the situation or object can trigger a panic attack. This can make a child feel even more anxious and upset.

Specific phobias in childhood, as distinguished from normal fears, are excessive and persistent. Children with phobias try to avoid the specific situations or objects they fear, and when confronted with the threatening stimulus, they often "freeze." A reaction may also be judged phobic when the threatening stimulus is benign, and fear is thus inappropriate, such as when a child who is phobic about snakes sees a picture of a snake in a book and "freezes." There are many different kinds of phobias common in childhood, such as the fear of failure, the dark, injury, small animals, death, and going to the dentist. One of the most common, however, is social phobia, in which a child is terrified of being embarrassed in front of other people. A child with a social phobia might feel afraid of talking to a teacher or of walking in front of the classroom on the way to the bathroom. A child with a social phobia can find it nearly impossible to give a book report in front of the class, or even enjoy a birthday party. Although it is normal to have some slight degree of nervousness in those situations, a child with a social phobia becomes so afraid that the phobia interferes with the enjoyment of life. A child with a social phobia is not just shy but absolutely unable to control the fear of being with others.

Agoraphobia is a phobia in which a child worries about having a panic attack in a place where leaving would be difficult or embarrassing. The fear of the panic is so strong that the child often avoids places such as crowds, highways, or a busy mall where a panic attack might occur.

Also, fears that may be normal for younger children may be considered phobic if experienced by an older child.

Cause

Scientists do not really know why some children become phobic, but experts suspect it may be genetic. For example, a child with a social phobia may have a parent with a similar fear. Sometimes a traumatic event in a child's life, such as the death of a parent or a divorce, can trigger a phobia.

About five out of every 100 Americans have at least one phobia. Most social phobias appear in adolescence, although any phobia can begin when children are much younger.

Treatment

If the phobias persist and interfere with a child's enjoyment of day-to-day life, professional help from a psychiatrist or psychologist who specializes in treating phobias can be helpful. Behavioral treatments have shown the greatest results in treating childhood phobias. Some of the most effective behavioral treatments are systematic desensitization, prolonged exposure, modeling, and cognitive self-management strategies.

Therapists suggest the best way to treat phobias is to expose a child to the source of the anxiety in small, nonthreatening doses. Under a therapist's guidance, for example, a child who is afraid of snakes might begin by talking about this fear and by looking at photographs or a videotape of snakes. Next, the child might watch a live snake from behind the safety of a window. Then, with a parent or a therapist at her side, the child might spend a few minutes in the same room with a small, docile snake. Eventually the child will be able to touch the snake. This gradual process is called desensitization, in which a child slowly becomes a little less sensitive to the source of the fear each time it is presented. Ultimately, the child will no longer feel the need to avoid the situation that has been the basis of the phobia.

While this process sounds simple, it should be done only under the supervision of a professional. It takes time for a child to confront and gradually overcome the anxiety.

What Parents Can Do

Since fears are a normal part of life, parents should be reassuring and supportive, acknowledging—without increasing or reinforcing—their child's concerns. Parents can point out what is already being done to protect the child and involve the child in identifying other things that can be done. Simple, sensitive, and straightforward parenting can resolve or at least ease most childhood fears. Parents can explain that many children have fears, but with support the child can learn to manage them. Parents should never ridicule a child's fears, particularly in front of the child's friends.

Parents also can encourage a child to progressively confront the feared object or situation. If the child is afraid of dogs, the parent can hold hands as the child watches a dog through a window. If a child is afraid of water, a parent could accompany the child as they wade together into a children's pool with the water reaching no farther than the knees. If every small success is praised, the next step will be easier. Attention should be focused on what the child has accomplished, not on the anxiety itself. Breathing and relaxation exercises can help children in stressful circumstances. Occasionally the pediatrician may recommend medications as part of the treatment program, although this should never be the only treatment method. Drugs may include antidepressants, which are designed to ease the anxiety and panic that often underlie these problems.

fear of animals One of the most common fears that children experience is the fear of animals—most often dogs. While the fear of animals affects almost all children, it seems to decrease as the child gets older. In the intervening years, a number of approaches can lessen a child's fears.

Treatment

A child who has been attacked by a animal should have professional therapy to help deal with the traumatic event. For most children, however, the fear of animals has not been triggered by violence, but by something as simple as a large dog running toward them. While the dog's intentions may have been to play, the sight of a large unknown creature heading directly toward the child can prompt some youngsters to be nervous toward all dogs.

It is important for parents to acknowledge, not belittle, a child's fear. Dogs can be unpredictable, and it is important that all children realize the potential danger that dogs can present. However, they must also be reassured that most dogs are perfectly friendly. A parent might say: "Dogs can be scary, but this little one lives across the street and he wants to be your friend."

Because the unknown intensifies fear, a child should be encouraged to learn about dogs and the proper way to behave around them. Allowing a child to tease or mistreat a dog in any way could result in a bite, which would only reinforce their fears. At the same time, a child should never be forced to pet an animal, no matter how cuddly the parents think the pet may be, nor should parents encourage hand-feeding animals whose bite may be bigger than the portion offered.

It may help to take a child to visit a neighbor who has a friendly, small dog that is good with children; regular visits will show the child that dogs can be friendly. At this point, the family of a child who is afraid of pets may want to consider getting a small dog or cat so the two can grow up together, and the child can help feed and care for the animal.

Eventually, children's fear of dogs may fade away as they get older.

Prevention

Many people develop a lifelong fear of an animal when they are bitten or growled at during childhood. To head off the development of such a phobia, parents should train their very young children how to handle animals in the following situations:

- *Do not disturb an eating animal* Children should understand that cats and dogs can become defensive when eating, so children should not startle an animal or put a hand near a bowl when the pet is eating.

- *Never take a toy or bone from a dog's mouth* Children should be taught that if a dog is unwilling to drop the toy, the child should have an adult retrieve it.

- *Pet nicely* Children should understand that pets are not toys, and that they should not pull an animal's tail or ears, poke its eyes, or throw things at it.

- *Never sneak up on a pet* Parents should teach children that dogs and cats can become defensive when frightened. They should approach a pet from the front with hands visible, speaking in a low, soft voice.

- *Observe body language* Children must be taught what it means when a dog raises its tail, with ears back, hair standing, teeth bared, and bark-

ing or growling—all signs that the dog should not be confronted. Children should avoid cats with hair standing, tail stiff, ears back, dilated eyes, and hissing.

- *Never run* Children must be taught that if they ever come face to face with a dog showing the above warning signs, they must not scream, run, or stare into the animal's eyes, because if they run the dog may chase and attack. A child should always walk away slowly, avoiding any eye contact with the dog.

- *Do not invade a dog's space* A child should never insert a hand into a car window or dog pen, because the dog might bite to defend its territory.

- *Do not separate fighting dogs* Children should be trained to get an adult to help break up a dogfight and not try to pry the animals apart.

- *Ask permission* No matter how friendly a dog appears to be, children should be trained to always ask the owner's permission before petting an unknown dog or cat.

fear of the dark Typically, a child who is afraid of the dark has developed a phobia because parents have insisted that the child must stay in a totally dark room at night. Parents need to recognize the fact that a room looks different to a child in the dark and take steps to reassure the child even if the fear seems completely irrational.

Experts agree that there is nothing wrong with allowing a child to use a night light, as long as it does not create frightening shadows. After the light has been turned out, the parent should stay in the room for a few minutes and talk about how different things look. The door to the child's room should be left slightly ajar, and the child should know the parent will be close by.

Treatment

Behavioral treatments have shown the greatest results in treating childhood phobias. Some of the most effective behavioral treatments are systematic desensitization, prolonged exposure, modeling, and cognitive self-management strategies.

fear of death At about age six or seven, as children develop an understanding about death, some youngsters can develop a fear of death—either their own or that of a loved one. Realizing that death will eventually claim everyone, and that it is permanent and irreversible, the normal worries about the death of family members or their own death can intensify. In some cases, this preoccupation with death can become disabling. It is perfectly normal that children should be curious about death, but the average child generally does not really fear death until facing the loss of a family member or pet.

What Parents Can Do

Parents should be willing to discuss death with the child in a reassuring way. Because it is a child's lack of knowledge that triggers fear, adults should be honest with the child when someone close to the family dies. Many children believe they may have caused the death, especially if they ever had angry thoughts about the person. It is vital that parents explain this is not the case.

Many experts feel that a child should be at least five years of age before being exposed to a funeral home or funeral service—and only then if he is willing. Parents may want to describe a funeral or viewing as a way of saying good-bye to the deceased. Under no circumstances should a child be forced to touch, kiss, or even approach the coffin of the dead person.

Parents may find it helpful to discuss their own childhood fears about death, explaining that they understand how scary such fears can be.

fear of school The fear of school, also called school phobia, is not unusual in young children, especially those entering kindergarten for the first time. Such a fear may be caused by a number of different fears, so dealing with school phobia centers on finding out what is causing the problem.

Some children are not really afraid of school but of leaving home. Others are not really fearful of school but of riding the school bus, getting lost, failing, or being teased. Each of these possibilities must be examined and dealt with individually. School fears can be eased by teaming the child up with a friend who can share the bus ride or play at recess.

A child who is really afraid of leaving home needs to feel that parents are comfortable with the idea of school, and that a parent will be at home when the child leaves school.

fear of separation See SEPARATION ANXIETY DISORDER.

febrile seizure See SEIZURES.

Federation for Children with Special Needs A center for parents and parent organizations to work together on behalf of children with special needs and their families. Organized in 1975 as a coalition of parent groups representing children with a variety of disabilities, the federation operates a Parent Center in Massachusetts that offers a variety of services to parents, parent groups, and others who are concerned with children with special needs.

The federation tries to provide information, support, and assistance to parents of children with disabilities, their professional partners, and their communities. The group is committed to listening to and learning from families and encouraging full participation in community life by all people, especially those with disabilities. (For contact information, see Appendix I.)

feeding problems Eating is a natural response to hunger, and the habits children develop early in life can influence their attitudes toward food for the rest of their lives. While a child who is reluctant to eat can be upsetting to parents, in fact most children go through at least one fussy-eating phase, refusing most of the foods they are offered. In most cases, these are just phases, and studies have found that while children may appear not to eat much over the course of a day, in fact over a week's time their intake is almost always adequate.

Most feeding problems can be resolved if parents simply provide a varied, appealing selection of healthy meals and snacks, allowing children to eat as much or as little as they wish. Mealtime battles are almost always a guaranteed losing proposition for parents, because in fact it is almost impossible to make a reluctant child eat.

Of course, guidelines about eating are still important. Excessive snacking interferes with normal appetite controls and can lead to weight gain and poor eating habits. Meals featuring healthy selections should be scheduled at regular intervals, and food should never be used as a bribe or reward. Just like adults, all children have likes and dislikes, and wise parents will respect their preferences where possible.

Infant Feeding Problems

A breast-fed baby under six months of age who is always restless and failing to gain weight even when emptying the breast may not be getting enough calories. A pediatrician should examine the baby and make recommendations for possible changes in diet or feeding methods. A bottle-fed baby who turns away from the bottle, or who vomits after most feedings, may in fact be getting too much food. Babies who avoid the bottle usually are full; persisting in trying to feed is not effective. However, if the infant vomits even after drinking less milk, a pediatrician should be consulted.

Some babies refuse solid food at first when it is introduced between ages four and six months. This is normal during the transition from a liquid diet. If the baby truly gets upset, solid foods should be stopped and then reintroduced a few weeks later.

Older Children

As babies enter toddlerhood, their growth slows down and they may eat and drink less. This is a normal appetite adjustment for this age group. Parents should serve smaller portions and not insist the child eat everything on the plate.

By the time children enter elementary school, they should have improved their eating habits and left their picky eating behind. For children this age who still refuse many foods, excessive snacks should be avoided and healthy meals offered on a regular basis.

At the other end of the eating problem spectrum are those children who seem to eat constantly, snack too much, or hoard food. These habits may develop as the result of stress, anxiety, or poor impulse control and can lead to overeating and weight gain. Parents should consult with a pediatrician about what is a normal, healthy weight for the child and offer healthy food in normal portions.

fetal alcohol syndrome (FAS)   A condition that describes the physical and mental birth defects in a child caused by the mother's excessive consumption of alcohol during pregnancy. Maternal use of alcohol during pregnancy may have been a factor for a substantial number of children receiving special education services.

More than 10 percent of children have been exposed to high levels of alcohol before birth. All will suffer varying degrees of effects, ranging from mild learning disabilities to major physical, mental, and intellectual impairment. It takes very little alcohol to cause serious damage; research has shown that even a single exposure to high levels of alcohol can cause significant brain damage in an unborn child.

Cause

Alcohol in a pregnant woman's bloodstream circulates to the fetus by crossing the placenta. There, the alcohol interferes with the ability of the fetus to receive enough oxygen and nourishment for normal cell development in the brain and other body organs.

Symptoms

A variety of problems are typically associated with fetal alcohol syndrome (FAS), including:

- *Growth deficiencies*   Small body size and weight, slower than normal development, and failure to catch up
- *Skeletal deformities*   Deformed ribs and sternum; curved spine; hip dislocations; bent, fused, webbed, or missing fingers or toes; limited movement of joints; small head
- *Facial abnormalities*   Small eye openings; skin webbing between eyes and base of nose; drooping eyelids; nearsightedness; failure of eyes to move in same direction; short upturned nose; sunken nasal bridge; flat or absent groove between nose and upper lip; thin upper lip; opening in roof of mouth; small jaw; low-set or poorly formed ears
- *Organ deformities*   Heart defects; heart murmurs; genital malformations; kidney and urinary defects
- *Central nervous system problems*   Small brain; faulty arrangement of brain cells and connective

tissue; mental retardation—usually mild to moderate but occasionally severe; learning disabilities; short attention span; irritability in infancy; hyperactivity in childhood; poor body, hand, and finger coordination

Diagnosis

Early diagnosis can help prevent secondary disabilities such as mental health problems, dropping out of school, trouble with the law, and substance abuse. After diagnosis, parents often find that their ability to cope with the child's behavior changes dramatically when they understand that the problems are most likely based on organic brain damage, rather than the child's choice to be inattentive or uncooperative.

Treatment

FAS is a lifetime disability with no cure; a child will not outgrow the problem. However, early and intensive intervention can make an enormous difference in the prognosis for a child. Up to about age 10 or 12 is the best time to intervene, since this is the period of greatest development of fixed neural pathways.

Prevention

FAS is preventable if a woman refrains from using alcohol during pregnancy. Studies suggest that drinking a large amount of alcohol at any one time may be more dangerous to the fetus than drinking small amounts more often. The fetus is most vulnerable to various types of injuries depending on the stage of development in which alcohol is encountered.

Because a safe amount of drinking during pregnancy has not been determined, all major authorities agree that women should not drink at all during pregnancy. Unfortunately, women sometimes wait until a pregnancy is confirmed before they stop drinking. By then, the embryo has gone through several weeks of critical development, a period during which exposure to alcohol can be very damaging. Therefore, experts urge women who are pregnant or anticipating a pregnancy to abstain from drinking alcoholic beverages.

fever An abnormal internal temperature of the body above 98.6°F due to disease, although the normal range depends on when and how the temperature is taken. Normal body temperature is lower in the morning and higher in the late afternoon and evening. Right after activity, a child's temperature may rise to 99°F. Rectal temperatures are up to a degree higher and under-the-arm temperatures are usually up to a degree lower than 98.6°F.

The thermal regulatory center in the brain is responsible for controlling the body's temperature. This setting rises during an infection, resulting in a fever, because white blood cells release certain proteins during the immune response. These proteins trigger the brain to release a chemical called prostaglandin, which causes the nerve cells to produce a feeling of coldness. This is why a patient experiences chills during the development of fever. In response to this coldness, the brain increases the body's temperature, speeding up the activities of the immune system against the invading germs. What this means is that a fever is actually not a thing to be avoided—it can actually help the body fight disease. Many parents do not understand this and become concerned as soon as a child runs a slight fever.

However, a very high fever can be uncomfortable and eventually—if it goes high enough—can lead to seizures and death.

Temperatures may be taken with either an oral or a rectal thermometer. Those who find a mercury thermometer hard to read may find a digital readout thermometer easier. While some doctors rely on this type of instrument, others insist that digital thermometers are not as accurate. Ear thermometers are also an option, although they should not be used in children under six months of age. A rectal thermometer is used for infants and young children who cannot hold an oral thermometer in their mouths. An oral thermometer should not be used to take a rectal temperature.

After each use, the thermometer should be cleaned using lukewarm soapy water and rinsed well with cold water. Hot water will break a mercury thermometer. The thermometer may be rinsed instead with alcohol followed by cold water.

The course of a fever depends on its cause. The degree of the fever does not really indicate how serious the illness is, however. Severe infections may only cause a low fever, and some mild infections can cause a high fever.

Treatment

Some parents prefer to treat a fever to lessen a child's discomfort or to head off the likelihood of febrile seizures. Treating a fever in children lessens the risk of seizures, which tend to run in families and occur in less than 3 percent of normal children up to six years of age. While they can be alarming to parents, febrile seizures last less than 15 minutes and do not cause brain damage or EPILEPSY.

Medication Medicines called "antipyretics" will bring down a fever. For example, aspirin and acetaminophen lower fever by slowing the production of prostaglandins. Because fevers are beneficial, however, most doctors recommend that a child should only take antipyretics for fevers over 101°F. Anything lower than this is considered to be a low-grade fever that may simply be a sign of a mild infection.

In an infant younger than three months of age, however, any fever over 100.4°F requires medical evaluation.

Aspirin should not be given to any child under age 18, because it has been associated with REYE'S SYNDROME, a very serious condition affecting the brain and liver, in children who have a viral infection such as INFLUENZA or CHICKEN POX.

Other methods If the fever is very high, a pediatrician may recommend a lukewarm tub bath or a wet sheet. A child should not be immersed in cold water, however, because this can lower the body temperature too quickly.

Children should not be rubbed with alcohol, since the fumes can be dangerous and there is evidence that alcohol can be absorbed through the skin.

When to Call the Doctor

Any child under three months of age with a rectal temperature higher than 100.4°F must see a doctor right away. Older infants and children should see a doctor right away if they have a fever above 102°F, a fever that lasts longer than three days, a fever that rises after two days, or if any of the following warning signs develop:

- unusual irritability, screaming, tense or stiff arms or legs

- extreme drowsiness (child hard to wake)
- confusion, delirium, hallucinations
- breathing problems (wheezing, crackling, high-pitched sounds)
- neck pain, stiff neck, holding neck in odd way
- seizures
- sunken or bulging soft spot on head (especially in front)
- vomiting after trying to drink fluids
- dry lips, tongue, and mouth
- no wet diaper or urination in 12 hours

A child should see a doctor within 24 hours for fever accompanied by:

- stomach pain
- sore throat, difficulty swallowing
- ear pain; pulling, tugging, or rubbing ear

fever blister   Another name for COLD SORE.

fifth disease   A viral infection that often affects red blood cells. Fifth disease is also known as "slapped cheeks disease" because of the telltale bright red rash across the cheeks. Named in 1899 as the fifth of six common childhood illnesses that cause a rash (after MEASLES, MUMPS, CHICKEN POX, and GERMAN MEASLES), it is the least well known.

Among healthy children the disease is mild; once the rash appears they are not contagious and may return to school.

Cause

This viral disease is caused by parvovirus B19, usually occurring in small outbreaks among young children in the spring. The virus itself was discovered in England in 1975, but it was not until 1983 that scientists realized it caused fifth disease.

In much the same way as a cold spreads, fifth disease is passed from one child to the next via mouth and nose secretions or from contact with contaminated objects. The virus also may travel through the air in small droplets and can be carried in the blood of infected patients, so a blood transfusion could pass on the disease.

Outbreaks occur from late winter through spring among school-age children. About 60 percent of adults have already been infected with the virus and have lifetime immunity, but adults who have never been exposed can catch the disease.

Symptoms
The illness begins with a headache, slight tiredness, or muscle pain followed in two or three days by a rash of rosy red spots on the cheeks which join to form one large red rash. Within a few days, the rash has spread over the body, buttocks, arms, and legs. There is often a mild fever in addition to the skin rash. About half the time, the rash will be itchy. Children with fifth disease appear to be contagious during the week before the rash appears; by the time the rash occurs, the person is probably beyond the contagious period.

Most babies born to mothers with the disease are normal and healthy, although the virus can cross the placenta and infect the fetus.

Children with sickle-cell disease do not get fifth disease. Instead, when these children are infected with the virus they develop a more serious infection called aplastic crisis in which their bone marrow stops making red blood cells.

Diagnosis
In most cases, the disease is diagnosed based on the appearance of typical symptoms. A specific blood test to confirm the diagnosis has recently become available but is not necessary in normally healthy children.

Treatment
There is no treatment for fifth disease. With bed rest, clear fluids, and acetaminophen to lower fever, the rash usually clears within 10 days. Red blood cells are given to sickle-cell patients. Fevers over 101°F should be treated; calamine lotion will ease the itch of the rash.

Complications
High-risk patients who contract fifth disease may experience chronic anemic conditions afterward. Those at high risk include anyone with sickle-cell anemia, HIV infection, or red blood cell abnormalities, who is undergoing immunosuppressive treatment for cancer, or who is an organ transplant recipient.

Prevention
As yet there is no way to control the spread of fifth disease.

fighting Toddlers and preschool-age children often fight over toys. Sometimes children are unintentionally rewarded for aggressive behavior. For example, one child may push another child down and take away a toy. If the child cries and walks away, the aggressive child feels successful since he or she got the toy. It is important to identify whether this pattern is occurring in children who are aggressive.

It is more effective to intervene in a disagreement when a parent sees the child frustrated or upset, before a child starts hitting. Young children who tend to fight should be supervised more closely. If one child hits another, the two should be immediately separated. Children should not be hit if they are hitting others, because this teaches them to use aggressive behavior.

If the fighting occurs between siblings, this should not be ignored by parents who assume that such disagreements are "normal." When hitting or fighting is frequent, it may be a sign that a child is sad or upset, has problems controlling anger, has witnessed violence, or may have been the victim of abuse at day care, school, or home.

Research suggests that children who are physically aggressive at a younger age are more likely to continue this behavior when they are older. Studies also indicate that children who are often exposed to aggression on TV or in videos or movies themselves act more aggressively.

Treatment
A young child who has a persistent problem with fighting, biting, or aggressive behavior should be taken to a child and adolescent psychiatrist or psychologist who specializes in the evaluation and treatment of behavior problems in very young children.

firearms Firearm injuries are the second leading cause of death for young people 10 to 24 years of age. For every child killed, four are wounded. According to the Centers for Disease Control and Prevention and the CENTER TO PREVENT HANDGUN

VIOLENCE, in 1994 nearly 90 percent of homicide victims aged 15 to 19 were killed with a firearm. Of violent deaths in schools, 77 percent are caused by firearms. About half all homes in the United States contain a firearm, and more than half of the handguns at home are loaded. In 1996 more than 1,300 children aged 10 to 19 committed suicide with firearms.

Many experts believe that the best way to protect children against gun violence is to remove all guns from the home. If guns are kept in the home, there will always be dangers, but the danger can be lessened by:

- storing all firearms unloaded and uncocked in a securely locked container whose whereabouts is known only to the parents
- guns and ammunition should be stored in separate locked locations
- a revolver should have a trigger lock or a padlock around the top strap of the weapon to prevent the cylinder from closing
- a pistol should have a trigger lock

A gun being handled or cleaned should never be left unattended, even for a moment. Parents who do not own a gun should check with other parents where their children play to make sure safety precautions are followed. Nearly 40 percent of accidental handgun shootings of children under 16 occurred in the homes of friends and relatives, most often when children were left unsupervised.

Children and adolescents with emotional or behavioral problems may be more likely than other children to use guns, against themselves or others. Parents who are concerned that their child is too aggressive or might have an emotional disorder may wish to seek an evaluation by a child and adolescent psychiatrist.

The average American child witnesses a great deal of violence on TV, in movies, and through computer games. Studies have found that children are more aggressive after extensive viewing of violence. Experts suggest that parents watch TV, movies, and videos with their children, ration TV, and disapprove of the violent episodes in front of the children, stressing the belief that such behavior is not the best way to resolve a problem.

fireworks   Each year fireworks injure thousands of American children and teenagers; in 1999, 3,825 children younger than 15 were treated in U.S. hospital emergency departments for fireworks-related injuries. Boys between five and 14 years of age have the highest fireworks-related injury rate. The hands (40 percent), eyes (20 percent), and head and face (20 percent) are the areas most often involved, and about a third of all eye injuries from fireworks result in permanent blindness.

Many types of fireworks are perfectly legal to use, but every type of legally available consumer firework has been associated with serious injury or death. Nearly two-thirds of fireworks-related injuries are caused by backyard class C fireworks such as firecrackers, bottle rockets, Roman candles, fountains, and sparklers, all of which are legal in many states. More than half of all fireworks-related injuries are associated with firecrackers, followed by bottle rockets and sparklers.

The most severe injuries, however, are usually caused by class B fireworks such as rockets, cherry bombs, and M-80s, which are federally banned from public sale. About 29 percent of all injuries are caused by illegal firecrackers.

In spite of federal regulations and varying state bans, class B and C fireworks are often easily bought by children. It is not uncommon to find fireworks distributors near state borders, where residents of states with strict fireworks regulations can take advantage of more lenient state laws next door.

How Accidents Occur

Bottle rockets can fly into a child's face and cause eye injuries, whereas sparklers can ignite clothing (sparklers burn at more than 1,000°F). Firecrackers also can injure a child's hands or face if they explode at close range. Injuries also may occur from standing too close to fireworks when they explode; for example, if a child bends over to look more closely at a firework that appears to be a dud, or when a misguided bottle rocket hits a nearby child.

Parental supervision is key to avoiding many accidents. One study estimates that children are 11 times more likely to be injured by fireworks if they are unsupervised. In addition, while many younger children lack the physical coordination to handle fireworks safely, they are often excited and curious around fireworks, which can increase their chances of being injured. Homemade fireworks also can lead to dangerous explosions.

Prevention

There are a number of simple guidelines that can make holidays safer for children:

- Only legal fireworks should be used, and only where they are allowed. Forest areas and national parks do not allow any fireworks.
- An adult should light the fireworks, and children should be supervised closely. Children aged 10 to 14 are most at risk, and boys suffer nearly three times the risk of injury.
- Fireworks should be used only in approved open areas and on flat, firm surfaces.
- Lighted fireworks should never be held in the hand, and used fireworks should cool before they are picked up. A bucket of water should be nearby to douse sparklers and other used fireworks before disposing of them.
- All warning labels and instructions should be followed carefully.
- If a lighted firework goes out or does not burn properly, consumers should not return immediately to check. After five minutes, an adult should carefully approach and place the firework into a bucket of water. The fuse should not be reignited.
- Fireworks, matches, and lighters should always be kept out of the reach of small children, who should never play with fireworks.

first aid kits Every home with a child should have a basic first aid kit available, one for the home and one for the car. Pharmacies sell prepared kits, or a family can assemble one themselves with the following important ingredients:

- acetaminophen chewable tablets or liquid for children
- adhesive tape (1-inch roll)
- antibiotic cream
- antihistamine tablets or liquid
- bandage: 3 inches wide
- bandage strips (adhesive)
- bandage tapes (butterfly) with thin adhesive strips
- calamine lotion
- cotton roll
- cotton swabs
- dressings, nonstick (4 inches square)
- elastic bandage (3 inches)
- flashlight
- hydrogen peroxide 3 percent
- petroleum jelly
- safety pins
- scissors
- soap
- thermometers (oral/rectal)
- tweezers

If the family assembles the kit themselves, they should periodically check the medications and replace items past their expiration date.

fish, contaminated High in protein, low in calories, fat, and cholesterol—and widely believed to protect against heart disease and cancer—this highly praised health food can also be vulnerable to contamination and spoilage. The problem is that fish readily soak up poisons and contaminants in water; tiny fish pick up contaminants from the plankton they feed on in polluted water, concentrating heavy metals in their organs. These fish are eaten by larger fish, further concentrating the toxins, and in big fish—such as swordfish and tuna—the contaminants may reach levels harmful to humans. The danger of fish contamination is not just with the contaminants they ingest. Because bacteria that live on fish are adapted to withstand the cold waters of lakes and oceans, they can thrive in temperatures cold enough to preserve other food. These microbes will quickly spoil the fish, unless it is kept at temperatures close to freezing. Even under the best conditions, fish lasts only seven to 12 days. It often takes about seven days for fish to get from the water to the supermarket, where it may sit for several more days.

Fish should look and smell fresh, with vivid skin and bright eyes, and no fishy or ammonia odor. It should be displayed on ice at the store; otherwise, fish is best selected from the bottom of the refrigerator case, where it is coldest. Once brought home, fish should be kept very cold and eaten within a day or two. It should be cooked thoroughly, although no amount of cooking will destroy contaminants.

5p-Society This nonprofit group was founded in 1986 by parents of children with 5p-syndrome (CRI DU CHAT SYNDROME), to provide information and support. The organization has no paid staff and relies on donations from its more than 600 members. (For contact information, see Appendix I.)

flatfeet A harmless orthopedic condition present in many babies that usually corrects itself as the child grows. Children who have flatfeet have an arch that never fully develops. Parents often first notice their child has what they describe as "weak ankles," in which the ankles seem to turn inward because of the way the feet are planted. This is simply a normal variation of human anatomy that does not usually cause any problems for the child. A child with flatfeet has just as much athletic potential as any other child.

Cause

A child's arch will usually develop whether the child wears shoes or goes barefoot, but one in seven children never develops an arch. Some normal arches are taller than others, but children usually have low arches because they are loose jointed, so that the arch flattens when they stand up. Usually, when the child does not put weight on the foot, the arch is apparent.

Treatment

Experts do not usually recommend special footwear (such as shoes with ankle or arch supports, or wearing a pad under the arch) because these treatments do not really affect arch development and may make the child uncomfortable. For children up to age three with flexible flatfeet, prescribing expensive shoe modifications and inserts is not necessary unless there is a strong family history of flatfeet persisting into adulthood. Even then, a prescription for orthopedic shoes probably treats the parents more than the child. Treatment is usually considered only if the condition becomes painful, in which case the pediatrician may recommend a heel cup or a shoe insert.

Surgery is not helpful for most children with flatfeet. Rarely, surgery may be considered if a child's flatfeet are caused by fused foot bones, and if shoe inserts and casts have not helped. However, a fixed or semirigid flatfoot usually involves bony and soft tissue structural changes that do not improve by simply altering footwear to relieve symptoms, and surgery is indicated in these children.

Consult a Doctor

A pediatrician might be concerned if the flatfoot is painful, so stiff that the toes do not bend up or down, or if the child seems to walk only on the inside of the foot instead of on the entire foot.

Healthy Footwear

Barefoot people have the healthiest feet, but children do need some protection to keep out the cold and ward off injuries. A child needs a flexible, soft shoe that allows freedom for the feet to develop normally. Fashion is not nearly as important as healthy feet, so parents should make sure a child's shoes meet the following guidelines:

- *Good fit* It is better for a shoe to be too large rather than too small. Shoes should be bought at least a half-inch longer than the child's feet, because children's feet grow quickly and because the toes need enough room to move.

- *Flexibility* Shoes with soles that are too stiff limit movement, which is necessary to develop strong legs, ankles, and feet.

- *Protection* A child's foot needs to be safe from cold and sharp objects, yet still move freely.

- *Good soles* A flat, rubber sole wears well and may prevent falls.

- *Soft material* Shoes should be made of soft materials that can "breathe," such as leather and canvas. This is especially important in hot weather.

• *Avoid*   Shoes with pointed toes and heels over 3/8″ high are poor choices. (See also BOWED LEGS; PIGEON TOE; TOE-WALKING; KNOCK-KNEES.)

flattened head syndrome   See POSITIONAL PLAGIO-CEPHALY.

flu   See INFLUENZA.

fluoride   A mineral that occurs naturally in all water sources (including the oceans) and that has been proven to reduce cavities in both children and adults. The fluoride ion comes from the element fluorine, the 17th most abundant element in the Earth's crust. Fluoride works to prevent cavities by strengthening teeth under the gums in the jawbone, and by strengthening tooth enamel on the surface of the teeth.

Fluoride's benefits for teeth were discovered in the 1930s when dental scientists noted remarkably low decay rates among people whose water supplies contained significant amounts of natural fluoride. Several studies conducted during the 1940s and 1950s confirmed that when a small amount of fluoride is added to the community water supply, decay rates among residents of that community decrease.

Children between six months and age 16 should take fluoride every day, but only at appropriate levels, according to the American Academy of Pediatric Dentistry (AAPD).

Two of the most common sources of fluoride are via tap water and fluoridated toothpaste. Although fluoride occurs naturally in all water sources, in most major municipalities it has been added to the water to help prevent tooth decay for the past 50 years. The recommended fluoride level in community water systems is 0.7 to 1.2 parts fluoride per million parts water.

However, as more parents turn to bottled water for drinking and food preparation, pediatric dentists are concerned about whether children will get enough fluoride. Most bottled water brands do not contain fluoride, although some types of bottled water do add fluoride to the final product and are safe for children of all ages.

Pediatric dentists recommend that children who regularly drink well water or unfluoridated bottled or tap water take fluoride vitamins, drops, or tablets.

Families who use water filters need to understand whether the devices filter out fluoride. Countertop filters and pitcher-type filters usually do not remove fluoride, but more sophisticated, point-of-use filters can. Consumers who want to filter tap water but keep fluoride can use a charcoal- or carbon-activated filtration pitcher (such as Brita) that offers better-tasting water without removing fluoride.

It is also possible to obtain professionally applied fluorides in the form of a gel, foam, or rinse applied by a dentist or dental hygienist during dental visits. These fluorides are more concentrated than the self-applied fluorides and therefore are not needed as frequently. The American Dental Association (ADA) recommends that dental professionals use any of the professional strength, tray-applied gels or foam products carrying the ADA Seal of Acceptance; there are no ADA-accepted professional fluoride rinses for use in dental offices.

While fluoride is important, it only works when used at the appropriate levels. Too much fluoride can cause a harmless discoloration of the teeth known as enamel fluorosis, which is usually caused when children take fluoride supplements despite the fact that their tap water is fluoridated. If there is enough fluoride in children's primary source of drinking water, they do not usually need supplements. Since it is impossible to know how much fluoride is in a child's primary source of drinking water without having it tested, a pediatric dentist should test the fluoride level of bottled, tap, or well water before supplements are prescribed. However, it is important to remember that a child may be drinking fluoridated water from sources other than the home water supply, such as school or day care, water in processed beverages, and foods prepared with fluoridated water.

Regardless of whether or not their water is fluoridated, children need to brush with a pea-sized amount of fluoridated toothpaste after breakfast and before bed. Parents need to supervise children's tooth brushing until age eight, when most children have the manual dexterity to accomplish this task on their own.

Children also need to visit the dentist early in life to assess fluoride needs. Exactly when to schedule that first dental visit is controversial, however. Pediatric dentists recommend scheduling a child's first dental visit when the first tooth appears or no later than the first birthday, to evaluate fluoride needs before the child's permanent teeth come in. But the American Academy of Pediatrics recommends that barring risk factors for tooth problems such as sleeping with a cup or bottle, teeth staining, or thumb sucking, the first visit to the dentist should be scheduled by the third birthday.

Parents should be careful in using toothpaste with children under age two, since children this age cannot spit the toothpaste out after brushing and tend to swallow it. Too much fluoride taken internally between the ages of two and four can lead to discolored teeth. Alternatively, younger children can use a nonfluoridated toothpaste such as Baby Orajel Tooth and Gum Cleanser until they can spit out toothpaste.

While some critics worry that fluoride may be linked to problems such as lower IQ in children, the Centers for Disease Control (CDC) calls the fluoridation of drinking water as one of the 10 greatest public health achievements of the 20th century. It notes that water fluoridation has helped improve the quality of life in the United States through reduced pain and suffering related to tooth decay, reduced time lost from school and work, and less money spent to restore, remove, or replace decayed teeth. Fluoridation, according to the CDC, is the single most effective public health measure to prevent tooth decay and improve oral health over a lifetime, for both children and adults.

Fluoridation to prevent tooth decay has been endorsed by the AAPD, ADA, American Academy of Pediatrics, American Medical Association, U.S. Public Health Service, and the World Health Organization.

food allergy An immune system response to a food that the body mistakenly believes is harmful. Once the immune system decides that a particular food is harmful, it creates specific antibodies to it in an attempt to protect the body. The next time the child eats that food, the immune system releases massive amounts of chemicals (including histamine) in order to protect the body. These chemicals trigger a cascade of allergic symptoms that can

affect breathing, the heart, the skin, or the gastrointestinal tract. Most food allergies trigger reactions such as itching, hives, and swelling, but in some cases a more serious response known as anaphylactic shock can occur. This leads to a loss of consciousness or even death.

Scientists estimate that between six and seven million Americans suffer from true food allergies. Many food allergies disappear as the child gets older; about a third of cases disappear in one to two years if the child carefully avoids the offending item. However, allergies to peanuts, nuts, fish, and shellfish often do not disappear with time.

Many different common foods may trigger an allergic reaction, including citrus fruits, dairy products, wheat, eggs, fish, cola drinks, artificial coloring, shellfish, berries, tomatoes, pork, and nuts. Infants prone to allergies may be especially sensitive to milk and milk products, wheat, eggs, and citrus fruits. Allergic reactions can be caused by even very tiny (even undetectable) amounts of the food. For example, a child who is allergic to peanuts could go into anaphylactic shock after eating a food that only has been touched by peanuts. Food additives also may cause problems. About 15 percent of children who are allergic to aspirin are also sensitive to Yellow Dye # 5 (tartrazine).

Although a child can be allergic to any food, the following eight foods account for 90 percent of all food-allergic reactions: milk, egg, peanuts, tree nuts (such as walnuts or cashews), fish, shellfish, soy, and wheat.

Milk There are a number of hidden sources of milk that can be of concern to children with food allergies:

- *Deli meats* Meat slicers are frequently used for both meat and cheese products and so could contaminate sliced meats.

- *Casein* Some brands of canned tuna fish contain a milk protein derivative called casein. Many nondairy products also contain casein, listed on the ingredient labels. Some meats also may contain casein as a binder.

- *Steaks* Many restaurants put butter on steaks after they have been grilled to add extra flavor. The butter is not visible after it melts.

- *Goat's milk*   Because goat's milk protein is similar to cow's milk protein it may cause a reaction in milk-allergic individuals. Goat's milk is not a safe alternative for children allergic to cow's milk.
- *Coffee drink foam*   Eggs and/or milk are used to create the foam topping on specialty coffee drinks; they are also used in some bar drinks.

Kosher symbols may help parents determine if a product is milk-free. A system of product markings is used to indicate whether a food is kosher (produced in accordance with Jewish dietary rules). A "D" or the word "dairy" on a label next to "K" or "U" (usually found near the product name) indicates the presence of milk protein; a "DE" on a label indicates that the food was produced on equipment shared with dairy. If the product contains neither meat nor dairy products it is Pareve (Parev, Parve). Pareve-labeled products indicate that the products are considered milk-free according to religious specifications. However, under Jewish law, a food product may be considered Pareve even if it contains a very small amount of milk, which means it could potentially have enough milk protein in it to cause a reaction in a milk-allergic individual.

A number of ingredients that may seem to include milk or dairy products in fact do not and can be eaten by a child with a milk allergy. These include:

- calcium lactate
- lactic acid
- calcium stearoyl lactylate
- oleoresin
- cocoa butter
- sodium lactate
- cream of tartar
- sodium stearyl lactate

Eggs   Influenza vaccines are grown on egg embryos and may contain a small amount of egg protein. The pediatrician should be notified before giving a flu shot to a child who is allergic to eggs. The recommendations of the American Academy of Pediatrics (AAP) acknowledge that the MMR vaccine can be safely administered to all children with egg allergy. The AAP recommendations are based in part on overwhelming scientific evidence supporting the routine use of one-dose administration of the MMR vaccine to egg-allergic patients, even among children with a history of severe, generalized anaphylactic reactions to egg.

Other egg sources include egg substitutes and pasta. Some commercial brands of egg substitutes actually contain egg whites. Most commercially processed cooked pastas (including those used in prepared foods such as soup) contain egg or are processed on equipment shared with egg-containing pastas. Boxed, dry pastas are usually egg-free. Fresh pasta also is usually egg-free. Read the label or ask about ingredients before eating pasta.

Peanuts   Children who are allergic to peanuts need to be particularly careful about the food they eat, because these types of nuts can cause severe allergic reactions in the tiniest doses. Although once considered to be a lifelong allergy, recent studies indicate that up to 20 percent of children diagnosed with peanut allergy may outgrow it.

All too often, peanuts are hidden in many foods so that it can be difficult to tell which ones contain nuts. All labels should be checked carefully. To be safe, children who are allergic to peanuts should avoid chocolate candies unless there is absolutely no risk of cross-contact during manufacturing procedures. African, Chinese, Indonesian, Mexican, Thai, and Vietnamese dishes often contain peanuts or are contaminated with peanuts during preparation of these meals. Many brands of sunflower seeds are produced on equipment shared with peanuts. In addition, foods sold in bakeries and ice cream shops often come in contact with peanuts. Therefore, experts recommend that peanut-allergic individuals avoid these types of foods and restaurants. In addition, peanuts may masquerade under other names; for example, *mandelonas* are peanuts soaked in almond flavoring, and *arachis oil* is peanut oil.

Most experts recommend peanut-allergic patients also avoid tree nuts (such as pecans or walnuts) as well (see below). Because many nut butters are produced on equipment used to process peanut butter, these butters are a somewhat risky alternative.

Studies show that most allergic individuals can safely eat peanut oil but not cold pressed, expelled, or extruded peanut oil, sometimes referred to as "gourmet oils."

If a pediatrician has prescribed injectable epinephrine (Epipen) it should always be carried by the child.

Tree nuts Tree nuts can cause severe allergic reactions, so if a pediatrician has prescribed injectable epinephrine (Epipen), it should always be carried with the child. Patients who have been diagnosed with an allergy to specific tree nuts should avoid all tree nuts to be safe; most experts advise tree nut-allergic patients to avoid peanuts as well.

In addition, tree nuts may be contained in a wide variety of products. Mortadella may contain pistachios, and natural and artificial flavoring may contain tree nuts. In fact, tree nuts have been used in many foods including barbecue sauce, cereals, crackers, and ice cream. In addition, hacky sacks, bean bags, and draft dodgers are sometimes filled with crushed tree nut shells.

A coconut is actually the seed of a drupaceous fruit and is not considered a tree nut. Therefore, coconuts are not typically restricted in the diet of a child who is allergic to tree nuts. However, some people have reacted to coconut, so potential reactions should be discussed with a doctor before introducing coconut to the child's diet. Likewise, nutmeg is obtained from the seeds of the tropical tree species *Myristica fragrans* and is considered to be safe for a child with a tree nut allergy.

Fish/shellfish Allergic reactions to fish and shellfish are commonly reported in children and can be severe. It is generally recommended that all types of fish should be avoided by children who have had an allergic reaction to one species of fish or positive skin tests to fish. The same rule applies to shellfish.

Fish-allergic individuals should be cautious when eating away from home and avoid fish and seafood restaurants because of the risk of contamination in the food-preparation area of their "non-fish" meal with a counter, spatula, cooking oil, fryer, or grill that was exposed to fish. In addition, fish protein can become airborne during cooking and cause an allergic reaction. In fact, some people have had allergic reactions just by walking through a fish market.

It is not always easy to spot fish or shellfish in food. For example, *caponata,* a traditional sweet-and-sour Sicilian relish, can contain anchovies, while Caesar salad dressings and steak or Worcestershire sauce often contain anchovies. Likewise, surimi (imitation crabmeat) often contains fish.

On the other hand, some products that may seem fish-related are not. Carrageenan (Irish moss) is not fish but a red marine algae that is used in a wide variety of menu items (particularly dairy foods) as an emulsifier, stabilizer, and thickener. It appears to be safe for most children with food allergies.

Despite common belief to the contrary, allergy to iodine, allergy to radiocontrast material (used in some lab procedures), and allergy to fish or shellfish are not related. A child with an allergy to fish or shellfish should not worry about cross-reactions with radiocontrast dyes or iodine.

Soy Soybeans have become a major part of processed food products in the United States, and it can be hard to avoid products made with soybeans. While soybeans alone are not a major food in the typical American diet, because they are contained in so many products, eliminating all those foods can result in an unbalanced diet. A dietitian should be consulted to help plan for proper nutrition. Soybeans and soy products are found in baked goods, canned tuna, cereals, crackers, infant formulas, sauces, and soups. At least one brand of peanut butter lists soy on the label.

Studies show that soy lecithin and soybean oil can be tolerated by most soy-allergic individuals.

Wheat It may not be obvious in what products wheat can be hidden, so labels should be read carefully. Wheat is contained in some brands of hot dogs, ice cream, and imitation crabmeat. Wheat flour is sometimes flavored and shaped to look like beef, pork, and shrimp, especially in Asian dishes. In addition, many country-style wreaths are decorated with wheat products.

There is a difference between CELIAC DISEASE and wheat allergy, which are two distinct conditions. Celiac disease (or celiac sprue) is a permanent sensitivity to GLUTEN, a protein contained in wheat flour. Those with celiac disease will not lose their sensitivity to this substance, but will have to restrict their intake of gluten all their lives. The major grains that contain gluten are wheat, rye, oats, and barley. These grains and their by-products must be strictly avoided by people with celiac disease.

On the other hand, children allergic to wheat have a reaction to wheat protein and must therefore avoid only wheat. Most wheat-allergic children outgrow the allergy.

Two alternatives to wheat are not safe for wheat-sensitive individuals. *Kamut* is a cereal grain related to wheat. *Spelt* is an ancient wheat that has recently been marketed as safe for wheat-allergic individuals, but this claim is untrue. Wheat-allergic patients can react as readily to spelt as they do to common wheat.

Symptoms

Symptoms of a food allergy include tingling sensations in the mouth, swelling of the tongue and the throat, breathing problems, hives, vomiting, abdominal cramps, diarrhea, low blood pressure, loss of consciousness, and death. Symptoms typically appear within minutes to two hours after the child has eaten.

Diagnosis

A food allergy is diagnosed following a detailed food history, physical exam, and pertinent tests; skin testing may help identify cases of food allergy in cases of acute itching. Skin testing is not usually helpful in diagnosing chronic itching due to food allergy. For these cases, a food diary and trial elimination of suspect foods may be effective in pinpointing the problem.

A child with a suspected food allergy should keep a food diary for one to two weeks detailing all ingested food and drinks, any symptoms, and when symptoms occurred. This information, combined with a physical examination and lab tests, will help the doctor determine what food is causing the symptoms.

The prick skin test or a blood test such as the RAST (radioallergosorbent test) are commonly used to determine if an allergy exists. A prick skin test is usually cheaper and can be done in the doctor's office. In this test, the doctor places a drop of the substance being tested on the child's forearm or back and pricks the skin with a needle, allowing a tiny amount to enter the skin. If the patient is allergic to the substance, a bump will appear at the site within about 15 minutes.

A RAST test requires a blood sample, which is then sent to a lab to be tested with specific foods to determine whether the patient has immunoglobulin E (IgE) antibodies to that food. The results are usually received within one week.

Although both tests are reliable, many doctors use a RAST for young children or patients who have eczema or other skin problems that would make it hard to read the results of a prick skin test. The results of either test are combined with other information, such as a history of symptoms and a food challenge, to determine whether a food allergy exists.

Treatment

Anaphylactic shock in reaction to food is a medical emergency, and the child should be taken to a doctor immediately. If the child's heart has stopped, cardiopulmonary resuscitation (CPR) should be started immediately. Epinephrine can be injected to treat anaphylaxis; antihistamines and steroids may be given to control hives and swelling.

Prevention

Eliminating or reducing access to the sensitive food can prevent the allergic response. Reading ingredient labels for all foods is the key to maintaining control over the allergy. If a product does not have a label, allergic individuals should not eat that food. If a label contains unfamiliar terms, shoppers must call the manufacturer and ask for a definition or avoid eating that food.

Drug therapy (antihistamines, corticosteroids, and cromolyn sodium) may be necessary for children with multiple food sensitivities that do not respond to elimination.

After a study found that severe reactions to food allergies were more likely to be caused by foods prepared outside the home, the National Restaurant Association (NRA) and the Food Allergy Network began a program to help restaurants understand food allergies. The NRA provides free information to restaurants about the proper way to handle food allergy problems via their hotline (202) 331-5900.

Food Allergy vs. Food Intolerance

Food allergy and food intolerance are not the same thing. A food intolerance is an adverse food-induced reaction that does not involve the immune system (such as lactose intolerance). A child with lactose intolerance lacks an enzyme that is needed to digest milk sugar, and will suffer from gas, bloating, and abdominal pain after ingesting milk.

A food allergy occurs when the immune system reacts to a certain food. The most common form of an immune system reaction occurs when the body creates immunoglobulin E (IgE) antibodies to the food. When these IgE antibodies react with the food, histamine and other chemicals cause hives, asthma, or other symptoms of an allergic reaction.

food poisoning   A toxic process caused by eating food contaminated by poisonous substances or by bacteria containing toxins. Children are particularly vulnerable to food poisoning, and an infection that would cause little concern in an adult can result in a serious illness in a young child.

More than 250 different diseases can be caused by contaminated food or drink, which makes food poisoning one of the most common causes of acute illness. The most common food-borne diseases are infections caused by bacteria such as campylobacter, the Norwalk family of viruses, and salmonella, which enters the body within contaminated foods such as poultry and eggs. Most food items which carry disease are raw or undercooked foods of animal origin, such as meat, milk, eggs, cheese, fish, or shellfish.

Food poisoning should be suspected in any illness that appears suddenly and causes stomach pain, vomiting, and diarrhea. Estimates of the number of food-borne illnesses have been ranged from a low of six million to a high of 81 million cases yearly, with 9,100 deaths, according to the Centers for Disease Control and Prevention. At least one-third of the cases have been traced to poultry and meat. According to the Food and Drug Administration (FDA), just about everyone experiences a food-borne illness at least once a year. Between 21 and 81 million cases of diarrhea related to food-borne illness are treated in the United States each year.

The greatest danger from food poisoning is not the toxin itself but the body's natural response to poison—vomiting and diarrhea—that robs the body of vital fluids. This is especially true in young children. If dehydration becomes serious, food poisoning victims need to be hospitalized and given fluids intravenously. In addition, however, poisoning from *E. coli* bacteria poses a unique and specific threat—severe infection that can include bloody diarrhea, leading to kidney failure. It is this type of food poisoning from improperly cooked hamburgers that killed several young children in 1993.

Symptoms

While the time between ingestion and onset of symptoms varies according to the cause of poisoning, symptoms usually develop between one and 12 hours for bacterial toxins, and between 12 and 48 hours for viral and salmonella infections. Symptoms also vary depending on how severely the food was contaminated, but there will often be nausea and vomiting, diarrhea, stomach pain, and—in severe cases—shock and collapse.

Treatment

In cases of food poisoning, symptoms should be treated much like a bout of INFLUENZA, including drinking fluids (water, tea, bouillon, and ginger ale) to replace fluid loss. Mild cases may be treated at home, with a soft diet, including some salt and sugar. Most cases of food poisoning are not serious, and recovery is usually within three days. Samples of any food left from recent meals should be saved for testing, if possible.

Governmental Overview

Governmental overview began in 1906 with the passage of the Pure Food and Drug Act and the Meat Inspection Act, designed to make American food as safe as possible. In addition, two different governmental agencies are responsible for regulating and monitoring the safety of the U.S. food supply. The U.S. Food and Drug Administration (FDA) is responsible for ensuring the safety and wholesomeness of all food except meat, poultry, and eggs. The Department of Agriculture monitors the safety of poultry, meat, and eggs and conducts inspections nationwide and inspects eggs and egg products.

If a child has:	It could be:
Ulcer pain, abdominal pain, fever, nausea, vomiting, and diarrhea one week after poisoning	Anasakiasis
Explosive watery diarrhea, abdominal cramps, dehydration	Asiatic cholera
Gastroenteritis, diarrhea, nausea/vomiting appearing one to six hours after eating	Bacillus cereus
Slurred speech, double vision, muscle paralysis appearing four to 36 hours after meal	Botulism
Cramps, fever, diarrhea, nausea/vomiting appearing one to five days after eating and lasting up to 10 days	Campylobacteriosis
Nausea, vomiting, and diarrhea within six to 12 hours after eating, followed by low blood pressure and heart rate; severe itching, temperature reversal, numbness/tingling of extremities that may last months	Ciguatera
Watery diarrhea, nausea/vomiting appearing within hours to a week after eating; severe cases include blood diarrhea; enterhemorrhagic infection includes bloody diarrhea and kidney failure	Enteric *E. coli*
Explosive diarrhea, foul-smelling, greasy feces, stomach pain, gas, appetite loss, nausea and vomiting; incubation period one to two weeks	Giardiasis
Fever, headache, diarrhea, meningitis, conjunctivitis, miscarriage appearing within days to weeks after ingestion	Listeriosis
Burning mouth/extremities, nausea, vomiting, and diarrhea within hours	Neurotoxic shellfish poisoning
Burning mouth/extremities, nausea/vomiting, diarrhea, muscle weakness, paralysis, breathing problems within minutes	Paralytic shellfish poisoning
Six–72 hours after eating: Diarrhea, rumbling bowels, fever, vomiting, cramps	Salmonellosis
Within minutes to hours: Itching, flushing cramps, diarrhea, nausea/vomiting, burning throat; severe infection includes low blood pressure and breathing problems	Scrombroid poisoning
One to seven days after eating: Gastroenteritis, diarrhea, nausea/vomiting, possible seizures	Shigellosis
Between 30 minutes and six hours after eating: Explosive diarrhea, cramps, vomiting, but not longer than a day (usually in baked goods)	*Staphylococcal* food poisoning
Diarrhea, nausea/vomiting, fever followed by muscle pain and stiffness two to three weeks later	Trichinosis (pork)
Gastroenteritis, explosive diarrhea, nausea/vomiting cramps eight to 30 hours after eating; *V. vulnificus* can lead to fatal blood infection	Vibrio food poisoning (*V. parahaemolyticus, V. vulnificus*)
One to two days after eating: Right lower quadrant pain, mimics appendicitis	Yersinia

Prevention

To prevent the spread of food-borne diseases, consumers should:

- make sure food from animal sources is thoroughly cooked or pasteurized; avoid eating such foods raw or undercooked
- keep juices or drippings from raw meat, poultry, shellfish, or eggs from contaminating other food
- not leave potentially contaminated food for extended periods of time at temperatures that allow bacteria to grow
- promptly refrigerate leftovers and food prepared in advance

The single most important way to prevent food-borne illness is thorough cooking, which kills most food-borne bacteria, viruses and parasites. In addition, proper food preparation—washing hands, cutting board, and knife with soap and water right after handling raw meat, poultry, seafood, or eggs—will help stop the spread of contamination. Anyone who is sick with diarrhea or vomiting should not prepare food for others.

HOW TO PREVENT FOOD POISONING

Meat, poultry, and eggs are most vulnerable to contamination during storage, preparation, cooking, and serving. To stay healthy, consumers should try to observe proper food handling and kitchen safety tips:

- *Proper refrigeration* Temperature in the refrigerator must be 40°F or below (0°F in the freezer). Cooling doesn't kill bacteria, but it stops their growth. Air should circulate around refrigerated items, and refrigerated food should always be wrapped to keep off bacteria in the air.

- *Clean hands* To avoid contamination by bacteria or other organisms when preparing food, hands should be washed thoroughly with soap and water before and after handling food.

- *Clean utensils* Cutting boards and utensils should be washed with hot soapy water before touching any other food with them.

- *Thawing* Meat and poultry should not be thawed at room temperature; instead, it can be thawed in a microwave oven or the refrigerator. Meat and poultry should be cooked right after thawing.

- *Marinades* Marinades from meat or poultry should not be served as sauces unless they have been cooked at a rolling boil for several minutes.

- *Serving* Meat and poultry should be served on a clean plate with a clean utensil to avoid contaminating the cooked food with its raw juices.

- *Leftovers* Poultry and meat should be cooled quickly when refrigerating leftovers; stuffed poultry should not stand for long periods. Stuffing should be removed after cooking and promptly refrigerated.

- *Eggs* Cracked eggs should never be used because they may contain *Salmonella* bacteria. However, because even an uncracked egg may contain bacteria, eggs should always be cooked thoroughly. Raw eggs (such as in homemade Caesar salad dressing, eggnog, hollandaise sauce, etc.) should not be used. Eggs should be refrigerated in their cartons in the coldest part of the refrigerator, *not* on the refrigerator door.

- *Mold* Any food with mold should be thrown away, except for cheese, which may be eaten after the mold is trimmed off.

- *Microwave* A turntable should be used to rotate dishes as they cook; because microwave ovens heat food unevenly, cold spots in a food may harbor dangerous bacteria.

- *Cleaning* Wooden salad bowls should not be seasoned with oil, which can eventually become rancid. Can openers and blenders should be kept clean, and the sink should always be scrubbed after working with poultry or meat. Sponges in the kitchen for wiping dishes or countertops should be discarded after one week; they should never sit in water, which encourages bacterial growth. Sinks and counters should be cleaned with detergent containing bleach to kill harmful bacteria.

KEEPING HOT FOODS SAFE

To keep hot foods safe, consumers should follow these guidelines from the U.S. Department of Agriculture:

- A meat thermometer should be used to make sure meats and poultry are cooked completely. The thermometer goes into the thickest part (avoiding fat and bone). Bacteria are killed at 160°F (poultry at 180°F or higher).

- Poultry should be cooked until it reaches 180 to 185°F or higher (or until the juices run clear or the leg moves easily in the socket). Poultry should not be cooked at a low temperature for a long period of time.

- Food should not be partially heated and then finished cooking later; half-cooked food may be warm enough to encourage bacterial growth but not hot enough to kill it. Subsequent cooking might not kill the bacteria.

- Consumers should allow at least one and a half times longer than usual to cook frozen foods that have not been pre-thawed.

- Hot foods must be kept at 140 to 160°F until serving time, especially those served in chafing dishes or warmers. Food should never be kept between 40° and 140°F for more than two hours, as this encourages bacterial growth.

- Leftovers should be thoroughly and evenly reheated; gravies should be brought to a rolling boil.

- The healthiest way to cook a steak is to precook it in a microwave on high for 30 to 90 seconds just before broiling or barbecuing, which reduces the formation of harmful amines. The juice should be discarded.

HOW TO REPORT CASES OF SUSPECTED FOOD POISONING

According to the U.S. Department of Agriculture's Safety and Inspection Service, parents should report possible food poisoning in three situations:

- if the food was eaten at a large gathering
- if the food was from a restaurant, deli, sidewalk vendor, or other kitchen that serves more than a few people
- if the food is a commercial product (such as canned goods or frozen food), since contaminants may have affected an entire batch.

When making a report, officials need to know:

- parents' name, address, telephone number

- a detailed explanation of the problem
- when and where the food was eaten
- who ate it
- name and address of the place where the food was obtained

If the food is a commercial product, parents should provide:

- the manufacturer's name and address
- product's lot or batch number
- the USDA inspection stamp on the wrapper if the tainted food is meat or poultry; this will identify the plant where the food was made or packaged.

Picnics are another potential trouble spot for food poisoning. Parents should use an insulated cooler with an ice block or frozen gel-pack on top, placing foods that need to be kept coldest on the bottom. Food should be packed into the cooler right from the refrigerator. Each item should be wrapped separately in plastic and should not be placed directly on ice that is not of drinking-water quality. Raw fish, meat, or poultry should be separated so that raw meat drippings do not contaminate other food. All hot foods should be kept hot in an insulated dish or vacuum bottle.

Once the family arrives at a picnic spot, the cooler should be kept in the shade with the lid on—not in the car's trunk. Utensils and food should be covered when not in use. Disposable wipes should be brought along to clean hands before and after food preparation. Food should not be unrefrigerated for longer than two hours or one hour if the temperature is above 85°F.

fractures   A break in the normal structure of a bone, which is among the most common injuries in children under age 12. Most bones are broken when children are playing or participating in sports. When children fall, the natural instinct is to throw the hands out in protection; this is why most fractures occur in the wrist, forearm, and above the elbow. Fractures generally cause fewer problems in children because the young bones are more flexible and better able to absorb shock. They also heal faster than adults' bones.

Children who participate in sports or are generally active are more likely to experience fractures. To reduce risks, the child should wear the recommended protective gear. Other children likely to sustain bone fractures are those with an inherited condition known as osteogenesis imperfecta, characterized by bones that are brittle and more vulnerable to fracture.

Types of Fractures
A fracture can range from a hairline crack in the bone to a complete break, in which the bone is shattered into two or more pieces. Fractures can be described in the following ways:

- *Complete fracture*   A bone that has broken into two pieces
- *Greenstick fracture*   A bone cracked on one side only, not all the way through
- *Single fracture*   A bone broken in one place
- *Comminuted fracture*   A bone that is crushed or broken into more than two pieces
- *Bending fracture*   A bone that bends but does not break, which occurs only in children

- *Open (or compound) fracture*   A broken bone that penetrates the skin. Open fractures need to be cleaned thoroughly in the sterile environment of the operating room before they are set because the bone's exposure to the air may lead to infection.

- *Closed fracture*   A broken bone that does not break the skin is called a closed fracture.

- *Buckle fracture*   A bone that bends on one side, raising a buckle; this occurs only in young children.

Diagnosis

A pediatrician often can tell whether a bone is broken just by checking the injured area for swelling or bruising, or a deformed limb. X rays are used to confirm a diagnosis, although some fractures can be difficult to detect even with X rays.

Treatment

Fractures heal at different rates depending upon the age of the child and the type of fracture. Young children may heal in as little as three weeks, although it may take six weeks for the same kind of fracture to heal in adolescents.

The bone begins to heal at the location of the fracture as the bones produce new cells and tiny blood vessels to rebuild the bone. These cells cover both ends of the broken part of the bone and eventually close up the break.

Setting the break   When a child breaks a bone, the doctor will first "set" the bone; this is known as a closed reduction. During a reduction, the doctor manipulates the fracture or displaced ends of the bone into proper alignment and then holds the realigned bone in place with a cast or pins.

Cast   After a bone has been set, the next step is usually putting on a cast to keep the bone in place for the one to three months it will take for the break to mend. Casts are made of bandages soaked in plaster of Paris or fiberglass material, which hardens to a tough shell. Plaster of Paris is easier to mold over difficult fractures, but it is heavier and less resistant to water. Synthetic material comes in many bright colors, is lighter and cooler, and is often used for less complicated fractures. Fiberglass casts with waterproof liners allow children to bathe and even swim during the healing process. The liner allows for evaporation of water and sweat, but it is fragile and must be protected to allow it to function properly. A doctor will determine if the fracture may be safely treated with a waterproof cast.

The problem with casts (especially plaster casts) are that they can be uncomfortable and itchy. A child suffering from itchy skin beneath a cast may find relief by having air blown into the cast with a hair dryer on a cool setting. Baby powder or oils should never be poured into a cast, nor should an itch be scratched with a pencil or hanger. These remedies could irritate a child's skin and cause an infection.

Traction   Certain fractures of larger long bones such as the thigh bone are hard to keep straight in a cast. Instead, some of these fractures are kept in traction for a few days until the fracture begins to show early healing; at this point, a cast can be applied to hold the bone straight until healing is complete. With breaks in larger bones, or more than two pieces, the doctor may put a metal pin in the bone to help set it.

When to Call the Doctor

A pediatrician or orthopedic surgeon should be called in the event of the following symptoms:

- redness, swelling, and inflammation
- temperature above 100.4°F
- toes (in a leg cast) or fingers (in an arm cast) that turn pale, blue, numb, or swollen
- increased pain in the fractured limb
- inability to wiggle the toes or fingers of the affected limb
- broken or loosening cast, or wet plaster

Prevention

Many broken bones could be prevented if parents and caregivers followed these simple safety measures:

- a baby should never be left alone on a changing table or bed
- children should always ride in well-secured car seats in the rear
- when playing sports, children should always wear protective gear (wrist guards, helmets, knee pads, mouth guards) that meet U.S. safety standards

- a child should always wear a helmet when rollerskating, biking, going in-line skating, or skateboarding

Soda and fractures Bone fractures are more than three times more common among girls who drink carbonated beverages, according to a 1998 Harvard University study. In physically active girls who drink cola—with or without other carbonated beverages—the risk of bone fractures is more than five times greater than the risk for active girls who do not drink carbonated beverages. This association between drinking carbonated colas and bone fractures among physically active teen girls confirms the findings of previous studies. Scientists suspect that soda may be linked to bone fractures because girls who drink soda may have poor dietary calcium intake and high phosphorus intake from the phosphoric acid contained in cola drinks. (See also GROWTH PLATE INJURIES.)

fragile X syndrome A hereditary condition that causes a wide range of mental impairment, from mild learning disabilities to severe MENTAL RETARDATION (mostly in boys). It is the most common cause of genetically inherited mental impairment. Also known as Martin-Bell syndrome, marker X syndrome, or Escalante syndrome, fragile X syndrome is associated with a number of physical and behavioral characteristics.

Cause

The biological cause of fragile X and the pattern of transmission of the disease are complex. Fragile X syndrome is transmitted from parent to child through the DNA in the sperm and eggs. Many inherited diseases (such as sickle-cell anemia and hemophilia) are caused by a single error in the genetic code in a person's DNA.

Fragile X syndrome, on the other hand, is not caused by a single change in DNA but by the multiplication of part of the genetic information. This is known as a trinucleotide repeat disorder.

In children who do not have fragile X syndrome, there is a section of the DNA in the FMR1 gene which is normally repeated a few times. Instead of having proteins repeated in order about 30 times, someone with the premutation of fragile X has 55 to 200 repeats in that part of the gene. Someone with the full mutation has 200 to 800 repeats.

Perhaps the most complicated part of the inheritance of fragile X syndrome is that the FMR1 gene can be unstable, which leads to frequent mutations. Because most genes have a very low rate of mutation, most children who inherit a disease have at least one parent who is a carrier for that disease since new mutations are rare. In contrast, once the FMR1 gene changes normal to unstable (called a "permutation"), it is highly likely that it will mutate from one generation to the next. This means that there can be a family with no history of fragile X syndrome in which the condition suddenly appears in a number of offspring.

Many children with fragile X syndrome have some cognitive weaknesses, and their overall potential may be lower than that of their peers and siblings, but they still may do very well with certain types of learning. Children may be both mentally retarded and learning disabled, meaning that their overall IQ is lower than average, but they may have strengths and weaknesses in various skills. Children with fragile X syndrome often have these varying patterns. Thinking skills are also affected by ATTENTION DEFICIT HYPERACTIVITY DISORDER (ADHD), seizure disorders, anxiety, speech, and language disorders, sensory motor problems, and other issues that may affect test taking and learning.

Many boys, and some girls, are described as mentally retarded. Children with fragile X syndrome progress at a slower developmental pace and with a lower end result than do normally developing children. Disabilities in adapting to the environment refer to delays in life skills, not just academics. However, many children with fragile X achieve more than would be expected based upon an IQ score alone.

Children with fragile X syndrome are often described as sweet and loving, with a strong desire for social interactions and humorous situations. At the same time, children with fragile X also often have some behavioral challenges.

Symptoms

Fragile X syndrome affects individuals in a wide variety of ways. Some children experience significant challenges, while the impact on others is so minor that they will never be diagnosed. In any case, boys and girls experience quite different physical, cognitive, behavioral, sensory, speech, and language problems. In general, however, girls with fragile X either do not have the characteristics seen in boys, or the characteristics show up in a milder form.

The difference is probably due to the fact that girls have two X chromosomes instead of the one that boys carry. This means that girls with fragile X have two sets of instructions for making FMRP (the fragile X mental retardation protein)—one that works and one that does not. Boys with fragile X have only one X chromosome with its nonfunctioning FMR1 (fragile X mental retardation 1) gene. It appears that girls are able to produce enough of the FMRP to fill most of the body's needs, but not all.

Anxiety in both boys and girls manifests itself in various ways. Some children with fragile X have trouble with changes in routine or stressful events such as fire drills. Parents often report that their children stiffen up when angry or upset, becoming rigid and very tense, or having tantrums. Crowds and new situations may cause boys to whine, cry, or misbehave so as to get out of the overwhelming situation. Many of the behavior problems of both boys and girls with fragile X syndrome overlap with the conversational problems they have in language. The poor eye contact and problems in keeping a conversation going cause many social weaknesses. Perseverative speech and self-talk may be symptoms of anxiety.

Some behaviors quite similar to AUTISM are common. Although most children with fragile X syndrome do not have all the characteristics of autism, about 15 percent are diagnosed as autistic. More often, children have "autistic-like" features, such as poor eye contact, hand flapping, and poor social skills.

Boys Several physical features are commonly associated with fragile X syndrome. Boys with fragile X often have distinctive facial features, connective tissue problems, and enlarged testicles that appear after the onset of puberty. However, none of these features occur in all boys with fragile X. The primary physical features of fragile X syndrome in boys are long faces and prominent, long ears—characteristics that are more common in boys over age 10. However, long ears are also common among mentally retarded boys who do not have fragile X syndrome. When compared to mentally retarded boys who do not have fragile X syndrome, those with fragile X have a larger head circumference, head breadth, and head length.

Up to 80 percent of boys with fragile X syndrome have delays in their cognitive ability; between 10 and 15 percent of boys tested may have IQs in the borderline or mild mental retardation range.

Up to 90 percent of boys with the condition are considered to be distractible and impulsive, with symptoms of attention deficit hyperactivity disorder (ADHD) or attention deficit disorder (ADD). They may have short attention spans and difficulty staying on task.

Many boys have unusual, stereotypic behaviors, such as hand flapping and chewing on skin, clothing, or objects, which may be connected to sensory processing problems and anxiety. Sensory processing problems may include tactile defensiveness, sensitivity to sound or light, and poor eye contact. About 90 percent of boys with fragile X syndrome are reported to have some type of sensory defensiveness.

Girls A premutation in the FMR1 gene typically has little or no effect on a girl's behavior and educational ability, but it may affect several facial characteristics such as prominent ears and prominent jaw. Girls with the full mutation may have some of the physical features associated with fragile X boys, including a long face and long ears. A number of girls with the full mutation have learning disabilities. About 30 percent of girls with the full mutation score above 85 on an IQ test, with the other 70 percent mostly in the borderline or mild mental retardation range.

Girls may show less hyperactivity but still have many symptoms of ADD. Girls with the full mutation of the fragile X gene appear to have some specific areas of concern in the area of behavioral and emotional difficulties. Shyness, anxiety, depression, and difficulties with social contacts are most often mentioned as characteristics of girls with fragile X.

Diagnosis

In the past, the only laboratory test for fragile X syndrome was a chromosome test, but in 1991 a DNA test (the FMR-1 gene test) was introduced as the first and most accurate way to detect fragile X syndrome. The chromosome test is still available through most labs, however, and is used for a variety of diagnostic purposes.

frostbite Exposure to very cold temperatures for a long period of time can freeze the skin and underlying tissues. The areas most likely to be affected are the feet, hands, nose, and ears. While anyone can become frostbitten, those with circulatory problems are at greatest risk.

Although it is theoretically possible for tissue to freeze in temperatures at about 32°F, the body's local internal temperature must fall to levels lower than that before freezing occurs at a specific area of the body. The danger of frostbite increases if a child is without adequate food, clothing, or shelter. Wind or wet skin also hasten the outward transfer of heat and increase the risk of frostbite.

Symptoms

Frostbitten skin looks firm, pale, and white, with a lack of sensitivity to touch. There may be a sharp, aching pain in the affected area. As the skin thaws, it becomes raw and painful. Frostbite damage that involves just the skin and subcutaneous tissue may be described as "superficial" (called "frostnip"). Deep frostbite affects the muscle, nerve, vessels, cartilage, and bone. In mild cases, the damage can be reversed, but if frostbite is severe the flow of blood to the area stops. Unless immediate treatment begins, the area will be irreversibly damaged and amputation of the extremity may be required.

Treatment

Normal body temperature should be restored before thawing any frostbitten flesh. A small area of frostnipped skin can be rewarmed by placing fingers or the heel of the hand over the affected area. Rapid thawing of the affected part in warm water baths is the current preferred treatment method for more extensive frostnip and for frostbite. If immediate emergency help is unavailable, severely frostbitten hands or feet should be thawed in warm, *not hot* water (between 100° and 105°F). Other heat sources (such as heating pads) should not be used because the frostbitten tissue can still be burned by temperatures that under normal conditions would not hurt the skin.

If the skin tingles and burns as it warms, circulation is returning. If numbness remains as the area is warmed, professional help should be obtained immediately.

A frostbitten area should never be rubbed as it thaws. If feet are affected, the child should not walk on them. In addition, neither bandages nor dressings should be used.

Thawing time is determined by the temperature of the water and the depth of freezing; it is complete when the extremity flushes pink or red. After rapid thawing, small blisters may appear, spontaneously rupturing in four to 10 days, followed by a black scab. Normal tissue may have formed beneath the scab. Constant exercises should be performed to preserve joint motion. Further treatment is designed to prevent infection and preserve function of the affected part.

In severe cases, antibiotics, bed rest, and physical therapy may be necessary after the affected part has been warmed. The best chance of successful healing after frostbite is if the affected part has not been frozen long, when thawing is rapid, and when blisters develop early. The outlook is more uncertain when thawing is spontaneous at room temperature, when the part is frozen for a long time, or if the frostbite occurred in an area of fracture or dislocation. A poor outlook is indicated if thawing is delayed or occurs due to excessive heat, if blisters are dark, or if thawing is followed by refreezing. Refreezing almost always ends in amputation.

Complications

Major complications include infection, tissue death, sensory loss, persistent deep pain, and limited joint movement. Permanent effects may include fixed scars, small muscle wasting, deformed joints, arthritic bone changes, and increased sensitivity to cold.

Prevention

Frostbite is theoretically simple to prevent by having children wear proper clothing in cold weather.

fungal infections Diseases of the skin that are caused by fungus and that can range from a mild to a fatal condition. Fungi are a phylum of plants including yeasts, rusts, slime molds, smuts, and mushrooms that are characterized by the absence of chlorophyll and the presence of a rigid cell wall.

A fungus is actually a primitive vegetable that can be found in air, in soil, on plants, and in water. There are more than 100,000 different species of fungi around the world, most of which are harmless or beneficial to human health (such as molds used to produce antibiotics, yeasts used in baking and brewing, edible mushrooms and truffles, and so on).

However, some fungi can invade and form colonies in the skin or underneath the skin, leading to disorders ranging from a mild skin irritation and inflammation to severe or fatal systemic infections. Only about half of all types of fungi cause disease in humans; those conditions are called mycoses. Mycoses can affect the skin, nails, body hair, internal organs (such as the lungs), or body systems such as the nervous system.

Fungi reproduce by sending out spores (cells that resemble plant seeds). When a spore lands in a moist place, it sends out small threads from which the fungus feeds. These moist places that support fungi include dead plant and animal matter and bacteria.

The *superficial* fungal infections include THRUSH (candidiasis) and TINEA (including ringworm and athlete's foot). *Subcutaneous infections* are rare; the most common is *sporotrichosis,* occurring after a scratch becomes contaminated; most examples of this type of condition occur in tropical climates.

Causes

Harmless fungi are present all the time on the skin, but they do not multiply there because of bacterial competition or because the body's immune system fights them off. Fungal infections of the skin are most common in those taking long-term antibiotics or those taking corticosteroid or immunosuppressant drugs, or in patients with an immune system disorder such as AIDS.

Treatment

Physicians use three classes of drugs to fight fungal disease, but in the past five years disease-causing fungi have begun to grow resistant to common drugs, just like some types of bacteria. Strains of fungi resistant to each of the three types of drugs are now common in hospitals that care for the sickest patients—especially patients with cancer and AIDS. This growing resistance appears to have developed for the same reasons that bacteria have grown impervious: the overuse of drugs to combat fungal infections.

High use of antifungal medications occurred because of the large number of people with impaired immune systems due to AIDS and chemotherapy. Between five and 10 percent of AIDS patients now have resistant fungi that cause oral CANDIDIASIS, a common mouth infection.

gastroenteritis Inflammation of the stomach and intestines that appears with a number of gastrointestinal disorders that can be caused by bacteria or viruses.

Symptoms
Sudden and violent onset of anorexia, vomiting, nausea, abdominal discomfort, and diarrhea.

Treatment
Bed rest, sedation, and fluids; intravenous fluids can be given if necessary. (See also GASTROINTESTINAL INFECTIONS.)

gastrointestinal infections A condition that usually causes diarrhea, caused by an infection with either viruses, bacteria, or parasites. How long the child is sick depends on the germ and the child. In cases of mild diarrhea caused by a virus, the diarrhea should pass after a few days; the child should recover completely with supportive care, rest, and plenty of fluids.

Cause
In developed countries such as the United States, outbreaks of diarrhea are more often linked to contaminated water supplies, improperly processed or preserved foods, or person-to-person contact in child-care centers. Diarrheal infections are contagious and can spread from child to child via dirty hands, direct contact with fecal matter, contaminated food or water, and some pets.

Viruses One of the most common diarrheal illnesses in American children is ROTAVIRUS, so widespread that almost all American children have had a rotavirus infection by the time they are four or five years old, although not all children show symptoms. The viruses can live for significant periods of time on toys and surfaces in play areas. Rotavirus commonly causes outbreaks of diarrhea during the winter and early spring months, especially in child-care centers and children's hospitals. Hand-washing in these places is very important to stop the rapid spread of outbreaks of rotavirus.

Another viral infection that causes diarrhea in children, especially during the summer months, is from ENTEROVIRUSES, particularly group A and B COXSACKIE VIRUSES.

Bacteria At least 13 different types of bacteria can cause diarrheal infections, including *Salmonella, Shigella, Escherichia coli*, and *Campylobacter*. In the United States, *Salmonella* bacteria cause between one and five million cases of diarrheal illness each year and are responsible for more than half the nation's food poisonings. *Shigella* bacteria, which commonly spread from person to person, are especially dangerous because they attack the intestinal wall and cause ulcers that bleed. As few as 10 *Shigella* bacteria are enough to cause an infection, so shigellosis spreads easily in families, hospitals, and child-care centers.

Five different classes of *E. coli* cause diarrheal infection in children, most often during their first few years of life. *E. coli* bacteria can cause diarrheal illness either by directly attacking the intestinal wall or by producing a toxin that irritates the intestines. One of the most dangerous *E. coli* infections is *E. coli* 0157:H7, which produces a toxin that can lead to HEMOLYTIC UREMIC SYNDROME—a severe illness that can seriously damage many organs and cause intestinal bleeding. Most *E. coli* infections are spread through contaminated food or water, especially in undercooked beef in hamburgers.

Parasitic infection Parasitic infections associated with gastrointestinal symptoms in the United States are most commonly caused by *Giardia*, which is easily spread through contaminated water supplies and human contact. This parasite can be spread in water parks and pools because it is resistant to chlorine treatment. It can also be transmitted through children's "touch tanks" in aquariums and museums. Bathing in and drinking water from contaminated streams or lakes can also lead to infection. GIARDIASIS can cause chronic diarrhea and malabsorption of food. Cryptosporidium, another parasitic organism, is another common cause of gastrointestinal illness in children that often occurs in diarrhea epidemics in child-care centers.

Symptoms

Incubation times before symptoms appear vary depending on the germ causing the infection. For example, the *Shigella* incubation period is usually 16 to 72 hours, but viral incubation periods can range from four to 48 hours. Parasitic infections generally have longer incubation periods; *Giardia* has an incubation period of one to three weeks.

Crampy, abdominal pain is followed by diarrhea that usually lasts a few days, but can last longer in some cases. When gastrointestinal upset and diarrhea last more than two weeks, the condition is known as chronic diarrhea. Some infants with chronic diarrhea either fail to grow, also called FAILURE TO THRIVE, or they begin to lose weight. Excessive loss of water, especially with explosive, frequent episodes of diarrhea, can lead to severe dehydration, especially in small children.

In addition, blood may appear in a child's stools, which indicates that the infectious germ is causing damage to the lining of the bowel. This is seen more often in certain bacterial infections caused by *Campylobacter jejuni, Salmonella,* certain strains of *E. coli,* and *Shigella,* in which case the stool may contain mucus as well as blood. One of the most common viral intestinal infections is ROTAVIRUS, which usually causes explosive, watery diarrhea. This is responsible for 35 percent of all hospital admissions in children with gastroenteritis.

Nonbloody diarrhea is usually caused by infections with other bacteria, viruses, or parasites, or by ingesting a toxin produced by bacteria. Many of the viruses, bacteria, and parasites that cause diarrhea also cause other symptoms, such as fever, loss of appetite, abdominal cramps, nausea, vomiting, weight loss, and dehydration.

Occasionally the germs that cause diarrheal infections may spread into the bloodstream, triggering infection in organs far away from the intestines. *Salmonella* bacteria, for example, can cause infections in the bones (osteomyelitis), joints (arthritis), brain (brain abscess), membranes covering the brain (MENINGITIS). This is especially common in children with chronic illnesses involving the spleen, such as SICKLE-CELL DISEASE.

When to Call a Doctor

A doctor should be consulted when a child has a severe or prolonged episode of diarrhea, fever, vomiting, or severe abdominal pain, or if the stools contain blood or mucus. Especially serious are signs of dehydration, which include dry lips and tongue, pale and dry skin, sunken eyes, listlessness or decreased activity, and decreased urination, such as fewer than six wet diapers a day in an infant.

Diagnosis

To determine the specific germ causing the problem, the doctor may take a sample of a child's bowel movement for lab tests.

Treatment

The immediate treatment goal for all diarrheal illnesses is to replace fluids and electrolytes (salt and minerals) that were lost by diarrhea, vomiting, or fever. They can be given by mouth or intravenously, if the child is severely dehydrated. Infants and small children should never be rehydrated with water alone because it does not contain enough sodium, potassium, or other important nutrients.

Depending on the amount of fluid loss and the severity of vomiting and diarrhea, the child may need to eat a milder diet for a day or two, together with special drinks to replace body fluids quickly.

For most diarrheal illnesses caused by bacteria and viruses, antibiotics or antiviral medications are not prescribed because most children recover on their own.

In very young children or in those with weakened immune systems, however, antibiotics are sometimes given to prevent a bacterial infection from spreading throughout the body.

Most parasitic infections are treated with antiparasitic medicines.

Prevention

Hand-washing is the most effective way to prevent diarrheal infections from passing from child to child. Dirty hands carry infectious germs into the body when a child bites nails or puts any part of the hands into the mouth. Children should wash their hands often, especially after using the toilet and before eating. Clean bathroom surfaces also help to prevent the spread of infectious germs.

Food and water also can carry infectious germs, so fruits and vegetables should be washed thoroughly before eating. Kitchen counters and cooking utensils should be washed thoroughly after they have touched raw meat, especially poultry. Meats should be refrigerated as soon as possible after bringing them home from the supermarket, and they should be cooked until they are no longer pink. After meals, cooked leftovers should be refrigerated as soon as possible.

When traveling, children should never drink from streams, springs, or lakes unless local health authorities have certified that the water is safe for drinking. Parents also should be careful when buying prepared foods from street vendors, especially if no local health agency oversees the operations.

Pets, especially reptiles, can spread germs if their feeding areas are not separate from family eating areas. Children should never wash pet cages or bowls in the same sink that is used to prepare family meals.

genital herpes   See HERPES, GENITAL.

genitourinary tract infections   See URINARY TRACT INFECTION.

German measles   The common name for rubella, this viral infection is not very similar to MEASLES, although it also causes a rash on the face, trunk, and limbs. Rubella, which causes a mild illness in children, is really serious only when contracted by pregnant women in the early months of gestation. During this time, there is a chance the virus will infect the fetus, which can lead to a range of serious birth defects known as rubella syndrome.

Although rubella was once found throughout the world, it is now much less common in most developed countries because of successful vaccination programs. The United States has tried to eradicate the disease by vaccinating all school-age children; in 1969 when the vaccine became available, at least 60,000 Americans had rubella. By 1993 the number had dropped to 192.

Cause

Rubella is caused by rubella virus that is transmitted by particles in the air when an infected person coughs or sneezes. It can also be transmitted on contaminated objects, where the virus can survive for a short period of time on tissues, doorknobs, phones, and so on. It infects only humans.

Before the development of the vaccine, rubella was common in spring and winter and peaked every six to nine years. There were huge rubella epidemics in the United States in 1935, 1943, and 1964.

Symptoms

In the past, the infection usually affected youngsters between ages six and 12 with a rash beginning on the face and spreading downward and outward to arms and legs. The rash typically runs together to make large patches, but it does not itch. It lasts for a few days, with a slight fever (less than 101°F.) and enlarged lymph nodes; some children may have a mild cough, sore throat, or runny nose before the rash appears. Sometimes the entire infection comes and goes without notice; at least 30 percent of children with rubella have no symptoms at all, although they are infectious to others.

Adolescents may have slightly more pronounced symptoms, including headaches, fever, body aches, eye infections, or a runny nose about one to five days before the rash. Swollen glands in the neck and ear typically appear seven to 10 days before the rash. The virus may be transmitted from a few days before the symptoms appear until a day after symptoms fade.

Incubation period ranges from 14 to 23 days; the average is 16 to 18 days.

Rubella may be confused with other conditions characterized by rashes, such as SCARLET FEVER or drug allergy.

Diagnosis

A lab test to confirm rubella is important, since the symptoms can be so mild they may be overlooked or mistaken for something else. Blood tests are available that reveal rubella immunity or an active rubella infection. If a person has been vaccinated, the blood test will show that the person is immune.

Treatment

There is no specific treatment for rubella, although acetaminophen may reduce the fever.

Complications

Congenital rubella is the most serious complication of rubella infection, since it can cause fetal death or miscarriage. The risk is highest when the pregnant woman is infected in the first 12 weeks of pregnancy (miscarriage rate is as high as 85 percent during this time). At 14 to 16 weeks, the risk drops to just 10 to 24 percent, and after 20 weeks the risk is almost nonexistent.

Infants who survive infection in the womb may be born with a variety of birth defects, including deafness, eye problems (including blindness), ear defects, MENTAL RETARDATION, growth retardation, and bleeding disorders.

Prevention

Any child with rubella must be kept at home until well past the infectious stage; babies born with rubella have the virus in their nose, throat, and urine for as long as a year.

Vaccination can provide long-lasting immunity. There is not usually any reaction to the vaccine, which is produced with a live virus that offers complete prevention to more than 95 percent of those who receive it. Rubella infection itself also provides immunity.

The recommended vaccine for all infants in the United States, is the MMR (measles, mumps, rubella), which is not effective when given earlier than 12 months because the baby may have maternal antibodies that will interfere with the vaccine's action. Therefore, the first dose of MMR is typically given to infants between 12 to 15 months; a booster is given at age four to six, before the child starts school. Older children who missed these shots should receive one dose of MMR.

Anyone who is not sure of having received the vaccine or having rubella should be vaccinated; there is no risk to receiving the vaccine if a person is already immune.

Children with a high fever or a severe allergy to neomycin should not be given the vaccine. There is no penicillin in rubella vaccine, and it is safe for those allergic to eggs.

giardiasis The most common cause of waterborne infection in the United States, this infection of the small intestine is caused by a protozoon found in the human intestinal tract and in feces. In recent years, outbreaks of giardiasis have been common among preschool children and in large public picnic areas. *Giardia* can easily be spread in the child's home, and parents and siblings may become infected.

Cause

Giardiasis is caused by *Giardia lamblia,* a type of protozoa found in the human intestinal tract and in feces. It causes foul-smelling, explosive diarrhea. The protozoa was named for the 19th-century French biologist Alfred Giard, who discovered it.

The protozoa are spread by contaminated food or water, or by direct personal hand-to-mouth contact. Children can spread the infection by touching contaminated toys, changing tables, utensils, or their own feces. For this reason, the infection spreads quickly through a day-care center or institution for the developmentally disabled. Unfiltered streams or lakes that may be contaminated by human feces are a common source of infection to campers. Infection is often spread by not properly washing hands after bowel movements, after changing diapers, or before preparing foods. In addition, outbreaks have also been linked to portable wading pools and contaminated water supplies.

Symptoms

The infection interferes with the body's ability to absorb fats in the intestinal tract, so the stool is filled with fat. Giardiasis is not fatal, and about two thirds of infected children have no symptoms. When they do occur, symptoms appear about one to three days after infection and include explosive diarrhea, foul-smelling and greasy feces, stomach pains, gas, loss of appetite, nausea, and vomiting. In some cases, the infection can become chronic.

Diagnosis

Giardiasis is diagnosed by examining three stool samples for the presence of the parasites. Because the parasite is shed intermittently, half of the infections will be missed if only one specimen gets checked. Stool collection kits are available for this purpose. A different test looks for the proteins of *Giardia* in the stool sample.

Treatment

Acute giardiasis usually runs its course and then clears up, but antibiotics will help relieve symptoms and prevent the spread of infection. Medications include metronidazole, furazolidone, and paromomycin. Occasionally, treatment fails; in this case, the patient should wait two weeks and repeat the medication. Anyone with an impaired immune system may need to combine medications. Healthy carriers do not need to be treated.

Complications

Some children get a chronic infection and suffer with diarrhea and cramps for long periods of time, losing weight, and growing poorly. Those most at risk for an infection are those with impaired immune function and malnourished children.

Prevention

While chlorine in water treatment will not kill the cysts, filtered public water supplies eliminate it. It can be prevented by thoroughly washing hands before handling food. In addition, children should:

- maintain good personal hygiene
- not eat unwashed fruit or vegetables unless they can be peeled
- stay home from a child-care center if they have severe diarrhea until the stool returns to normal.

See also FOOD POISONING; GASTROINTESTINAL INFECTIONS.

gingivitis See GUM DISEASE.

gluten sensitivity A mixture of two proteins found in wheat and rye that is important for baking properties; when mixed with water, it becomes sticky and helps trap air in the dough. Sensitivity to gluten leads to CELIAC DISEASE in children.

gonorrhea The most commonly reported communicable disease in the United States, most often affecting the genitourinary tract and sometimes the pharynx, eyes, or rectum. Sexual abuse should be strongly considered when a gonorrheal infection is diagnosed in a child older than newborn and prior to puberty. A sexually transmitted disease may be the only physical evidence of sexual abuse in some cases.

Reported rates of gonococcal infection range from 3 percent to 20 percent among sexually abused children. A gonococcal infection may be diagnosed in the course of an evaluation of a medical condition such as conjunctivitis, in which no suspicion of abuse existed, or it may be diagnosed during an assessment for possible sexual abuse. In preteens, gonococcal infection usually occurs in the lower genital tract, and vaginitis is the most common symptom. PELVIC INFLAMMATORY DISEASE occasionally occurs. Infections of the throat and rectum typically do not have symptoms and may go unrecognized.

By law, all known cases of gonorrhea in children must be reported to the local health department and to a child protective services agency. An investigation should be conducted to determine whether other children in the same environment who may be victims of sexual abuse are also infected.

In addition, a child with a positive culture for the agent that causes gonorrhea should be examined for the presence of other sexually transmitted diseases (STDs) such as SYPHILIS, CHLAMYDIA infection, HEPATITIS B, and HIV infection.

Cause

The disease is caused by a circular bacterium, *Neisseria gonorrhoeae,* that is always grouped in pairs. It is passed from one person to the next only during sex with an infected person. It is not possible to get gonorrhea from toilet seats or swimming pools.

A girl who has unprotected sex with an infected man has an 80 to 90 percent chance of being infected herself—a much higher rate than with other STDs—but a boy who has unprotected sex with an infected girl has only a 20 to 25 percent chance of becoming infected. Boys have less risk because it is harder for bacteria to enter the body through the penis than through the vaginal walls.

Symptoms

Between three to five days after exposure, the symptoms will appear in the genital area, rectal area, or in the throat, depending on the sexual activity. Up to 80 percent of infected boys experience painful urination, frequent urge to urinate, and white or yellow thick pus from the urethra. About half of infected girls have massive swelling of the vagina, abnormal green-yellow vaginal discharge, vaginal bleeding between periods, pelvic discomfort (itching and burning), and pain when urinating.

As the infection spreads—which is more common in girls than boys—there may be nausea and vomiting, fever, and rapid heartbeat or peritonitis. Inflammation of the tissues surrounding the liver also may occur, causing pain in the upper abdomen. Severe spread of the disease is also more common in girls and is characterized by signs of blood poisoning with tender lesions on the skin of the hands and feet and inflammation of the tendons of the wrists, knees, and ankles. If the disease spreads to the conjunctiva of the eyes, there may be scarring and blindness.

In both girls and boys, infection in the throat causes a mild, red sore throat.

Diagnosis
Culture of the organism from a smear of bodily fluids.

Treatment
For many years, penicillin was the drug of choice, but in the late 1970s the bacteria became resistant; most resistant strains are in New York, California, and Florida, but resistance is seen in all states and most of Canada.

Today treatment involves two antibiotics, a shot of ceftriaxone and doxycycline pills. The pills will also cure chlamydia, which has similar symptoms to gonorrhea. Alternatively a doctor may give a single dose of cefixime. An infant born with the symptoms of gonorrhea must be hospitalized and given ceftriaxone.

Complications
Pelvic inflammatory disease develops in almost 40 percent of untreated girls and causes scars in the tubes, infertility, and tubal pregnancies. Babies born to infected mothers may have gonorrhea conjunctivitis during delivery; if the baby is not treated, it will be blind. For this reason, drops are placed in all babies' eyes at birth to prevent gonorrhea and

chlamydia conjunctivitis. In boys, untreated gonorrhea can lead to infections of the testicles, or scar the urethra, which can lead to sterility.

group A strep   See STREPTOCOCCAL INFECTIONS.

group B strep   See STREPTOCOCCAL INFECTIONS.

Group B Strep Association   A nonprofit organization formed in June 1990 by parents whose babies were victims of group B strep (GBS) infections. The association hopes to increase public awareness of the importance of prenatal screening and prevention of GBS disease and regularly lobbies government agencies. The association has provided information about group B strep, counseling, and support to more than 100,000 families nationwide. (For contact information, see Appendix I.)

growing pains   Relatively severe pain in the legs and behind the knee that occur in elementary school children, often after a strenuous day of activity. Growing pains occur at night while a child is in bed but always pass in time and should never be a cause for concern. Most experts believe there is little connection between the pain and growth spurts except for the fact that they usually occur during a period of rapid growth.

Growing pains generally strike at two periods during early childhood: among three to five year olds, and again in eight to 12 year olds. Growing pains typically affect about a quarter of all children, and although the pains are not serious, they can be upsetting to a child. Growing pains do not mean that a child is too active or doing anything wrong. Perfectly healthy children have these pains, which occur slightly more often in girls.

Causes
No firm evidence exists to show that growth of bones causes pain, and so a child is not actually feeling the bones grow. Instead, the pain is probably due to the strain caused by vigorous daytime activities on growing muscles and bones. These pains should disappear by the time she is a teenager. The pains can occur after a child has had a particularly athletic day.

Symptoms

Although growing pains often strike in late afternoon or early evening before bed, there are occasions when pain can wake a slumbering child. The intensity of the pain varies from child to child, and most kids do not experience the pains every day.

Growing pains usually last for 30 minutes to an hour as the child is going to sleep, and they always affect both sides of the body the same way. The pain is usually deep in the muscles of the calves and thighs, or sometimes behind the knees. Growing pains are often intermittent, coming once a week or even more infrequently, and always appear in the muscles rather than the joints. While joints affected by more serious diseases are swollen, red, or warm, the joints of children experiencing growing pains appear normal.

One important difference between growing pains and other diseases is that children in pain due to a serious medical disease do not like to be handled, whereas children with growing pains feel better when they are held, massaged, and cuddled.

Diagnosis

Doctors can diagnose growing pains simply by ruling out other conditions with a thorough history and physical examination. In rare instances, blood and X-ray studies may be needed before a diagnosis of growing pains is made.

Treatment

Massage, stretching, heat, acetaminophen (Tylenol), or ibuprofen (Advil) may help to relieve the pain. Support and reassurance that growing pains will pass as children grow up can help them relax.

When to Call a Doctor

Pains in the shoulders, arms, wrists, hands, fingers, neck, or back, or pain associated with a particular injury, are not due to growing pains and should be evaluated by a child's doctor. Since growing pains always affect both legs, pain in just one leg and never the other is unusual and should be seen by a physician. And since growing pains are always gone by morning, pain that is still present when the child wakes up could signal something more serious.

A doctor should be consulted if any of the following symptoms occur along with the growing pain:

- swelling
- redness
- fever
- unusual rashes
- loss of appetite
- weakness and fatigue

A child should see the doctor if the pain is severe and coming from one particular spot; the doctor may want to do a bone scan to rule out a bone infection or tumor. If the child cannot put weight on a red, swollen limb and there is a fever, the child could have an infection or a fracture. A blood test will reveal any infection and an X ray will diagnose a potential fractured bone. If the child's pain is in a joint and it cannot be easily moved, or the joint is swollen, there is a slight chance the child could have juvenile rheumatoid arthritis or an autoimmune disorder.

If the child has a great deal of pain in one hip, thigh, or knee and has trouble putting weight on that leg, the doctor may want to x-ray the thighbone to rule out Legg-Calve-Perthes disease. In this condition, the blood supply to the bottom of the thigh bone gets cut off so that the tip dies. The bone will regenerate within a few years, but the child may need bed rest or a cast to relieve pressure until the area begins to heal. Usually this disease affects boys between age four and puberty.

growth charts Charts used by a pediatrician to compare a child's measurements with those of other children the same age. It is important to be able to evaluate a child's growth, tracking change over time and monitoring the development in relation to other children. Therefore, the growth charts used by pediatricians are a standard part of any well-child checkup.

There are two sets of standard growth charts for boys and girls—one for infants up to 36 months of age, and another for children aged two to 20 years. Boys and girls are plotted on different charts because their growth rates and patterns differ. The charts include a series of percentile curves that show the distribution of growth measurements of children from across the country.

The growth charts most commonly used in the United States were developed in 1977 by the National Center for Health Statistics; these were recently updated to reflect better cultural and racial diversity. The original infant charts were based on data from one study of middle-class, formula-fed Caucasian infants from southwestern Ohio. Because almost all the children studied were white, middle class, and formula-fed, the charts fail to reflect several differences in growth among different children. For example, healthy breast-fed babies tend to gain weight more slowly than their formula-fed counterparts. Asian children are often smaller than Caucasian children. As a result, a pediatrician may mistakenly conclude that a particular child is not growing or gaining weight adequately. Equally problematic is the fact that two different groups of children were used for the overlapping charts covering children from birth to 36 months and from two years to 18 years.

This meant that the same 24- to 36-month-old child can measure in a different percentile when progressing from one chart to the next, often leading to misdiagnoses and expensive clinical tests. Finally, the charts developed to compare weight for stature ended at 10 for girls and 11 for boys, making it difficult to follow the growth of teenagers.

To correct these problems, several nutritionists, pediatricians, and statisticians at the National Center for Health Statistics, the National Institutes of Health, and the Centers for Disease Control and Prevention compiled a large sampling of new data from several recent annual national health and nutrition surveys based on millions of children. Their comprehensive data, covering children from birth to 20, better reflect the country's racial and ethnic diversity and include formula-fed and breast-fed babies. The new charts are significantly more accurate for monitoring the growth of infants, children, and adolescents.

The most important feature of the new growth charts is the inclusion of a measure called body mass index (BMI), which is calculated by dividing the weight by the height squared. BMI is commonly used to determine if adults are overweight and correlates well with a person's total body fat. Nutrition experts have long advocated that BMI be applied to children and teenagers because a major-

ity of overweight adults start as overweight children. The researchers found that by the age of eight it is possible to predict with great precision which child is likely to be overweight later in life.

At each well-child visit, the doctor records certain measurements in the child's medical record. For an older child, for example, a doctor may plot height for age, weight for age, weight for height, and body mass index (BMI). An infant usually is measured for length, weight, weight for length, and head circumference for age. Weight for height (or length) compares someone's weight at his height to other children's weight at that same height (or length). Although weight for height charts can be useful for assessing body weight in children two years and older, the Centers for Disease Control and Prevention have stressed that the recently released body mass index charts are preferred for this purpose.

Head circumference measures the distance around an infant's head at the widest point. Doctors take these measurements for premature infants, too. They correct for prematurity on the growth charts until age two years by subtracting the missed months of gestational time from the child's chronological age—so an eight-month-old baby who was born two months early will be plotted as a six-month-old. Known as "corrected age," this reflects the fact that a premature eight-month-old has been growing for two fewer months than an eight-month-old who was born on time. (By the time they are two years old, premature kids usually catch up to other children in growth.)

A growth chart has seven curves, each representing a different percentile: 5th, 10th, 25th, 50th, 75th, 90th, and 95th. The 50th percentile line represents the average value for age. There are also charts that show 3rd, 10th, 25th, 50th, 75th, 90th, and 97th percentiles. Doctors sometimes use these when they plot measurements that fall to the very outer edges of one or more growth curves. A child's growth measurements will be plotted among these percentile curves.

Parents should not assume that a high or low reading means that there is a problem. A baby whose head circumference is in the 90th percentile might also fall in the 90th percentile for weight and length. The child whose weight falls in the 10th percentile may have parents who are a bit below average for height and weight; therefore, for this child, being in the 20th percentile is an entirely normal reading. Sometimes, however, a child's measurement increases or falls sharply, or is at one extreme of the growth chart. For example, children who fall below the 5th percentile on the weight for height chart are considered underweight; children at or above the 85th percentile on this chart are considered overweight (and at risk for obesity); and those at or above the 95th percentile are considered to be obese. Generally, if a measurement exceeds the 95th percentile or crosses two percentile curves (such as climbing from the 40th percentile to the 75th percentile, thereby crossing the 50th and 75th percentile curves), there may be some cause for concern. On the other hand, if a measurement falls below the 5th percentile or crosses two percentile curves (dropping from the 50th to the 20th percentile, for instance), the doctor will also consider the possibility of a health problem. The growth chart should be viewed as a trend, not a fixed impression. What is more important is the examination of a growth chart reading over time to reveal a pattern of development. That pattern reveals how a child is growing in relation to other children.

growth disorders Any type of problem in children that prevents them from meeting realistic expectations of growth. Growth disorders may include FAILURE TO THRIVE in infancy, failure to gain height and weight in young children, and short stature or delayed sexual development in teens.

Shorter parents tend to have shorter children, which is a condition known as familial (or genetic) short stature; in this case, the short child does not have any symptoms of diseases that affect growth. Children with familial short stature still have growth spurts and enter puberty at normal ages, but they usually will only reach a height similar to that of their parents.

Children with constitutional growth delay are small for their ages but are growing at a normal rate. They usually have a delayed "bone age,"
which means that their skeletal maturation is younger than their chronological age. (A child's bone age is measured by taking an X ray of a child's hand and wrist and comparing it to standard X-ray findings seen in children of the same age.) These children, who do not have any symptoms of diseases that affect growth, tend to reach puberty later than their classmates. On the other hand, these children tend to continue to grow until an older age, eventually catching up to their peers when they reach adult height. Often in these cases, one or both parents or other close relatives also experienced a similar delayed growth pattern.

Because children with familial short stature or constitutional growth delay often face social problems because they are short or lagging behind in sexual maturity, they may need help in coping with teasing.

Other Causes of Growth Disorders

Diseases of the kidneys, heart, gastrointestinal tract, or lungs also may lead to growth disorders, which may be the first sign of a problem in some of these conditions. Endocrine diseases involving too little or too many hormones can cause growth failure during childhood and adolescence. Growth hormone deficiency is a disorder that involves the pituitary gland, which may not produce enough hormones for normal growth. Hypothyroidism is a condition in which the thyroid gland fails to make enough thyroid hormone, which is essential for normal bone growth.

One of the most common genetic growth problems is Turner syndrome, which occurs in girls when there is a missing or abnormal X chromosome. In addition to short stature, girls with Turner syndrome usually do not experience normal sexual development because their ovaries do not function normally.

Diagnosis

A child who has stopped growing or is growing more slowly than expected will often need additional testing to uncover signs of the many possible causes of short stature and growth failure. These tests may include:

- *Blood tests* To look for hormone and chromosome abnormalities and eliminate other diseases

- *Bone age X ray*
- *Brain scans*   To check the pituitary gland for abnormalities
- *Growth hormone stimulation test*   To measure how well the pituitary gland produces growth hormone by giving medication to trigger the secretion of growth hormone, and then checking growth hormone levels

Treatment

Treating a growth problem is usually not urgent, but early diagnosis and treatment of some conditions may help children achieve a more typical adult height. If an underlying medical condition is identified, specific treatment may improve growth. Growth failure due to hypothyroidism, for example, is usually simply treated by replacing thyroid hormones.

In addition, growth hormone injections for children with growth hormone deficiency, Turner syndrome, and chronic kidney failure may help them reach a more normal height. Human growth hormone is generally considered safe and effective, although full treatment may take many years and not all children will have a good response.

growth plate injuries   The growth plate is the area of growing tissue near the end of the long bones in children and adolescents. Each long bone has at least two growth plates, one at each end. The growth plate determines the future length and shape of the mature bone. When growth stops during adolescence, the growth plates close and are replaced by solid bone.

Growth plate injuries occur in children and adolescents because the growth plate is the weakest area of the growing skeleton, weaker than the nearby ligaments and tendons that connect bones to other bones and muscles. In a growing child, a serious injury to a joint is more likely to damage a growth plate than the ligaments that stabilize the joint. An injury that would cause a sprain in an adult can be associated with a growth plate injury in a child.

About 15 percent of all childhood fractures involve injuries to the growth plate. They occur twice as often in boys as girls, with the greatest incidence among 14- to 16-year-old boys and 11- to 13-year-old girls. Older girls experience these fractures less often because their bodies mature at an earlier age than boys. As a result, their bones finish growing sooner, and their growth plates are replaced by stronger, solid bone.

About half of all growth plate injuries occur in the lower end of the outer bone of the forearm at the wrist. These injuries also occur frequently in the lower bones of the leg and in the upper leg bone or in the ankle, foot, or hip bone.

While growth plate injuries are usually caused by an accident such as a fall or a blow, chronic injuries can also result from overuse. For example, gymnasts, long-distance runners, or baseball pitchers can all have growth plate injuries. Most growth plate injuries in children are caused by falls, usually while running or playing on furniture or playground equipment. Competitive sports, such as football, basketball, softball, track and field, and gymnastics, account for a third of all growth plate injuries. Recreational activities, such as biking, sledding, skiing, and skateboarding, make up another fifth of all growth plate fractures, while car, motorcycle, and all-terrain-vehicle accidents accounted for only a small percentage of fractures involving the growth plate.

Whether an injury is acute or due to overuse, a child who has pain that persists or affects athletic performance or the ability to move or put pressure on a limb should be examined by a doctor. A child should never be allowed or expected to work through the pain. Children who participate in athletic activity often experience some discomfort as they practice new movements. Some aches and pains can be expected, but a child's complaints always deserve careful attention. Some injuries, if left untreated, can cause permanent damage and interfere with proper growth of the involved limb.

Although many growth plate injuries are caused by accidents that occur during play or athletic activity, growth plates are also susceptible to other disorders, such as bone infection, that can alter their normal growth and development.

Child abuse also can cause skeletal injuries, especially in very young children who still have years of bone growth remaining. One study reported that half of all fractures due to child abuse were found in children younger than age one, whereas only two percent of accidental fractures occurred in this age group.

Injury from extreme cold, such as FROSTBITE, can also damage the growth plate in children and result in short, stubby fingers or premature degenerative arthritis. Both radiation and chemotherapy used to treat certain cancers in children may damage the growth plate. The same is true of the prolonged use of steroids for rheumatoid arthritis.

Children with certain neurological disorders that result in sensory problems or muscular imbalance are prone to growth plate fractures, especially at the ankle and knee. Similar types of injury are seen in children who are born with insensitivity to pain. In addition, the growth plates are the site of many inherited disorders that affect the musculoskeletal system. Scientists are just beginning to understand the genes and gene mutations involved in skeletal formation, growth, and development. This new information is raising hopes for improving treatment of children who are born with poorly formed or improperly functioning growth plates.

Diagnosis

After learning how the injury occurred and examining the child, the doctor will use X rays to determine the type of fracture and decide on treatment. Because growth plates have not yet hardened into solid bone, they do not show on X rays but appear as gaps between the shaft of a long bone and the end of the bone. Because injuries to the growth plate may be hard to see on X ray, an X ray of the noninjured side of the body may be taken so the two sides can be compared. Magnetic resonance imaging (MRI), which is another way of looking at bone, provides useful information on the appearance of the growth plate. In some cases, other diagnostic tests, such as computed tomography (CT) or ultrasound, will be used.

Treatment

For all but the simplest injuries, the doctor may recommend that the injury be treated by an orthopedic surgeon or a pediatric orthopedic surgeon. Treatment should be started as soon as possible after an injury, and it generally involves a mix of the following:

- *Immobilization*   The affected limb is often put in a cast or splint, and the child must limit any activity that puts pressure on the injured area.

- *Manipulation or surgery*   If the fracture is displaced, the doctor will have to put the bones or joints back in their correct positions either by hand or during surgery. After the procedure, the bone will be set in a cast to enclose the injured growth plate and the joints on both sides. The cast is left in place for between a few weeks to two or more months. The need for manipulation or surgery depends on the location and extent of the injury, its effect on nearby nerves and blood vessels, and the child's age.

- *Strengthening and range-of-motion exercises*   These treatments may also be recommended after the fracture is healed.

- *Long-term followup*   Evaluation includes X rays of matching limbs at three- to six-month intervals for at least two years. Some fractures require periodic evaluations until the child's bones have finished growing.

Most growth plate fractures heal without any lasting problems. However, if the injury was severe and the blood supply was cut off, growth can be stunted. If the growth plate is shifted, shattered, or crushed, a bony bridge is more likely to form and the risk of stunted growth is higher. An open injury in which the skin is broken carries the risk of infection, which could destroy the growth plate.

gum disease   Infection at the roots of the teeth that causes bleeding, receding gums that—if unchecked—can lead to tooth loss.

New research at the University of Michigan School of Dentistry showed that it is possible to treat severe root-level bacterial infections with antibiotics, not surgery. Until recently, most dentists treated gum disease by scraping or planing away the root-level plaque and tartar caused by bacteria. In severe cases, oral surgeons made cuts at the gum line to improve access to the affected roots.

The new treatment includes drug capsules to be taken for two to four weeks (depending on the severity of the problem), followed by as many as three rounds of topical antibiotics by temporarily gluing on experimental drug-impregnated cellulose film into the root surface. Using this regimen, researchers avoided surgery or extraction for 88 percent of patients, including 67 percent of those with teeth identified by other dentists as too infected to save.

habit   A strong behavior pattern that is repeated again and again. Five of the most common habits of children that often annoy parents include nail-biting, thumb sucking, hair twirling, nose picking, and breath holding. Although a child's habits may be irritating to parents, in most cases a habit is just a phase in the normal developmental process and no need for alarm. Habits also tend to occur in clusters, so it is not unusual to see a child chewing on her nails while entwining her other hand in her hair.

Some studies estimate that 40 percent of children between the ages of five and 18 chew on one or more nails; occasionally a child also may bite his toenails. Both boys and girls appear equally prone to the habit in earlier years, but as they get older, boys are more likely to be nail-biters.

Hair-twirlers are likely to be girls who spend time twisting, stroking, or pulling their hair, usually beginning in early childhood and lasting until adolescence. In some girls, the behavior may first appear during the teen years.

Nose picking appears to be a habit that usually begins in childhood but may actually linger into adulthood. In fact, a 1995 study of adults found that 91 percent picked their noses on a regular basis.

Thumb sucking is another popular habit that probably begins when an infant's thumb brushes the mouth as the result of random movements. Some children also suck their fingers or their entire fists. Most thumb suckers are younger children, but while about 45 percent of two year olds suck their thumbs, only about 5 percent of 11 year olds do.

Breath holding is yet another popular habit. Actually watching a child try to stop breathing can be a frightening experience, but it is more worrisome to parents than dangerous for the child.

Breath holding may begin in infants as young as six months old and tends to occur in tense and overly active children. In a few cases, the child may hold his breath so long that he passes out; rarely, breath holding may trigger a seizure. Most often, children try holding their breath about once a week, although in some children it can happen several times a day.

Causes

Experts admit that they are not always sure what causes a habit, but they know it is a learned behavior that usually provides a positive experience for the child. Habits may develop as entertainment for a bored child, or as a coping mechanism to soothe an anxious one. Biting nails or twirling hair might be one way a child relieves tension, just as a parent might try to relax by having a cocktail or exercising.

Studies also suggest that nail-biting may have a strong genetic component. Other habits may be holdovers from infancy, such as thumb sucking as a common self-comfort behavior that has pleasurable associations with feedings and cessation of hunger. The behavior may linger into childhood because of its positive associations. Hair twirling, too, may be an attempt by a child to regain the feelings associated with close contact with the mother's body or clothes.

Still other children will engage in habits to attract attention or as an attempt to manipulate their parents. If your child feels that you are ignoring him, he may engage in the annoying habitual behavior because he knows that it will provoke a reaction from you. A child who does not want to go to bed early may holds his breath to frighten his parents into allowing him to stay up longer. This is a learned behavior that may signal a child who is trying to gain control of his environment. Breath holding is said to be more likely to occur if parents are overprotective or insistent upon rigid schedules.

Treatment

Most habits eventually disappear. Often if a parent ignores a habit, the behavior will eventually stop when the child no longer needs it or outgrows it. Many habits, in fact, do disappear when a child reaches school age.

Habits vs. Mental Problems

In rare instances, a habit may be due to a physical or psychological problem. For example, a child who picks his nose may do so because he has stuck an object in his nose. A child who constantly sucks her thumb might be feeling extremely anxious. Most habits are harmless, but they can sometimes lead to injury. For example simple hair twirling is a common habit, but a child who pulls her hair out in patches may have trichotillomania, a more serious condition in which a child intentionally pulls out her hair. Habits that affect a child's social relationships or interfere with daily life are considered obsessive behaviors, such as those seen in obsessive-compulsive disorder. When a person imposes some control over an obsessive behavior, he begins to feel increasing anxiety until he displays the behavior again.

Haemophilus influenzae type B (Hib) A type of rod-shaped bacterium not to be confused with the influenza virus that causes the flu. Haemophilus influenzae type B (Hib) is a bacterium that causes potentially deadly MENINGITIS, PNEUMONIA, and blood infection (bacterial sepsis). *H. flu* meningitis is a serious infection characterized by inflammation of the brain and spinal cord that may be fatal.

According to the Centers for Disease Control (CDC), from the 1980s more than half of the estimated 20,000 Americans aged five years or younger who contracted HIB disease each year developed bacterial meningitis. This disorder was the leading cause of acquired mental retardation in the United States, leaving many youngsters blind, deaf, or paralyzed. More than two-thirds of all bacterial meningitis victims are children younger than five. The condition is serious because nearly one

child in every 20 who gets meningitis dies, and up to 35 percent of those who live develop permanent brain damage. However, widespread use of a vaccine licensed for infants in 1990 has dramatically reduced the incidence of a deadly disease that only 10 years ago killed 800 infants each year in the United States. According to the CDC, the incidence of invasive Hib infection has dropped by almost 98 percent among infants and children since the introduction of the vaccine. Although the disease is not yet completely eradicated, the vaccine has been stunningly effective.

Cause

Hib disease is caused by the *Haemophilus influenzae* type B bacteria, which has several different strains, each with a different capsule around the bacterium. Type B was the most common cause of meningitis in children before the vaccine; the other types are rare. One strain (non-typeable) is a common cause of ear infections in children. Other illnesses caused by *H. influenzae* type B bacteria include epiglottitis, septic arthritis, CELLULITIS, bacteremia, and pneumonia.

The bacteria enters a child's nose and will cause meningitis if the bacteria travels through the blood into the membrane covering the brain (the meninges). Healthy children can carry the bacteria in their nose and throat secretions; the infection is spread by kissing or sharing possessions, drinks, food, and so on. Child-care workers can also spread the bacteria.

Symptoms

If a child is going to develop symptoms, they will appear within two weeks after exposure. All types of meningitis may appear in children either gradually or suddenly. The gradual type is harder to diagnose because the symptoms (at least at first) are vague. Much more common is the abrupt onset variety of meningitis, in which symptoms appear in less than 24 hours, with a sudden high fever (100°F to 106°F), chills, vomiting, stiff neck, intense headache in the front of the head, or a seizure. There may be muscle spasms and photophobia (eye pain when exposed to light).

Some children exhibit unusual behavior as the infection begins, including aggressiveness, irritability, agitation, delirium, or screaming, following by lethargy or coma. Some may experience a cold or ear infection before the onset of meningitis.

A baby from age three months to two years may exhibit fever, vomiting, irritability, seizures, and a high-pitched cry. The baby may suddenly become rigid, and the soft spot on the front of the head may become hard or bulging.

Diagnosis

A lumbar puncture (spinal tap) is necessary to sample the fluid around the spinal cord and check for bacteria, white cells, sugar, and protein. This will help determine what sort of virus or bacteria is causing the meningitis. Bacterial meningitis causes cloudy fluid, with a high amount of certain types of white blood cells, low sugar, and high protein. Bacteria will grow in blood or spinal fluid in 24 to 48 hours; rapid tests on fluid or blood give results in just a few hours, and are often helpful in identifying the type of bacteria.

Recent antibiotic treatment prior to getting meningitis may make diagnosis more difficult. Lumbar puncture is a safe procedure when done in a large emergency room or in an experienced pediatrician's office, and it is imperative in correctly diagnosing meningitis.

Treatment

Without treatment, a child can die from *H. flu* meningitis; with antibiotics, about 95 percent of children recover. Any child with possible *H. flu* meningitis will be admitted to the hospital for IV antibiotics. A baby or child would also receive dexamethasone before the first dose of antibiotic and continue to take it for two to four days to prevent hearing problems.

Children should rest in a darkened, quiet room; any fever higher than 101°F should be treated with acetaminophen and sponge baths.

A child with *H. flu* meningitis is considered to be infectious until after receiving 24 hours of antibiotics; however, even after recovery some children will carry bacteria in nose and mouth. Rifampin is given to eliminate this bacteria. Healthy carriers are infectious for a few weeks to a few months, and should also be given rifampin.

Children who recover from this type of meningitis, as well as those who are vaccinated, are immune.

Complications

Increased pressure on the brain from fluid buildup is a serious complication; signs of this include changes in head measurement, activity, vision, breathing, pupils' response to light, or decrease in urine.

The most common long-lasting complication is hearing impairment. Recent studies suggest that children over six weeks of age who received dexamethasone immediately had less hearing loss than those who did not receive the steroid.

Other, less common complications include blindness, hydrocephalus, arthritis, seizures, and permanent developmental delays.

Prevention

The best prevention for Hib is vaccination for all infants. Optimal protection is achieved when children receive their vaccines as early as possible within the recommended schedule. It is recommended as a four-dose series, with three doses given to infants at two, four, and six months of age, followed by a booster dose at 12 to 18 months. DTaP/Hib combination products should not be used for primary immunization in infants at ages two, four, and six months but can be used as boosters following any Hib vaccine. In late 1990 the Food and Drug Administration (FDA) approved two new vaccines for use in children two months of age and older.

The Hib vaccine is one of the safest of all vaccine products, and it cannot cause meningitis. About one in every eight children who receive the vaccine may have some slight redness, swelling, or tenderness at the injection site. About one in every 140 children will develop a fever higher than 102°F. The reactions begin within 24 hours of the shot and quickly pass.

Before the vaccine, as many as 5 percent of healthy preschoolers carried *H. flu* type B, but did not get sick. Vaccinated children, however, cannot become carriers.

The antibiotic rifampin is used to prevent cases of Hib after exposure; if all babies and young children in a home or child-care group are vaccinated, preventive medicine after an exposure is not necessary. Rifampin will temporarily get rid of *H. flu* from the noses and throats of healthy carriers about 95 percent of the time. It helps prevent any exposed child in a day-care center or a family from getting *H. flu* meningitis.

hand, foot, and mouth disease   A common viral disease of toddlers that produces blistering of palms, soles, and the inside or the mouth. The condition often sweeps through day-care centers in the summer. There is no connection to the cattle disease known as hoof-and-mouth disease.

The child is infectious wherever the rash or sores appear; the virus will be present in stool and digestive tract for several weeks. Infected children do not need to be isolated, however, because most adults are immune and the illness is not severe. Many children are infected but do not exhibit symptoms; they develop immunity without illness.

Cause

The disease is caused by the coxsackievirus and is spread by contact with nose and mouth secretions. While infection bestows immunity for life, it is possible to get this disease a second time from a different type of coxsackievirus.

Symptoms

Symptoms usually appear within four to six days after infection. The mild illness usually lasts only a few days and includes ulcers inside the cheeks, on gums, or tongue, together with a fever, achiness, sore throat, headache, and poor appetite. Two days later, a rash on palms, fingers, soles, and diaper area appear; this is the signal that the virus is abating.

Diagnosis

Tests are unnecessary to diagnose this condition, but if the child is very ill, samples can be taken for culture from the lesions or stool.

Treatment

There is no treatment other than painkillers to relieve blister discomfort, although Benadryl solution may help. Acetaminophen is given for fevers above 101°F or for headaches. Small sips of soothing foods and fluids will ease mouth sores, with the use of frozen or diluted juice, lukewarm broth, soft noodles, or gelatin desserts.

Complications

Complications are extremely rare.

Prevention

Hand-washing is the only way to prevent this disease. This is especially important in a day care or nursery school. Family members can be protected by washing the towels, washcloths, and bedding used by a sick child.

hantavirus pulmonary syndrome   A respiratory illness caused by a new strain of hantavirus (a group of viruses carried by rodents) that causes its victims to gasp for air as their lungs fill with fluid. It kills about half the people it infects, usually within a week. Hantaviruses can be found throughout the world, where more than 170 names have been given to the hantavirus infections, including the often-fatal hemorrhagic fever. The syndrome was first diagnosed in the United States in 1993 at a Navajo reservation in the Four Corners area of New Mexico, Colorado, Utah, and Arizona.

Until 1993, hantaviruses around the world had been linked to the development of hemorrhagic fever, but the strain that was discovered in Four Corners provoked a new disease, with debilitating flu-like symptoms and respiratory failure. Today the number of infections with the hantavirus in the United States is rising, reaching 131; almost half have been fatal, according to the Centers for Disease Control and Prevention. More than 50 of the 131 cases occurred before the Navajo reservation outbreak. Since the Navajo outbreak, more than 100 cases of hantavirus pulmonary syndrome have been reported in 21 states (including New York). In addition, seven cases have been diagnosed in Canada and four in Brazil.

Cause

The hantaviruses are a group of viruses carried by rodents responsible for a variety of diseases including hantavirus pulmonary syndrome and hemorrhagic fever. They are not passed directly from human to human. The severity of the illness it causes depends on the strain.

Each hantavirus infects primarily one type of rodent. The Hantaan, Seoul, Puumala, Prospect Hill, and Porogia strains are five viruses within the *Hantavirus* genus, the newly added fifth genus within the *Bunyaviridae* family. The Hantaan virus was isolated in a Korean lab in 1976 from the lungs of a striped field mouse. The Seoul virus infects domestic rats, and the Puumala virus affects the bank vole. Deer mice carry the U.S. strains.

Hantavirus pulmonary syndrome (HPS) is caused by a hantavirus named Muerto Canyon (Valley of Death) virus for the spot in New Mexico where it was isolated. The disease can be spread by several common rodent species (deer mice, white-footed mice, and cotton rats) and has been found in 24 states; it is most common in New Mexico, which has had 28 cases; in Arizona, with 21 cases, and in California, with 13 cases. Hantaviruses are not passed directly from human to human.

Scientists believe the outbreak was triggered by climate irregularities associated with the most recent El Niño (the occasional warming of waters in the tropical Pacific). While it is believed that the mice who carry the virus probably were infected for years, the climate-induced explosion in the deer mouse population may have fueled the spread of the disease in humans.

People can become infected with the virus after being bitten by rodents, and many people who have developed the disease live in mice-infested homes. Researchers do not know why some people are susceptible to the infection while others are not. The hantavirus does not appear to be highly infectious, and it almost always occurs in isolated cases. There were only four instances in which more than one case occurred at the same time and place.

Symptoms

Hantavirus pulmonary syndrome begins as a flu-like illness with fever and chills, muscle aches, and cough; it can be easily misdiagnosed as HEPATITIS or an inflamed pancreas. The virus goes on to damage the kidneys and lungs, causing an accumulation of fluid that can overwhelm the lungs. The disease is fatal in 40 percent of cases.

Treatment

There is no treatment approved specifically for hantavirus. However, if the infection is recognized early and the child is taken to an intensive care unit, some may do better. In intensive care, patients are intubated and given oxygen therapy to help them through the period of severe respiratory distress. The earlier the child is brought in to intensive care, the better. Patients experiencing full distress are less likely to survive.

Children who have been around rodents and have symptoms of fever, deep muscle aches, and severe shortness of breath should see a doctor *immediately.* Parents should be sure to inform the doctor that the child has been around rodents, which will alert the physician to look closely for any rodent-carried disease such as HPS. Although the antiviral drug Virazole (ribavirin) is effective in a related disease (hemorrhagic fever) caused by Old World hantaviruses, it is not effective against HPS and is not recommended. Ribavirin is not available for this use under and existing research protocol.

Prevention

For the first time, in October 2003 scientists demonstrated that an experimental vaccine against hantavirus pulmonary syndrome (HPS) triggered a strong antibody response—a response that is key to preventing the virus from causing infection. In addition, the antibodies, produced in nonhuman primates that received the vaccine, protected hamsters from disease even when administered five days after exposure.

The Centers for Disease Control (CDC) cautions homeowners about rodent excretion, even though hantavirus is a rare disease. People should assume that all rodent excretions are infected and should handle the droppings only after spraying them with disinfectant and wearing gloves.

hay fever   The common name for allergic rhinitis, this is the most common respiratory allergy in children, caused by the immune system's response to an airborne allergen. Those with a family history of allergies or personal history of other allergies are more likely to develop hay fever.

Cause

Hay fever is caused by a wide variety of allergens, but in babies and young children, mold, animal dander, and dust are more likely the allergens than pollen.

Symptoms

Most victims suffer only moderate discomfort. Allergic rhinitis should be suspected if the following symptoms last longer than the typical cold:

- runny nose
- sneezing
- watery, itchy eyes

- stuffy head
- clogged sinuses
- headache
- ticklish or sore throat from postnasal drip
- cough

Consult a Doctor

A doctor should be consulted if the child:

- has trouble breathing
- is wheezing severely
- has green or yellow nasal discharge
- is miserable due to the symptoms
- has symptoms that become much worse

Diagnosis

A child with severe allergies should see an allergist to determine the actual substances that cause the allergic reactions. Skin or blood tests may be recommended to determine the specific allergen.

Treatment

An antihistamine can help relieve symptoms by blocking the allergic reaction, and a brief course of decongestants can help open up the nasal passages. The child should gently blow mucus from the nose but should not blow hard because that could lead to an ear infection or bloody nose. The child may need more rest when suffering from an allergy. In haled steroids and antihistamine eye drops can help ease stuffy noses and itchy eyes.

The home (especially the child's bedroom) should be kept as clean as possible. The child's nose and mouth should be covered with a mask while doing things that may trigger the allergic reaction. Children with an animal-dander allergy should not have pets in the bedroom; otherwise, the pet should be kept clean and well groomed. Families of children with a mold allergy should use an air conditioner with an electrostatic filter during the summer. Children with a pollen allergy should be kept indoors as much as possible during pollen season, especially on dry, windy days.

Prevention

Avoiding the known allergens is the best course of action. A series of injections to help the child become less sensitive to the allergen may help.

headache   Headaches are an uncomfortable reality not just for adults but also for up to 20 percent of children from about age five to 17. Typically, chronic headaches in childhood occur most often as a result of tension (15 percent), although five percent of the time headaches are migraines. By the time they reach high school, most teenagers have experienced some type of headache, but less than 5 percent are due to serious problems such as a tumor or head injury.

If a child who has only had a headache once or twice a month suddenly starts experiencing them three or four times a week, the headaches have become chronic and a doctor should be consulted. A few children have their first headaches before they reach elementary school. If a young child cries or stops eating or has been restless or irritable, a doctor should be consulted.

Migraines

Migraines can occur in children as young as four years of age; most boys will outgrow migraines by their early teens. Girls, however, usually experience more migraines as they enter adolescence as a result of hormonal changes. Most children who have migraines have inherited the tendency, especially if they also experience motion sickness.

Cause   Migraines are often called "vascular headaches" because they occur when the blood vessels constrict or expand. Although constricting blood vessels do not cause pain, they can temporarily affect vision or balance. It is when blood vessels dilate, however, that their expansion triggers pain.

In some children, certain things trigger a migraine, such as stress, a change in routine or sleep patterns, bright lights, loud noises, or certain foods and beverages.

Symptoms   Unlike adults, children experience a migraine on both sides of the head, along with nausea, vomiting, dizziness, blurred vision, sensitivity to light and sound, and changes in temperament and personality. Unlike an adult's experience, a child may suffer with a migraine in only an hour, or for no longer than a day. About 15 percent of children also experience an "aura" several minutes before the onset of the migraine, featuring blurred vision, blind spots, or seeing colored or flashing lights, or wavy lines. A few children also may stumble or may have trouble expressing themselves.

Migraine variants In addition to traditional migraines, other less common forms of migraines can affect children. *Hemiplegic migraine* causes weakness of the arm or leg on one side of the body before, during, or after the actual headache. The weakness usually goes away within 24 hours. Oral contraceptives may increase the frequency of this migraine variant.

Ophthalmoplegic migraine is a rare headache that occurs in children, affecting the nerves and characterized by drooping eyelids, dilated pupils, and paralysis of the eye muscles along with a severe headache. It may last for weeks.

Basilar artery migraines can occur in younger people and generally last just a day. Symptoms are caused by a diminished blood supply to the parts of the brain supplied by the basilar artery and include dizziness, vertigo, nausea, double vision, unsteady gait, slurred speech, confusion, and weakness.

Confusional migraines occur in adolescents, triggering headache, confusion, and disorientation that may last up to 12 hours. Rarely, teens may experience a prolonged stupor or comatose state that may last up to seven days.

Paroxysmal vertigo is a condition that occurs in children between two and six years of age in which a sudden, intense episode of loss of balance and dizziness last for a few moments.

Alice-in-Wonderland syndrome is a very rare condition in which a child experiences bizarre visual illusions and spatial distortions associated with migraines. Children describe objects that seem smaller than their actual size (micropsia) or larger than their actual size (macropsia) and other perception distortions.

Treatment Several types of medication can ease the symptoms of migraine. Acetaminophen or ibuprofen can ease migraine pain for children and adolescents, and pediatricians may prescribe a sedative to help a child rest. Young children who experience very frequent migraine attacks that interfere with school and other activities might be given preventive medications such as cyproheptadine, propranolol, tricyclics, or calcium-channel blockers.

Adolescents who have occasional migraines without an aura may take medications to stop the migraine, including ergotamine tartrate and caffeine (Cafergot); a combination medication (Midrin); and triptans (Imitrex, Zomig, Amerge, and Maxalt). Teens whose migraines are more frequent might be given preventive medications such as propranolol, tricyclic antidepressants, calcium-channel blockers, or anticonvulsants, such as divalproex sodium (Depakene, Depakote). None of these medications is approved for migraine treatment in children.

In addition to medication, many migraine sufferers find biofeedback and relaxation techniques may be helpful. Relaxation techniques such as deep breathing exercises, progressive muscle relaxation, mental imagery relaxation, or relaxation to music can be very effective in alleviating a migraine headache. Instruction for these techniques is available on audio tapes and CDs, and some record shops and bookstores carry them.

Prevention The best way to prevent migraines is to identify what triggers their onset:

• *Stress* Exercise, rest, and hobbies can reduce stress. Some children can reduce migraines by learning biofeedback techniques to control stress.

• *Good diet* Children should always eat three balanced meals, because skipping meals lowers the blood sugar level and can cause migraines.

• *Caffeine* Suddenly cutting back on caffeine can trigger a migraine, as can drinking too many caffeinated beverages. Cutting back on caffeine should be done slowly.

• *Food* Certain foods or additives can trigger a migraine in some children, including aged cheeses, pizza, luncheon meats, sausages or hot dogs containing nitrates, chocolate, yogurt, and MSG (monosodium glutamate).

• *Sleep* Children should have consistent sleep schedules and avoid lack of sleep, which can trigger migraines.

• *Hormones* Ovulation and menstruation can trigger migraines or increase their frequency.

Tension-Type Headaches

Tension headaches can either be episodic or chronic, and occur far more frequently in children than do migraines. The episodic headache can occur several times a month, while a child may suffer with chronic headaches almost every day.

Symptoms Episodic tension headaches produce a moderate pain that feels like a band of pressure around the head. These headaches often begin gradually in the middle of the day, lasting anywhere from a half hour to all day.

Conversely, chronic tension headaches seem to be ever-present with a dull throbbing on the front, top, and sides of the head, together with a band of pressure and soreness.

Cause Children's tension headaches are often caused by stress, depression, or insufficient rest, but they are not inherited and are not caused by disease.

Treatment Heat or an ice pack on the head can ease the pain. Because tension headaches are triggered by emotional stress related to family, school or schoolmates, or friends, the best way to eliminate the pain is to work on easing the stress. A nap, walk, or warm bath or shower may help. Relaxation techniques such as deep breathing exercises, progressive muscle relaxation, mental imagery relaxation, or relaxation to music can be very effective in reducing or eliminating the tension that produces a headache.

Counseling can help a child or adolescent better understand and appreciate where the headaches are coming from and can help children and their families to identify and manage stressful situations. Headaches also can be managed by using biofeedback, in which sensors are connected to the body to monitor changes in muscle tension, blood pressure, or heart rate. Feedback is displayed on a computer screen, so that a child can learn to recognize the signs of tension and apply a relaxation technique to ease stress.

Nonprescription medications such as acetaminophen (Tylenol), ibuprofen (Advil or Motrin), or naproxen sodium (Aleve) can ease the symptoms of either episodic or chronic headaches. Children under 14 should not take aspirin because of its connection to REYE'S SYNDROME.

Some doctors may prescribe medications to reduce the frequency and severity of chronic tension headaches. Preventive medications include antidepressants with a sedating effect, such as amitriptyline (Elavil).

Organic Headaches

Fortunately, fewer than 5 percent of children's headaches are caused by serious disease or physical problems such as an abscess, head injury, tumor, blood clots, intracranial bleeding, or MENINGITIS. Nevertheless, a physician will want to rule out these causes.

Other Conditions

A fever may produce a headache, which can be the result of INFLUENZA or a bacterial infection. A fever, headache, and neurological symptoms together can also signal a central nervous system infection. Rarely, a high fever and severe headache are signs of meningitis or encephalitis, especially if these symptoms are accompanied by a stiff neck, weakness, seizures, vision changes, lethargy, personality changes, nausea, and vomiting. It is urgent that these diagnoses be made as quickly as possible, because delays can cause serious complications.

Most children bump their heads occasionally, but a few suffer more serious head injuries that may affect the brain. In this case, the child will probably have a headache and maybe nausea or vomiting at first. However, if the headache continues for more than a few days or gets worse, the child should be immediately examined by a physician.

Sinus infection, temporomandibular jaw syndrome (TMJ), and dental problems also may cause headaches. Although headaches can accompany TMJ, most of these are actually undiagnosed tension headaches or migraines.

Diagnosis When an organic cause is suspected, lab tests can be used to form a diagnosis. Both a computed tomography (CT) scan or a magnetic resonance imaging scan (MRI), reveal problems within the brain. Unless a child has abnormal movements or has lost consciousness, an electroencephalogram (EEG) is usually unnecessary, and a skull X ray will not provide much helpful information. While these tests may reveal tumors, abscesses, fractures, or other organic problems, they cannot diagnose a migraine or tension-type headache.

Call a Doctor

Parents should call a doctor if their child has a headache and also if the child:

- has a seizure or loses consciousness
- experiences a personality change
- loses balance or becomes uncoordinated
- experiences nausea and vomiting or visual problems
- has a stiff neck and fever in addition to headaches

head injury Even the mildest bump on the head is capable of damaging the brain. More than a million of these head injuries every year are sustained by children, 30,000 of whom will suffer permanent disabilities. In fact, 60 percent of patients who sustain a mild brain injury continue to have a range of symptoms called "post-concussion syndrome" as long as six months after the injury. These symptoms can result in a puzzling interplay of behavioral, cognitive, and emotional complaints that can be difficult to diagnose and that can cause ongoing discomfort and destroy personal lives.

Boys are twice as likely to be injured as girls, especially between the ages of 14 and 24. Children are more likely to incur traumatic brain injury during the spring and summer. Traffic accidents account for almost half of the injuries in school-age children and teens; about 34 percent occur at home and the rest in recreation areas. In young children, abuse is the primary cause of head injury; 64 percent of babies under age one who are physically abused have brain injuries, usually caused by shaking. In children under age five, half of all head injuries are related to falls.

The kind of injury the brain receives in a closed head injury is determined by the type of accident: whether or not the head was restrained on impact, and the direction, force, and velocity of the blow. If the head is resting upon impact, the maximum damage will be found at the impact site; a moving head will experience damage on the side opposite the point of impact. A closed head injury can cause widespread damage as the force of impact causes the brain to smash against the opposite side of the skull, tearing nerve fibers and blood vessels. This type of injury may affect the brain stem, causing physical, intellectual, emotional, and social problems. The entire personality of the child may be forever changed.

Symptoms
The signs following head injury may be elusive, but it is important to understand that symptoms tend to get worse over time. If a child begins to play or run immediately after getting a bump on the head, for example, serious injury is unlikely, but the child should still be closely watched for 24 hours.

Symptoms after a head injury may be caused both from the direct physical damage to the brain and from secondary factors such as lack of oxygen, swelling, and blood flow disturbances.

Both kinds of injuries can cause swirling movements throughout the brain, tearing nerve fibers and causing widespread vascular damage. There may be bleeding in the brain, and swelling may raise pressure inside the skull and block oxygen to the brain.

After a head injury, there may be a period of impaired consciousness followed by a period of confusion and poor memory with disorientation, and problems with the ability to store and retrieve new information. The physical and emotional shock of the accident interrupts the transfer of all short-term memory information just before the accident. This is why some children can remember information several days before and after an accident but not information right before the accident occurred. Indeed, brain scan research indicates that contusions and diffuse injuries associated with mild head injury are likely to affect those parts of the brain that relate to memory, concentration, information processing, and problem solving.

There may be a temporary amnesia following head injury that often begins with memory loss over a period of weeks, months, or years before the injury, diminishing as recovery proceeds. Permanent amnesia, however, may extend for just a few seconds or minutes before the accident; in very severe head injuries, however, the permanent amnesia may cover weeks or months before the accident.

A small minority of children are plagued by symptoms, including headache, dizziness, confusion, and memory loss, which may continue for months. Obvious warning signs include:

- lethargy
- confusion
- irritability

- severe headaches
- changes in speech, vision, or movement
- bleeding
- vomiting
- seizure
- coma

More subtle signs of head injury may also appear gradually, and may include:

- long- and short-term memory problems
- slowed thinking
- distorted perception
- concentration problems
- attention deficits
- communication problems (oral or written)
- poor planning and sequencing
- poor judgment
- changes in mood or personality

Sometimes, certain behavior may appear long after the traumatic brain injury occurs. These behaviors may include overeating or drinking, excessive talking, restlessness, disorientation, or seizure disorders.

Diagnosis
In the past, diagnostic tests were not sensitive enough to detect the subtle structural changes that can occur and persist after a mild head injury. While computerized axial tomography (CAT) scans are widely available in emergency rooms to help diagnose brain bruises, many experts believe these scans may not pick up the subtle damage after a mild head injury. Magnetic resonance imaging (MRI) and PET scan are more sensitive in pinpointing many brain lesions and may be more sensitive in detecting the diffuse shearing and contusions as well.

In many children, however, brain scans cannot detect the microscopic damage that occurs when fibers are stretched in a mild, diffuse injury, as brain axons lose some of their covering and become less efficient. This mild injury to the white matter of the brain reduces the quality of communication between different parts of the brain. In this case, a quantitative electroencephalogram (EEG)—that measures the time delay between two regions of the brain and the amount of time it takes for information to be sent from one region to another—may help to reveal damage. Evoked potential brain tests are not generally used in children with mild head injury because they are not sensitive enough to document physiological abnormalities unless testing is done within a day or two of injury.

Treatment
Only a small percentage of children with mild head injury are hospitalized overnight, and instructions upon leaving the emergency room usually do not address behavioral, cognitive, and emotional symptoms that can occur after such an injury. Patients who do experience symptoms should be seen by a specialist. Unless doctors are thoroughly familiar with medical literature in this new field, experts warn that there is a good chance that patient complaints will be ignored. Parents of children with continuing symptoms after a mild head injury should call the local office of the Brain Injury Association (see Appendix I for address) for a referral to a specialist.

Prevention
Head injuries can be prevented by taking appropriate safety precautions, such as insisting that children wear helmets when biking, riding a scooter, skating, sledding, or skiing. Children also should wear seat belts and ride in the backseats of cars.

head lice   See LICE.

hearing, normal development   Because normal hearing is so crucial to the development of language, it is important to understand whether an infant can hear correctly. At the age of birth to three months, a baby should:

- look startled if there is a sudden loud noise
- stir in sleep, wake up, or cry if someone makes a noise
- recognize the sound of a parent's voice, usually quieting down and becoming calm when the voice is heard

At the age of three to six months, a baby should:

- respond to a parent's voice
- move the eyes to search for an interesting sound
- turn eyes toward a parent who calls the child's name

At the age of six to 12 months, a baby should:

- turn toward a parent who calls the child's name from behind
- turn toward an interesting sound
- look around when hearing new, interesting sounds
- understand simple words like "no" and "bye-bye"

If a baby cannot do some of these things, a pediatrician should be consulted. The earlier a baby's hearing loss is diagnosed, the better for the child.

hearing problems The lack of early detection of hearing problems in children is one of the most serious public health problems in the United States today. Hearing loss affects about 3.5 percent of all children up to age 17. Hearing is a critical part of a child's development; even a mild or partial hearing loss can affect a child's ability to speak and to understand oral language. Yet the average age at which moderate-to-severe hearing loss is detected in children is two to three years of age, although these problems can and should be identified and treated much sooner.

If hearing loss is detected early enough, babies can be fitted with hearing aids or be exposed to sign language. Because children learn language by being exposed to it, it is hard for these children to develop adequate speech or sign without experiencing either spoken or sign language.

Types of Hearing Loss
Conductive hearing loss is caused by an interference in the transmission of sound to the inner ear. Infants and young children frequently develop conductive hearing loss due to ear infections. This loss is usually mild, temporary, and treatable with medicine or surgery.

Sensorineural hearing loss involves malformation, dysfunction, or damage to the inner ear (cochlea).

It usually exists at birth. It may be hereditary or may be caused by a number of medical problems, but often the cause is unknown. This type of hearing loss is usually permanent. The degree of sensorineural hearing loss can be mild, moderate, severe, or profound. Sometimes the loss is progressive (hearing gradually becomes poorer) and sometimes unilateral (one ear only). Because the hearing loss may be progressive, repeat audiologic testing should be done. Sensorineural hearing loss is generally not medically or surgically treatable, but children with this type of hearing loss can often be helped with hearing aids.

A *mixed hearing loss* occurs when both conductive and sensorineural hearing loss are present at the same time. A central hearing loss involves the hearing areas of the brain, which may show as difficulty "processing" speech and other auditory information.

Prenatal Causes of Hearing Loss
Between 7 percent and 20 percent of deaf and hard-of-hearing people lost their hearing before birth. The three major threats to the hearing mechanism of a woman's unborn baby are viral diseases, drugs that harm hearing (otoxic drugs), and poor condition of a woman's uterus during pregnancy.

The most common cause of prenatal deafness is viral disease contracted by the mother. Of these, the most dangerous is rubella; other viral diseases that can harm hearing include INFLUENZA, MUMPS, TOXOPLASMOSIS, CYTOMEGALOVIRUS, and HERPES simplex. Of course, almost any severe infection can damage a baby's hearing, especially during the first trimester when the fetus seems to be especially vulnerable. Of all potential viruses, only the common cold appears to carry no threat at all to the hearing of an unborn child.

Bacterial infections are also a concern. If a mother contracts a bacterial infection before giving birth, she can transmit the infection to her baby. Other infectious agents that might be in the amniotic fluid can be swallowed by a fetus and then pumped up the eustachian tube into the tiny middle ear, where they can create an ear infection.

Cytomegalovirus Of all children born with cytomegalovirus (CMV), 95 percent do not show any symptoms. Among those who do, 60 percent will develop hearing loss. Those who don't have the symptoms rarely develop neurological problems, but 10 percent of those infants remain at risk for hearing loss nevertheless.

Each year in the United States, about 4,000 children acquire hearing loss linked to CMV. It is suggested that the virus may interfere with the fetal development of the ear. The hearing loss usually centers in the high-frequency sounds, with equal loss in both ears. There is no known treatment.

Rubella   In the United States, rubella among pregnant women is rare; when it does occur, it leads to deafness between 25 percent and 50 percent of the time. Hearing loss related to rubella is profound in 55 percent of cases, severe in 30 percent, and mild to moderate in 15 percent of cases. The hearing loss affects all frequencies, but the middle frequencies cause the most problems. Recent research suggests that congenital rubella is progressive and continues to damage the ears even after infancy.

Toxoplasmosis   Infection with *Toxoplasma gondii* during birth has been related to hearing loss, although the reason behind the problem is not well understood. Women can be infected after handling the litter of infected cats or by eating contaminated food. Up to 45 percent of American women carry the organism, although most may not have symptoms. One baby out of every 800 will acquire toxoplasmosis from the mother; the infection causes hearing loss in about 17 percent of children infected in the womb.

Many pregnant women do not have any symptoms of infection, which can include fatigue and muscle pain. A doctor cannot confirm the disease unless the mother had a negative toxoplasmosis test early in the pregnancy. Infection in the mother can be treated with medication, but an infection early enough in the pregnancy can cause a miscarriage. Even if a mother does become infected while pregnant, most babies do not develop the infection themselves. Some babies may not show evidence of the infection right away, but many doctors advise treatment anyway. Treatment with pyrimethamine, sulfadiazine, or spiramycin is effective.

Bacterial meningitis   One of the most common causes of acquired sensorineural deafness in newborns is bacterial meningitis, an infection of the covering of the brain. Bacterial meningitis in infants is usually caused by *Escherichia coli (E. coli)* bacteria, which can cause a hearing loss ranging from mild to profound. About half the infants who contract this disease will have a profound hearing loss that is usually permanent. Meningitis can cause a sudden, profound, and irreversible deafness in both ears. Often the cochlea is damaged when bacteria is transmitted along the cochlear nerve from the covering of the brain. Prognosis for infants who contract bacterial meningitis is poor; about half of those who live will have severe problems, including hearing loss, retardation, and seizures. Because this type of deafness is incurable, doctors usually try to prevent or treat meningitis early to head off such complications. Recent studies indicate that *Haemophilus influenzae* type B (Hib) meningitis patients who received dexamethasone right away had less hearing loss than those who did not. Because of vaccination, *H. flu* is no longer a major cause of hearing loss in the United States.

Group B strep   By 1964 doctors recognized group B strep as a threat to a newborn's health and hearing. Today it is responsible for most of the serious illnesses in babies younger than two months of age. Group B streptococcus is a round bacterium grouped in chains. While there are several different groups of streptococci, group B seems to infect pregnant women and newborns. The bacteria occur in soil and vegetation and are found normally in humans and many animals. However, between 4 percent and 40 percent of pregnant women experience a group B infection in the genital area. About half of these women will give birth to babies affected by group B strep, but only one in 100 of these newborns will have symptoms.

Most experts recommend screening all pregnant women for group B strep at 26 to 34 weeks of pregnancy. Some suggest giving antibiotics during delivery to all mothers who have a positive group B strep culture.

About 99 percent of babies born to mothers with group B strep in the vaginal area will still be born healthy. Of those babies who are born with an infection, about half will experience long-term hearing loss.

Syphilis   Scientists have known for a long time that congenital syphilis is a cause of hearing loss. It is caused by a spirochete transmitted from infected mother to child during pregnancy; it may cause an inner ear hearing loss in the child either during the first two years of life, or at puberty. In fact, 35 percent of affected newborns will eventually go on to experience some degree of hearing loss. This eventual hearing loss is hard to quantify, however, since the deafness may show up suddenly later in childhood or even in adulthood. Children with syphilis tend to experience sudden hearing loss in both ears; if it appears before age 10, the deafness is usually profound.

Syphilitic labyrinthitis is usually caused by congenital syphilis and results in a sudden, flat sensorineural hearing loss or a sudden, increasing fluctuation of sensorineural hearing loss. Incidences of congenital syphilis today are very rare. When they do occur, they can be treated with antibiotics.

HIV infections   Studies have reported that up to 49 percent of HIV-infected patients have some degree of sensorineural hearing loss, as a possible result of infection of the cochlea or the hearing center in the brain or both. Patients with HIV-associated hearing loss also may experience vertigo and facial nerve palsy. Drug treatment does not seem to affect the hearing loss.

Other Factors

If a mother has Rh-negative blood and she gives birth to a child with Rh-positive, the resulting *Rh-factor incompatibility* can led to deafness in subsequent fetuses. The cells from the first baby trigger the development of antibodies to the Rh-positive blood in the mother; while this will not harm the first baby, subsequent pregnancies carry a risk of damaging the hearing mechanism of the fetus when the antibodies attack the red blood cells of any Rh-positive fetus.

This incompatibility can injure the ears or nervous system of the newborn during the first few days of life, either directly or as a result of jaundice. This type of jaundice is caused by abnormal destruction of red blood cells at or shortly after birth. As the hemoglobin is broken down, it produces bilirubin, which can cause jaundice as it builds up in certain areas of the brain. The auditory system is one of the systems that is likely to be injured by this bilirubin buildup.

Prompt massive transfusions for the baby can ease the problems, but a transfusion done too early or too late will not prevent permanent injury to the hearing mechanisms. Hearing problems for newborns due to Rh-sensitization are becoming rare since the development of Rh (D) immune globulin; when injected into the mother 72 hours before delivery, it prevents 99 percent of the incidences of sensitization.

Cerebral palsy   CEREBRAL PALSY (CP) is a general term for nonprogressive disorders of movement, posture, or speech caused by brain damage during pregnancy, birth, or early childhood. Between two and six infants out of every 1,000 develop CP shortly before or after birth. Of these, between 25 percent and 30 percent will have hearing problems.

Kernicterus   Extremely high levels of bilirubin in a newborn that occur as a result of jaundice can sometimes lead to a condition called kernicterus that can damage the cochlear nuclei in the brain, causing hearing loss.

Loss of oxygen   During birth, a complete loss of oxygen and reduced oxygen are the two most common causes of damage to the organ of Corti, the body's hearing organ. Any disturbance of the infant's breathing or circulation can cause a loss of oxygen to the blood and brain.

About 6 percent of newborns experience a sensorineural hearing loss ranging from mild to severe if deprived of oxygen at birth. In premature infants, about 5 percent will experience some type of mild-to-severe sensorineural hearing loss.

The complete loss of oxygen is very rare, but it can kill cells unless corrected quickly. This loss of oxygen can be caused by a long labor, heavy sedation of the mother, obstruction of the baby's respiratory passages, poor lung development, or heart defects. The only way to prevent oxygen loss is to prevent these conditions.

Smoking   Evidence suggests that smoking cigarettes during pregnancy may triple a child's risk of developing an ear infection at birth, perhaps by interfering with the baby's immune system. Children of women who smoked during pregnancy were far more likely to suffer middle ear infections or require ear surgery by age five than were those whose mothers did not smoke.

Atresia   In about one of every 30,000 live births, a baby is born with a poorly developed or absent portion of the ear (atresia). This usually occurs during development of the external or the middle ear and usually affects only one side. Surgery can repair the ear's appearance; if the canal is closed, surgery can restore hearing by creating a passage for sound to reach the inner ear. Complete external and middle-ear atresia in one ear usually causes only a 60-decibel (dB) hearing loss for speech. Hearing loss after surgery depends on the severity of the ear's malformation, but half the time there is at least a 20-dB improvement.

Cleft palate   A number of children with cleft palate also have mild to moderate conductive hearing loss because of the cleft condition of the mouth; this loss is usually medically treatable. A hearing assessment is generally given during speech tests to find out if a hearing loss is present.

Down syndrome   DOWN SYNDROME is a chromosome disorder that results in mental retardation and physical deformities that also can lead to a hearing loss. Children born with this syndrome often have irregularities in the middle and inner ears and are susceptible to middle-ear infections that can lead to conductive hearing loss.

Low birth weight   Premature infants with a low birth weight (less than 3.3 lbs) are at risk for sensorineural hearing loss ranging from mild to severe. Approximately 5 percent of these low-weight infants will have hearing problems. However, full-term babies who do not weigh much are not at risk for this hearing loss.

Fetal alcohol syndrome   Evidence suggests that FETAL ALCOHOL SYNDROME may cause a sensorineural or conductive hearing loss in up to 64 percent of infants born to alcoholic mothers.

Otoxic drugs   Certain drugs taken by a pregnant mother can affect the hearing mechanism (especially the cochlea) of a developing fetus. They are particularly damaging to the developing baby during the sixth or seventh week of gestation. These drugs include:

- *Streptomycin*   This drug, which is almost never used anymore, can cause a sensorineural hearing loss in the baby ranging from mild problems hearing high-frequency sounds to a severe hearing loss in both ears.

- *Aminoglycosides and diuretics*   Aminoglycosides include kanamycin, neomycin, gentamicin, tobramycin, and amikacin, which only occasionally cause prenatal deafness. They cause deafness only when mothers received diuretics for kidney problems and also took aminoglycosides.

- *Aspirin*   High doses of aspirin and other salicylates can cause ringing of the ears and a hearing loss of up to 40 decibels, both directly related to the amount of the drug in the blood. Both hearing loss and tinnitus are reversible when the drug is stopped.

Acquired Deafness in Childhood

Almost any of the infectious diseases of childhood also may affect the inner ear. In these cases, often only one ear is damaged, although it is possible for both ears to be affected.

Ear infections   These infections are the most common cause of hearing loss in the United States. They may lead to a fluctuating hearing loss that disappears and reappears from time to time, related to allergies and the common cold. This type of hearing loss is not easy either to detect or to treat, since sometimes the child appears to have normal hearing and other times there seems to be a real problem.

Ear infections are responsible for 30 million pediatrician visits each year in the United States. Almost all American children will have at least one infection by the time they are six, although they are most likely to be infected before age two. Children are prone to these infections because their eustachian tubes are shorter, straighter, narrower, and more horizontal, making it easier for bacteria to enter from the back of the throat. Some children have recurring infections through age 10.

Infections of the middle ear occur in the cavity between the eardrum and the inner ear that can produce pus, fluid, and hearing loss. A child with a cold may experience swelling and blocking of the eustachian tube, the passage that connects the back of the nose to the middle ear. This tube may become blocked by the infection or by enlarged adenoids. Fluid produced by the inflammation cannot drain off through the tube and instead collects in the middle ear. This accumulation allows bacteria and viruses drawn in from the back of the throat to breed, causing infection.

The most common type of bacteria that cause ear infections normally live in a child's throat, including *Streptoccus pneumoniae, Haemophilus influenzae,* and *Moraxella catarrhalis.* During the winter, both viruses and bacteria may lead to ear infections.

Ear infections cause a sudden, severe earache, hearing problems, ringing of the ears, sense of fullness, and fever. Chronic untreated infection can cause hearing loss due to constant irritation. In some cases, acute infection never fully clears.

Lyme disease   The agent that causes LYME DISEASE (*Borrelia burgdorferi*) has been linked to hearing loss in about 2 percent of children with the disease, usually involving low-frequency sound waves. The reason behind the deafness is not clear, but researchers suspect the loss occurs as a result of damage to the auditory center of the hearing nerve. Doxycycline or amoxicillin can be given to patients over age nine; younger children should receive amoxicillin, penicillin V, or erythromycin. Those with hearing loss in the high frequencies are more likely to see improvement with antibiotics.

Measles   About one in every 1,000 cases of measles leads to hearing loss in childhood as a result of complications of ear infections or ENCEPHALITIS. Sensorineural hearing loss associated with measles is usually sudden and occurs in both ears, primarily in the higher frequencies; there may also be vertigo and ringing in the ears. This hearing loss tends to be permanent. Once very common around the world, today measles appears much less often in developed countries because of vaccinations.

Mumps   Hearing loss as a result of mumps infection occurs in about five of every 10,000 cases and is the most common cause of severe, one-sided deafness. It usually appears suddenly and happens without ear pain, and it may go unnoticed for many days or years after it occurs. Often, a patient will say he only recently noticed deafness in one ear. Close examination and history reveal that the deafness has in fact been present since an attack of mumps in childhood.

The deafness is usually profound and permanent and usually occurs in the higher frequencies. There also may be ringing of the ears, sensation of fullness in the ear, vertigo, nausea, and vomiting. Deafness due to mumps usually causes complete loss of hearing in one ear by irreparably destroying the inner ear without affecting the balance mechanism. If any hearing does remain in the affected ear, the deafness does not become progressive.

The deafness occurs when the mumps virus spreads to the lining of the brain. There have been fewer cases of mumps-related deafness in the United States since vaccination was introduced in 1967.

Chicken pox   Chicken pox is a common, mild childhood infectious disorder that has been known to cause sudden severe deafness in one ear. Related to the herpes family of viruses, chicken pox is caused by the varicella-zoster virus. After infection, the virus lies dormant within nerve tissues and may erupt as herpes zoster (shingles) later in life. One episode of the viral disease confers lifelong immunity. Chicken pox is heralded by a rash on the body, face, upper arms and legs, under the arms, inside the mouth, and sometimes in the bronchial tubes. While children usually have only a slight fever, adults may become quite ill with severe pneumonia and breathing problems.

Complications include encephalitis (brain inflammation), which can lead to central hearing loss. While the incidence of deafness and other complications related to chicken pox is small, the American Academy of Pediatrics recommends that all children receive the vaccine against chicken pox.

Tuberculosis   While it is uncommon to find infection with *Mycobacterium tuberculosis* in the middle ear, it may sometimes be the first symptom of tuberculosis (TB). Such infection causes multiple perforations of the eardrum and chronic ear inflammation. Anti-TB drugs treat this condition.

Fungal infections   Fungal infections of the ear can cause either a conductive or sensorineural hearing loss. A variety of antifungal drugs can be used to treat the problem, but there are no studies that prove that they work.

Encephalitis   This inflammation of the brain can cause central hearing problems in children. The hearing loss is usually the result of problems with the brain, not problems with the hearing apparatus, although sometimes there may be a problem with the cochlea. Encephalitis is usually caused by an infection; viruses are the most common, although the disease can result from many different kinds of organisms, including bacteria, protozoa, or worms, or by chemicals. There are two types of viruses that cause encephalitis: viruses (such as rabies) that invade the body and do not cause trouble until they are carried to the brain cells in the blood, and other viruses (such as herpes simplex, herpes zoster, and yellow fever) that first harm non-nervous tissue and *then* invade brain cells.

Hearing Tests

Ideally, doctors should identify infants with hearing loss before three months of age, so that intervention can begin by six months of age. Because prompt diagnosis of hearing problems could help offset lapses in language development, the American Academy of Pediatrics now recommends that all newborns be checked for hearing loss.

Although hearing loss is far more frequent than other disorders that are now assessed at birth, screening for hearing loss is only required in 10 states.

Newborn screening Screening tests for newborns are noninvasive and painless and usually include either tests of the small hair cells in the cochlea or the use of ear cuplets and sensors on the baby's head to measure brain response to sound.

In the past, only newborns in certain high-risk categories were tested for hearing problems. These high-risk categories included babies who were exposed to infections such as rubella or herpes, lack of oxygen at birth, bacterial meningitis, defects of the head or neck such as cleft palate or ear malformations, severe jaundice requiring transfusion, family history of childhood hearing loss, and low birth weight. Among these high-risk infants, the chance of having a congenital hearing problem is between one out of 20 to one out of 50.

Parents are usually the first to suspect a hearing loss. Most newborn infants startle or "jump" at sudden loud noises. By three months, a baby usually recognizes a parent's voice, and by six months an infant should turn the eyes or head toward a sound. By 12 months, a child should imitate some sounds and produce a few words, such as "Mama" or "bye-bye." If a child fails to follow these developmental patterns, a hearing evaluation may be a good idea. Hearing tests are also helpful if a young child has limited, poor, or no speech; seems frequently inattentive; has difficulty learning; or has

any signs of hearing loss, such as boosting the television volume.

In conjunction with any behavioral symptoms, hearing assessment also may be necessary if there are certain risk factors for hearing loss, such as childhood hearing loss in family members, severe complications at birth, frequent ear infections, or infections such as meningitis or cytomegalovirus. A parent with any doubts about slower-than-normal sound and speech-language development should discuss them with a pediatrician.

Behavioral testing A behavioral test is a better measure of hearing and usually should be used first in most children and older infants. In sound field audiometry, the child is placed in a soundproof booth and exposed to sound, because even an infant of one or two months will startle after a loud noise. An infant who does not show a startle reaction may have a hearing problem. However, relying on startling alone may not identify infants with smaller but still significant losses.

In a type of test called visual response audiometry, older infants will turn their head toward noise that gets their attention. Eventually they can learn that a stuffed animal will light up when there is noise, and they will look for the animal when they hear the noise. If they do not look, they did not hear it.

Conditioned play audiometry is a type of test that teaches toddlers up to age three or four to put a toy in a box when they hear the noise. Failure to put a toy in the box is an indication that they did not hear the noise.

In an *air conduction audiometry* test, children with a developmental age over four are given earphones and asked to raise their hands when they hear a sound.

Older children can respond to a bone vibration, which helps to determine whether a hearing problem is in the middle ear or inner ear, in cases where both ears are not the same. This is called *bone conduction audiometry.*

Brain stem evoked response testing This testing method is not a direct measure of hearing but a measure of hearing nerve activity. It is used with children who cannot respond in a soundproof booth—because in this type of test, no responses are required from the child. As the child sleeps (with or without sedation), earphones and electrodes record activity from the hearing nerve. The test, which measures high-pitched sounds better than low-pitched sounds, is often used by hospitals to test newborns.

As nerve impulses pass through the lower levels of the brain from the auditory nerve on their way to higher brain centers, they make connections in the brain stem near the base of the skull. The auditory brain stem response (ABR) test measures this electrical activity in the brain stem to see how well certain portions of the auditory system in the brain respond to a presented tone or beep. Clicks or tone pips are fed into the ear and a computer then analyzes brain activity to see if the brain waves change. Rather than a true test of the entire process of hearing, the ABR determines whether sound signals are reaching the brain.

By repeating the stimulus up to 100 times and averaging the response by computer, the responses can be enhanced while eliminating random background electrical activity. This way, auditory thresholds can be established that are quite close to those that can be obtained in conventional audiometry.

Otoacoustic emissions This test is a new method of testing hearing that also can be used with a child who cannot respond to behavioral testing. This rapid test can be used for screening in the newborn nursery; it is based on the fact that the ear not only hears noise but also makes noise. By measuring the very faint noises made by the ear, the test estimates how well the ear hears. An ear that does not hear will not make the expected noises. These noises are much too faint to be heard by human ears, but there are machines that can measure the sounds.

Central auditory processing testing A child must be able to speak in full sentences and have reasonably advanced language to take the central auditory processing test, so they must be at least over age five. The test assesses the ability to process the sounds children hear. Some children hear very well but have trouble deciding what to do with the sound once they hear it. These children are typically intelligent but have trouble following directions in school (especially in noisy environments). They may have had many ear infections when they were younger and developed difficulty dealing with sound as a method of communication. (See also HEARING PROBLEMS, GENETIC.)

hearing problems, genetic Deafness may be caused by a wide variety of inherited abnormalities, most of which are present at birth and do not improve. These genetic types of deafness are responsible for about half of all types of deafness in children. There are about 200 different types of genetic hearing problems ranging in degree from mild to profound. Although some types of hearing loss are associated with other physical characteristics or medical problems (such as changes in the eye or hair color), most types of genetic hearing loss do not involve other types of physical changes. The ability to hear is just one of many different physical traits that are handed down in families.

There are several ways that genes can influence a child's ability to hear. Each child receives half of its genetic material from each parent. There are many different gene locations that affect hearing and many different varieties of genes. Different forms of deafness may involve different gene locations.

Research has found mutations in several genes that are linked to deafness. The gene called Connexin 26 may be responsible for as many as 40 percent of cases of inherited hearing loss. Most of these children are born to parents with normal hearing. About 40 percent of children with this genetic mutation will have a profound hearing loss. Another gene (GJB2) mutation is the predominant cause of inherited moderate-to-profound deafness in the Midwest. Although there are many deafness-causing mutations in the GJB2 gene, one mutation causes the most cases of deafness. Couples who have had one child with GJB2-associated deafness have a 17.5 percent chance of having a second deaf child.

Scientists also have found a gene that plays a significant role in the development of cells essential to hearing. The gene (Math 1) sends a signal that triggers certain ear cells to mature into hair cells in the inner ear. Hair cells are responsible for both hearing and balance, and loss of these cells is a common cause of deafness. Once these cells have been destroyed, they cannot be re-created.

Genetic Diseases

There are a number of diseases that can be passed down in families that will result in hearing loss in children, including ALPORT'S SYNDROME, Cogan's syndrome, Penred's syndrome, Refsum's syndrome, and Usher's syndrome.

Alport's disease This genetic condition causes kidney inflammation in childhood, followed by a sensorineural hearing impairment in young adulthood. It is more common among boys than girls. There is no clear relationship between the extent of kidney disease and the onset of deafness. Treatment is supportive, since glucocorticoids and cytotoxic agents do not help.

Cogan's syndrome This condition involves an inflammation of the cornea that also can damage new bone formation around the round window and destroy the organ of Corti and cochlear nerve cells, leading to vertigo, tinnitus, and severe sensorineural hearing loss. Treatment with steroids is often effective in suppressing disease activity; in some patients, drugs may be tapered off and stopped, while others require maintenance-level treatment.

Penred's syndrome An inherited condition that causes deafness usually at birth. Children with the syndrome have different degrees of hearing loss, but it is severe for more than half. The syndrome is probably the most common form of deafness that appears with another condition (in this case, goiter). Research suggests that Penred's syndrome may be related to a gene mutation that produces a defective form of the protein pendrin and associated problems in transporting chloride ions that are normally found in the inner ear. This could lead to abnormal electrolyte concentrations that may make it impossible for the inner ear to properly transfer sound waves to the brain.

Refsum's syndrome A rare, genetic neurological disease of fat metabolism that is associated with hearing loss that begins in childhood and very slowly progresses. In 1997 the gene for the disease was identified on chromosome 10. While the syndrome can be treated with dietary changes, once the deafness appears the damage cannot usually be repaired.

Infantile Refsum's disease An unrelated condition affecting infants that leads to a buildup of phytanic acid in tissue and blood. It causes hearing loss that begins in infancy, and there is no cure. Death usually occurs in the 20s.

Usher's syndrome type II A condition that begins with a profound congenital deafness followed by a gradual loss of vision that often reaches complete blindness. This is one form of retinitis pigmentosa, in which pigment is deposited in and damages the light-sensitive portion of the eye. Originally described in 1959, the syndrome may account for 10 percent of all cases of congenital deafness. Although there is no treatment, regular exams by an ophthalmologist are recommended for all deaf children, as they can help identify Usher's syndrome early (usually before age six). Scientists have identified genes causing all three types of Usher syndrome to five different places on the chromosomes.

Waardenburg's syndrome A rare genetic syndrome. About half of all patients have a nonprogressive sensorineural hearing loss ranging from mild to severe in one or both ears. Only about one out of five patients have a hearing loss severe enough to require some aid to verbal communication. But some with the gene are totally deaf, and others are deaf in one ear yet have completely normal hearing in the other.

heart problems While most people think of heart disease as an adult problem, more than 40,000 American children are born with a heart defect each year, and others develop heart disease in childhood. Congenital heart defects are the most common birth defect and are the number one cause of death from birth defects during the first year of life. Nearly twice as many children die from congenital heart disease in the United States each year as die from all forms of childhood cancers combined. At present at least 35 different heart defects in children have now been identified.

Still, the outlook for children born with heart disease is slowly improving. The risk of dying after congenital heart surgery has declined from 30 percent in the 1970s to 5 percent today.

Congenital Heart Disease

Most heart disease in children is congenital, which means that a structural problem with the heart was present at birth. Eight out of 1,000 infants will be born with a congenital heart defect—about 35,000 babies each year. Defects range in severity from simple problems—holes between heart chambers, abnormal valves or connections of heart vessels, abnormally narrow heart vessels—to very severe malformations, such as the complete absence of one or more chambers or valves.

Defects appear when a mishap occurs during heart development soon after conception—often before the mother realizes she is pregnant. These defects are usually but not always diagnosed early in life.

Severe heart disease generally becomes evident during the first few months after birth. Some problems trigger very low blood pressure shortly after birth; others cause breathing difficulties, feeding problems, or poor weight gain. Minor defects are most often diagnosed on a routine medical checkup, since these defects rarely cause symptoms. While most heart murmurs in children are normal, some may be due to defects.

Cause   The cause of congenital heart problems is often unknown. Although the reason most defects occur is presumed to be genetic, only a few genes have been discovered that have been linked to the presence of heart defects. Rarely the ingestion of some drugs and the occurrence of some infections during pregnancy can cause defects. A maternal viral infection may also produce serious problems. For example, if a pregnant mother gets GERMAN MEASLES (rubella), the infection may interfere with the baby's heart as it develops or may lead to other malformations. Other viral diseases also may cause defects before birth. Certain conditions that affect multiple organs, such as DOWN SYNDROME, also can involve the heart.

Acquired Heart Disease

Acquired heart disease develops at some point during childhood as a result of infection—a much more unusual type of heart disease. This includes conditions such as KAWASAKI DISEASE, RHEUMATIC FEVER, and infective endocarditis. Children also can develop heart rate problems such as slow, fast, or irregular heart beats, known as "arrhythmias."

Diagnosis

The echocardiogram is a noninvasive procedure that uses ultrasound to image the structures of the heart. Doctors can obtain much more echocardiographic information in children than in adults. The structure of these hearts is often extremely different from the normal adult heart. Heart surgery texts often devote five times as many chapters to congenital heart problems as they do to adult heart diseases.

Catheterization, a common procedure for evaluating adult heart conditions, is used less often in children because inserting a catheter into a child's tiny artery carries a much higher risk. Only about one in four children must have the procedure for diagnosis.

Treatment

Because most childhood heart problems require sophisticated care, it is important that these children be treated in a center that specializes in pediatric cardiology. These centers can provide the highly skilled technical expertise needed, specialized diagnostic equipment designed for children, and the social and emotional support needed by the families.

Surgery itself involves much more sophisticated techniques than for adults, because the structure of a child's heart is so small. Of equal significance is the degree of care necessary to support the child under anesthesia, where medications must be administered precisely matched to the child's weight.

In the past repairs to a child's heart were often delayed because the risks were so significant, but today doctors realize delay can interfere with growth and cause FAILURE TO THRIVE. Modern doctors believe that preserving heart function as soon as possible permanently improves the quality of life. Half of all heart repairs in children are now done less than one month following birth.

Prognosis

Virtually all children with simple defects survive into adulthood. Although exercise capacity may be limited, most lead normal or nearly normal lives.

heat cramps   See HEAT ILLNESSES.

heat illnesses   Children normally cool themselves by sweating and releasing heat through the skin. Under certain circumstances, such as unusually high temperatures, high humidity, or vigorous exercise in hot weather, this natural cooling system may begin to fail, allowing internal heat to build up to dangerous levels. The result may be heat illness, which can be in the form of heat cramps, heat exhaustion, or heatstroke.

Heat Cramps

These brief, severe cramps in the muscles of the leg, arm, or abdomen may occur during or after vigorous exercise in extreme heat; they are painful but not serious. Children are particularly susceptible to heat cramps when they have not been drinking enough fluids. Most heat cramps do not require special treatment other than a cool place to rest. Fluids should ease the child's discomfort, and massaging the muscles may help.

Heat Exhaustion

Heat exhaustion is a more severe heat illness than heat cramps. It can occur when a child in a hot climate or environment has not been drinking enough fluids. A child can lose up to a quart of sweat during a two-hour sports game, and children are more susceptible to DEHYDRATION and heat exhaustion than adults; active children who do not drink enough are most at risk.

Symptoms   Symptoms can include dehydration, fatigue, weakness, clammy skin, headache, nausea and/or vomiting, rapid breathing, or irritability.

Treatment   The child should rest in a cool area, drink fluids, and be encouraged to eat. Clothing should be loosened or removed, and the child should be sponged with cool (not cold) water. A doctor should be called for more advice.

If the child is too exhausted or ill to eat or drink, intravenous fluids may be necessary. If left untreated, heat exhaustion may escalate into heatstroke, which can be fatal.

Heatstroke

Heatstroke is the most severe form of heat illness and is a life-threatening emergency. When significantly overheated, the body loses its ability to regulate its own temperature and fever can soar to 105°F or even higher, leading to brain damage or even death if not quickly treated. Prompt medical treatment is required to bring body temperature under control.

Risk   Overdressing for the climate and extreme physical exertion in hot weather with inadequate fluid intake increase the risk of heatstroke. Heatstroke also can occur if a child is trapped in a car on a hot day. When the outside temperature is 93°F, the temperature inside a car can reach 125° in just 20 minutes, quickly raising a child's body temperature to dangerous levels.

Symptoms   Emergency medical help should be obtained immediately if a child has been outside in the sun for a long time and shows one or more of the following symptoms of heatstroke:

- headache
- dizziness or weakness
- disorientation, agitation, or confusion
- sluggishness or fatigue
- seizures
- hot, dry skin
- temperature of 105°F or higher
- loss of consciousness.

Treatment   A child with any of the above symptoms should be moved indoors or into the shade, undressed, and sponged or doused with cool (not cold) water.

heat rash   An irritating skin rash also known as prickly heat that is associated with obstruction of the sweat glands and accompanied by prickly feelings on the skin. The medical term for prickly heat is *miliaria rubra,* the Latin term for "red millet seeds," which refers to the appearance of the rash. A milder form of the condition, known as *miliaria crystalline,* sometimes appears first as clear, shiny, fluid-filled blisters that dry up without treatment.

Symptoms

Numerous tiny, red, itchy spots cover mildly inflamed parts of the skin where the sweat collects, especially in the waist, upper body, armpits, and insides of the elbows. With prickly heat, the child is comfortable sleeping only in cool surroundings. Lack of sleep and intense skin irritation can make the child irritable.

Cause

While doctors are not completely sure of the reason behind the development of prickly heat, it is believed to be associated with trapped sweat.

Treatment

Frequent cool showers and sponging the area will relieve the itch. Calamine lotion and dusting powder may also help to ease the discomfort. Clothes should be clean, dry, starch-free, and loose to help sweat evaporate.

Prevention

Slow acclimation to hot weather will reduce the chance of prickly heat. Avoiding strenuous activities in the heat will also help prevent the problem.

heatstroke   See HEAT ILLNESSES.

Heimlich maneuver   The Heimlich maneuver is a series of abdominal thrusts designed to create an artificial cough, which forces a foreign object out of the airway. More than 2,600 children die from accidental choking each year in this country, according to the American College of Emergency Physicians (ACEP).

These accidents are usually attributed to food, liquid, balloons, marbles, or other foreign objects that lodge in the airway and result in suffocation. Children are more susceptible to choking because their airways are narrower than adults' airways. Foods commonly implicated in choking incidents include nuts, grapes, hot dogs, popcorn, chunks of meat, hard candy, and peanut butter.

The Heimlich maneuver can be performed on an older child or adolescent using this method:

1. The helper stands behind the child and locates the bottom rib with the hand.
2. The helper moves the hand across the abdomen to the area above the navel, and makes a fist. The thumb side of the fist is kept on the child's abdomen.
3. The helper places the other hand over the fist, pressing into the child' s stomach with a quick upward thrust until the foreign object is dislodged. The force of the thrust should be adjusted according to the child's physique. A

heavy 15-year-old girl needs a firmer thrust than would a six-year-old child.

4. The helper should have someone else call 911 after the Heimlich maneuver begins, or if the child has lost consciousness. The Heimlich maneuver should be continued until the object is dislodged.
5. If the child stops breathing, loses a heartbeat, and becomes unresponsive, cardiopulmonary resuscitation (CPR) should be started immediately until help arrives.

Heimlich Maneuver on a Baby

The Heimlich maneuver should not be performed on a baby if the baby can cough strongly and breathe, cry, or make a normal voice sound. If the baby cannot do any of these things, there may be a serious airway blockage.

No one should try to attempt to retrieve the object blocking the airway unless it is visible in the mouth. If visible, the object can be swept out with a finger. By attempting to retrieve an object that is not visible, a helper risks pushing it farther down the baby's windpipe. Someone should call 911 while the helper begins the Heimlich maneuver this way:

On an infant less than a year old:

1. The baby should be held face down in the helper's forearm, with the forearm extended out in front, making sure the baby's head is lower than its feet.
2. With the palm of the other hand, hit the baby's back, gently but firmly, five times between the shoulder blades.
3. Turn the baby face up in the helper's arm, and perform five chest thrusts, using the third and fourth fingers of the other hand. Repeat steps two and three until the object is expelled.
4. If the baby becomes unresponsive, stops breathing, or loses a heartbeat, infant CPR should be started until help arrives.

Helicobacter pylori   A type of bacteria that can cause digestive illnesses, including inflammation and infection of the stomach lining, and peptic ulcer (sores on the lining of the stomach or small intestine). Experts believe that most such infections produce no symptoms, so a child can have an infection without knowing it. When the bacteria do cause symptoms, they are usually either symptoms of gastritis or peptic ulcer disease. Scientists suspect that *H. pylori* infection may be contagious, because the infection seems to run in families and is more common where people live in crowded or unsanitary conditions.

Symptoms

In children, symptoms of gastritis may include nausea, vomiting, and pain in the abdomen, in addition to stomach ulcers. In older children, the most common symptom of stomach ulcers is a gnawing or burning pain in the abdomen, usually in the area below the ribs and above the navel. This pain typically gets worse on an empty stomach and improves with food, milk, or an antacid medicine.

About 20 percent of children with this condition have bleeding ulcers, causing bloody vomit or black, bloody, or tarry stools. Younger children with stomach ulcers may not have symptoms as clear-cut as those of older children, and their illness may be harder to diagnose.

H. Pylori *vs.* Campylobacter Pylori

H. pylori was once grouped with the *Campylobacter* species of bacteria, *Campylobacter pylori*. Medical researchers have now placed *H. pylori* in its own category, noting its role in causing gastritis, stomach ulcers, and possibly two types of stomach cancer. In industrialized countries, the infection is rare in children, although risk of infection is higher for persons who live in overcrowded or unsanitary conditions.

Diagnosis

Doctors can make the diagnosis of an *H. pylori* infection by using many different types of tests. They may look at the stomach lining directly with an endoscope, and take samples of the lining to be checked in the laboratory for microscopic signs of infection and for *H. pylori* bacteria. They may also conduct blood or a breath test.

Treatment

Doctors treat *H. pylori* infections using antibiotics. Because the bacteria may not be killed with a single antibiotic, a combination of antibiotics may be given. The doctor will probably also prescribe antacid medication and medicine to block production of stomach acid. If a child has symptoms of bleeding from the stomach or small intestine, these symptoms will be treated in a hospital. Over time, with proper treatment *H. pylori* gastritis and stomach ulcers (especially ulcers in the duodenum, a portion of the small intestine) can often be cured.

H. pylori infection can be cured with antibiotics. The pediatrician may also give antacids or acid-suppressing drugs to neutralize or block production of stomach acids. One way to help soothe the abdominal pain of *H. pylori* infections is by following a regular meal schedule. This means planning meals so that a child's stomach does not remain empty for long periods. Eating five or six smaller meals each day may be best, followed by some time to rest after each meal. Aspirin, ibuprofen, or anti-inflammatory drugs should be avoided because these may irritate the stomach or cause stomach bleeding. If a child vomits blood or has vomit that looks like coffee, a doctor should be called immediately.

Prevention

There is no vaccine against *H. pylori*. Although research suggests that infection is passed from person to person, scientists do not really know exactly how this happens, so it is difficult to present prevention guidelines. However, it is always important to wash hands thoroughly, eat food that has been properly prepared, and drink water from a safe source.

When to Call the Doctor

Stomachaches are quite common in children, and most are not caused by *H. pylori* bacteria. Still, a doctor should be consulted if a child has any of the following symptoms:

- severe abdominal pain
- bloody vomit
- bloody, black, or tarry stool
- persistent gnawing/burning pain below the ribs that improves after eating, drinking milk, or taking antacids

hemangioma A benign tumor or birthmark caused by an abnormal number of blood vessels in the skin. Hemangiomas may be either superficial, superficial and deep, or deep.

Superficial hemangiomas, known as STRAWBERRY BIRTHMARKS, are bright red protrusions that develop shortly after birth. At about the age of six months the tumor begins to subside and the red color slowly fades; by age seven, the hemangioma completely disappears.

Deep hemangiomas are blue and never clear up by themselves. These are found most often in young children, usually on the head and neck. Deep hemangiomas are composed of dilated veins rather than capillaries and are distinguished by their slow growth and by the fact that they do not disappear.

Treatment

Superficial hemangiomas do not require treatment for any medical reason, but if the marks appear on the face there may be psychological reasons to remove these tumors. Superficial hemangiomas may be removed by pulsed dye lasers, which are most successful in young patients.

Deep hemangiomas subject the child to profound psychological stress and can permanently rob children of their sight, or distort their facial features if present for too long. Systemic corticosteroids may help the lesions shrink, and cryotherapy, electrodessication, carbon idoxide, or argon laser treatments can successfully remove the growths.

hemolytic uremic syndrome (HUS) This serious disorder—once considered to be a rare form of kidney disease—in recent years has become more common as a complication of food-borne infection of *ESCHERICHIA COLI* 0157:H7. In very young children, between two and seven percent of *E. coli* 0157:H7 infections lead to this complication. In fact, hemolytic uremic syndrome (HUS) is the main cause of kidney failure in American children.

Symptoms

As the bacteria enter the kidneys, causing bleeding and destroying red blood cells, the child becomes pale and tired, with a fever and rising blood pressure. The kidneys shut down and urine is no longer produced.

Treatment

HUS is a life-threatening condition that must be treated in a hospital intensive care unit, where the child receives blood transfusions and is placed on kidney dialysis to allow the organs to recover. Most patients do recover at this point, but a small percentage (about 15 percent) do not and thus require permanent dialysis or a kidney transplant.

Even with intensive care, the death rate from this complication is still between 3 and 5 percent. One-third of the survivors will have abnormal kidney function years later and a few need long-term dialysis. Another 8 percent suffer with other complications, including high blood pressure, seizures, blindness, and paralysis for the rest of their lives. (See also ESCHERICHIA.)

hemophilia A bleeding disorder caused by a deficiency in blood clotting factors. Hemophilia A (often called classic hemophilia) is a hereditary disorder in which the clotting ability of the blood is impaired, which can lead to excessive bleeding. This type accounts for about 80 percent of all hemophilia cases. Although minor injuries and punctures are usually not a problem, uncontrolled internal bleeding can cause pain, swelling, and permanent damage to joints and muscles.

Hemophilia A occurs in about one out of 10,000 live male births. About 17,000 Americans have hemophilia, most of whom are men. Very rarely does it occur in girls and women. The only way a woman could ever have hemophilia is if her father has the disease and her mother carries the gene. With proper treatment, most boys with hemophilia will grow up to lead relatively normal lives.

Symptoms

Severity of symptoms can vary. Prolonged bleeding is the hallmark of hemophilia A, often first appearing when an infant is circumcised. Additional bleeding incidences appear as the baby begins to move around. Mild cases may go unnoticed until later in life, when the child experiences excessive bleeding and clotting problems after surgery or accidents. Internal bleeding may happen anywhere, and bleeding into joints is common.

The severity of the symptoms of hemophilia A depends on how a particular gene abnormality affects the activity of clotting factor VIII. When the activity is less than 1 percent of normal, episodes of severe bleeding recur for no apparent reason. Symptoms may include bruising, spontaneous bleeding, bleeding into joints, and associated pain and swelling, gastrointestinal tract and urinary tract hemorrhage, blood in the urine or stool, and prolonged bleeding from cuts, tooth extraction, and surgery.

Children whose clotting activity is 5 percent of normal may have only mild hemophilia with only rare unprovoked bleeding episodes. However, surgery or injury may cause uncontrolled bleeding, which can be fatal. Milder hemophilia may not be diagnosed at all, although some people whose clotting activity is 10 percent to 25 percent of normal may still have prolonged bleeding after surgery, dental extractions, or a major injury.

Typically, the first bleeding episode occurs after a minor injury before 18 months of age. A child who has hemophilia bruises easily, so that even an injection into a muscle can cause a large bruise. Recurring bleeding into the joints and muscles can ultimately lead to crippling deformities. Bleeding can swell the base of the tongue until it blocks the airway, making breathing difficult, or a bump on the head can trigger substantial bleeding in the skull, causing brain damage and death.

Cause

Hemophilia A is caused by an inherited sex-linked recessive trait with a defective gene on the X chromosome. Females are carriers of this trait. Half of the male offspring of female carriers have the disease and half of their female offspring are carriers. All female children of a male with hemophilia are carriers of the trait.

However, a third of all children with hemophilia A do not have a family history of the disorder. In these cases, hemophilia develops as the result of a new or spontaneous gene mutation.

Genetic counseling may be advised for carriers, who can be identified by genetic testing. A girl or woman is definitely a hemophilia carrier if she is:

- the biological daughter of a man with hemophilia
- the biological mother of more than one son with hemophilia
- the biological mother of one hemophilic son who has at least one other blood relative with hemophilia

A woman may or may not be a hemophilia carrier if she is:

- the biological mother of one son with hemophilia
- the sister of a male with hemophilia
- an aunt, cousin, or niece of an affected male related through maternal ties
- the biological grandmother of one grandson with hemophilia

Diagnosis

A laboratory analysis of blood samples can determine whether the child's clotting is abnormally slow. If it is, the doctor can confirm the diagnosis of hemophilia A and can determine the severity by testing the activity of factor VIII.

Treatment

Hemophilia is treated by giving the child the missing clotting factor. How much clotting factor is given depends upon where and how much the child is bleeding and the size of the patient. In the past, mild hemophilia A was typically treated with an infusion of a substance that triggered the release of factor VIII stored within the lining of blood vessels.

Clotting factors are found in plasma and in plasma concentrates. Some plasma concentrates can be used at home, either on a regular basis to prevent bleeding or when bleeding first starts. Both the dose and frequency depend on the severity of the bleeding problem, and the dose is adjusted according to the results of periodic blood tests. During a bleeding episode, more clotting factors are needed.

Prevention

To prevent a bleeding crisis, children with hemophilia and their families can be taught to administer clotting factor concentrates at home at the first signs of bleeding. People with severe forms of the disease may need regular preventive infusions.

Depending on the severity of the disease, clotting factors may be given before dental extractions and surgery to prevent bleeding. Immunization with hepatitis B vaccine is necessary because of the increased risk of exposure to hepatitis due to frequent infusions of blood products.

Children with hemophilia should avoid situations that might cause bleeding and take good care of their teeth so they will not need to have teeth pulled. Children with hemophilia also should avoid drugs that worsen bleeding problems, including aspirin, heparin, warfarin, and painkillers such as nonsteroidal anti-inflammatory drugs.

Complications

Complications of hemophilia include chronic joint deformities caused by bleeding into the joint or brain hemorrhage. Some children with hemophilia develop antibodies to transfused clotting factors so that the transfusions become ineffective. If antibodies are detected in blood samples, the dosage of the plasma concentrates may be increased, or different types of clotting factors or drugs to reduce the antibody levels may be used.

In the past, plasma concentrates carried the risk of transmitting blood-borne diseases such as hepatitis and AIDS. About 60 percent of people with hemophilia treated with plasma concentrates in the early 1980s were infected with HIV. Today, however, the risk of transmitting HIV infection through plasma concentrates has been virtually eliminated by using screened and processed blood and a genetically engineered clotting factor VIII (Recombinant).

New Research

Researchers are studying ways to use gene therapy to treat hemophilia by using a genetically engineered virus to deliver beneficial genes. Gene therapy is a novel form of disease treatment in which the active agent is a sequence of DNA, instead of the proteins or small molecules now used as drugs.

hemorrhagic colitis   See *ESCHERICHIA COLI* 0157:H7.

hepatitis   The description for inflammation of the liver. Children most commonly are diagnosed with hepatitis A, which is considered to be a food-borne illness. However, a number of specific viruses cause different versions of hepatitis that have been given alphabetical names to distinguish them, beginning with A and ending in G. Although the viruses are unrelated to each other, they act in similar ways, attacking and damaging the liver.

The various hepatitis viruses differ in their likelihood of producing chronic infection. For example, hepatitis A infection is not usually serious, whereas hepatitis B and C can lead to liver failure and death. When the liver is damaged, it cannot excrete the waste substance called bilirubin, which then builds up in the blood. This causes a yellow tinge to skin and eyes, called JAUNDICE.

Hepatitis A

The most common type of hepatitis in children, hepatitis A is spread by eating food or drinking water contaminated with the hepatitis A virus that is shed in the stool. Formerly known as "infectious hepatitis," hepatitis A tends to occur in cycles. In the United States, cases peaked from 1961 to 1971, declined, and then peaked again from 1983 to 1991; numbers dropped again after 1992. Food has been implicated in more than 30 outbreaks since 1983. It was implicated in 2004 in a large out break at a Pennsylvania Chichi's Restaurant, later traced to tainted scallions from Mexico.

Hepatitis A belongs to the enterovirus group of the picornaviruses, which include POLIO virus, COXSACKIE VIRUS, echo virus, and rhinovirus. The virus enters through the mouth, multiplies in the body, and is passed in the feces; it can then be carried on an infected child's hands and spread by direct contact, or by eating food or drink handled by that person. While anyone can get hepatitis A, it occurs most often among children, most of whom become infected either from close personal contact between family members or in nursery schools or child-care centers.

The virus is hardy and spreads easily. Unlike many other viruses, it can live for more than a month at room temperature on kitchen countertops, children's toys, and other surfaces. It can be maintained indefinitely in frozen foods and ice. To inactivate the virus, food must be heated at 185°F for one minute.

A food handler can spread the disease by touching food that is not cooked before it is eaten, such as sandwiches or salads. Well water contaminated by improperly treated sewage also has been implicated, since hepatitis A can live for a long time in untreated water. It is possible to get hepatitis A from eating raw or undercooked foods, such as shellfish, especially oysters. Shellfish filter large amounts of water as they eat, and if it is contaminated with hepatitis A, the virus will be concentrated in the shellfish.

Outbreaks of hepatitis A among children attending day care have occurred since the 1970s. Because infection among children is usually mild or asymptomatic and patients are infectious before they develop symptoms, outbreaks are often only recognized when adult contacts (usually parents) get sick. Poor hygienic practices among staff who change diapers and prepare food contribute to the spread of hepatitis A. Outbreaks rarely occur in child-care settings serving only toilet-trained children.

Symptoms   Infants and young children tend to have very mild symptoms; three-quarters of children have no symptoms. The rest have low fever and achiness, but rarely jaundice. In the rest, the disease is characterized by fever (100 to 104°F), extreme tiredness, weakness, nausea, stomach upset, pain in the upper right side of the stomach, appetite loss. Within a few days, a yellowish tinge appears in the skin and whites of the eyes. Urine will be darker than usual and the stool is light colored. Anyone over age 12 may become quite sick for a week or two. Once the jaundice appears, patients begin to feel better. The disease is rarely fatal and most children recover in a few weeks without any complications. The incubation period ranges from 15 to 50 days, and children are most infectious in the two weeks before symptoms develop.

Diagnosis   Blood tests showing antibodies to hepatitis A are the best diagnosis. Symptoms of hepatitis A are so similar to other diseases that a doctor needs a test to make the correct diagnosis.

Treatment   There is no drug treatment for hepatitis A. While symptoms appear, children should rest and eat a low-fat, high-carbohydrate diet in small amounts (such as crackers, noodles, rice, or soup). Antiemetics may be prescribed for severe nausea. Headaches or body aches may respond to acetaminophen. Normal activities may be resumed when the acute illness is over.

Complications   Rarely hepatitis A develops into fulminant hepatitis in which the child's liver cells are completely destroyed. As liver function stops, toxic substances build up and affect the brain, causing lethargy, confusion, combativeness, stupor, and coma. This can often be fatal, although the patient may live with aggressive treatment. If the child does not die, the liver is able to regenerate and resume function and the brain recovers.

Prevention   A new vaccine said to be 100 percent effective after a single primary dose became available in 1996 in the United States for children two years of age and older. The hepatitis A vaccine currently is recommended for children living in areas with consistently higher rates of hepatitis A, including 11 states where the prevalence of hepatitis A is more than twice the national average: Alaska, Arizona, California, Idaho, Nevada, New Mexico, Oklahoma, Oregon, South Dakota, Utah, and Washington. Routine vaccination also can be considered in six states where the prevalence of hepatitis A is less than twice, but still higher than the national average: Arkansas, Colorado, Texas, Missouri, Montana, and Wyoming. In addition, the vaccine is recommended for children traveling to countries where the disease is highly prevalent, including all countries and regions other than Canada, Japan, Australia, New Zealand, Scandinavia, and Western Europe. The vaccine is also recommended for children with chronic liver disease or blood-clotting disorders.

Although hepatitis A outbreaks sometimes occur in child-care settings, these outbreaks do not happen often enough to make it necessary for child-care providers or children in child care to be routinely vaccinated against hepatitis A. However, workers in child-care centers where there are diapered children must maintain strict rules about frequent hand-washing and procedures for diaper changing.

In addition, cooking contaminated food kills the virus. Shellfish from contaminated areas must be cooked (boiled) for at least eight minutes to be considered safe for eating.

Those who are exposed to hepatitis A can prevent infection by getting a shot of immunoglobulin (Ig), which is pooled human blood plasma that contains protective antibodies against the disease. People who need a shot of Ig include:

- all household members of someone with hepatitis A
- close friends of an infected school-age child
- if three or more children in day care or their families have hepatitis A, family members of the other children need Ig as well
- unimmunized travelers to developing countries

Hepatitis B

Formerly known as serum hepatitis, this is the most common preventable infectious disease in the United States. The virus can destroy the liver and is 100 times more transmissible than the AIDS virus. It is believed that there are 300,000 cases a year, of which only about 15,000 are reported; about 1.25 million Americans are carriers, which means they are infectious for the rest of their lives.

Almost 6,000 Americans each year die from acute hepatitis B or complications of the infection; around the world, the fatality rate is two million. It can be prevented by vaccine, but of the group who accounts for the most infections—those aged 15 to 39—only about 5 percent ever get vaccinated.

Cause   The hepatitis B virus (HBV) is carried in the blood and is also found in saliva, semen, and other bodily fluids. It is transmitted much the same as the AIDS virus, but hepatitis B is even easier to catch. One drop of infected blood contains hundreds of thousands of virus; one drop of blood with HIV virus is not infectious. However, it is not spread by casual contact. The virus must get into a person's blood to cause infection, but it can survive on dried surfaces for days. It enters the blood via sexual contact, blood transfusions, dirty needles, or sharing toothbrushes, razors, or eating utensils.

It is also possible for an infected mother to pass the virus to the fetus during the final three months of pregnancy, during delivery, or during nursing. There is less danger of passing on the infection if the mother contracts the disease in the early stages of pregnancy. All pregnant women should be tested for hepatitis B.

Symptoms   Incubation period ranges from six weeks to six months. Only about 10 percent of children who become infected with hepatitis B have any symptoms. When children do have symptoms, they may be similar to those for hepa-

titis A: fatigue, loss of appetite, jaundice, dark urine, light stools, nausea, vomiting, and abdominal pain. However, hepatitis B is a much more serious infection.

After infection with hepatitis B, chronic infection develops in 70 percent to 90 percent of infants, 15 percent to 25 percent of one to four-year-old children, and 5 percent to 10 percent of older children. Children who develop chronic hepatitis B infection may remain infectious for the rest of their lives.

The virus can be found in blood and body fluids several weeks before symptoms appear and several months after. Once antibodies appear in the blood, the child is no longer infectious. People who are chronic carriers (about 10 percent of those infected) do not develop antibodies and are always infectious although they do not appear to be ill. Those who recover are immune for life.

Diagnosis   Hepatitis B can be diagnosed by blood tests; other tests (that look for markers) can differentiate hepatitis B from other types of hepatitis. Liver function tests can measure enzymes produced by the liver that will be elevated in all forms of hepatitis.

Treatment   Hepatitis B is treated with alpha-interferons or infection-fighting proteins if the patient has a chronic hepatitis B infection. Short-term side effects include fever, chills, appetite loss, vomiting, muscle aches, and sleep problems; these disappear after a few weeks. Bed rest and a high-carbohydrate, low-fat diet are important. After recovery, patients need blood tests to see if they have developed antibodies. If they have not, they may become a chronic carrier; if so, they need to be tested to see if they carry the *antigen*. Those who do are extremely infectious and are at higher risk of developing complications. About 10 percent of these chronic carriers lose the antigen each year.

Complications   Between 10 percent and 85 percent of babies born to infected mothers will develop hepatitis themselves; of those, 90 percent become chronic carriers, at risk for eventually developing cirrhosis or liver cancer as adults. Twenty-five percent of them will die of liver disease as adults. Chronic carriers have a 100 times greater risk of developing liver cancer, which is almost always fatal, and are also at greater risk for developing cirrhosis of the liver because of the continual damage by the virus. Some people may be saved by liver transplants. Occasionally hepatitis B can lead to fulminant hepatitis, in which the liver cells are completely destroyed. As the liver function stops, toxic substances build up and affect the brain, causing lethargy, confusion, combativeness, stupor, and coma. This can often lead to death, although the patient may live with aggressive treatment. If the victim does not die, the liver is able to regenerate and resume function, and the brain recovers.

Prevention   While hepatitis B is completely preventable, thousands continue to come down with the disease each year. The vaccine, introduced in 1983, was made from blood plasma; a few years later a vaccine from synthetic products was introduced. A third synthetic vaccine was produced in 1991. All infants should receive the first dose of hepatitis B vaccine soon after birth and before hospital discharge; the first dose may also be given by age two months if the infant's mother tests negative for hepatitis B. The second dose should be given at least four weeks after the first dose, except for HIB-containing vaccine, which cannot be administered before age six weeks. The third dose should be given at least 16 weeks after the first dose and at least eight weeks after the second dose. The last dose in the vaccination series (third or fourth dose) should not be administered before age six months. Infants born to hepatitis B-positive mothers should receive hepatitis B vaccine and hepatitis B immune globulin (HBIG) within 12 hours of birth at separate sites. The second dose is recommended at age one to two months, and the vaccination series should be completed (third or fourth dose) at age six months. Infants born to mothers whose infection status is unknown should receive the first dose of the hepatitis B vaccine series within 12 hours of birth. Maternal blood should be drawn at the time of delivery to determine if the mother has been infected; if the test is positive, the infant should receive HBIG as soon as possible (no later than age one week). As of November 1991, the vaccine was recommended for all infants; boosters are not currently recommended. Unlike some vaccines, there is no apparent risk of serious side effects from the hepatitis B vaccine. Reactions seem to be limited to a sore arm at the site of injection or a slight fever.

Carriers should follow standard hygienic procedures to make sure their close contacts are not directly contaminated. Carriers must not share toothbrushes or any other object that may become contaminated with blood. In addition, household members should be immunized with hepatitis B vaccine.

Hepatitis C

The virus that causes hepatitis C was identified in 1988 and was first known as "non-A, non-B" hepatitis. In the United States, hepatitis C virus is linked to 20 percent of all clinical hepatitis cases and is the leading cause of chronic hepatitis. It causes liver cancer, kills up to 10,000 Americans a year, and causes almost half of all deaths from liver failure. More than half of all patients exposed to the virus become carriers, and up to 20 percent of these carriers develop cirrhosis, a severe liver disease.

About five out of every 100 infants born to HCV-infected women become infected at the time of birth. There is no way to prevent this from happening. Most infants infected with hepatitis C at birth have no symptoms and do well during childhood; scientists do not know if these children will have problems from the infection as they grow older.

Cause   Most children are infected at birth from infected mothers. There is no evidence that breast-feeding spreads hepatitis C, but infected mothers should consider abstaining from breast-feeding if their nipples are cracked or bleeding. Otherwise, hepatitis C is spread primarily through blood-related sources, such as transfusions and kidney dialysis. It is the cause of most cases of post-transfusion hepatitis. The risk of sexual transmission appears to be small, and there is no evidence that this type of hepatitis can be spread by casual contact, through food or by coughing or sneezing. Some people carry the virus in their bloodstream and may remain contagious for years.

Symptoms   About 25 percent of those infected with the virus will become sick with symptoms including appetite loss, fatigue, nausea and vomiting, stomach pain, and jaundice within two weeks to six months after exposure. Usually, symptoms appear by two months.

Diagnosis Children should not be tested for antibodies to hepatitis C before 12 months of age, as the antibodies from the mother may last until this age. If testing is necessary before 12 months of age, it could be performed at or after an infant's first well-child visit at age one to two months.

Treatment There are no licensed treatments or guidelines for the treatment of infants or children infected with hepatitis C. Children with elevated liver enzyme levels should be referred for evaluation to a specialist familiar with the management of children with hepatitis C-related disease.

Prevention At the present time, there is no hepatitis C vaccine. Hope for such a vaccine faded, according to the National Institute of Allergy and Infectious Disease, when their studies showed that exposure to the virus does not protect against reinfection.

Hepatitis D Virus (HDV)

An uncommon version of the hepatitis virus in the United States, it infects about 15 million people around the world. In the United States, hepatitis D infection occurs more often among adults than children. However, children from underdeveloped countries where hepatitis D is endemic are more likely to contract the virus through breaks in the skin.

Cause The virus requires the presence of hepatitis B virus to produce infection, so the frequency of hepatitis D closely parallels hepatitis B. Transmission from mother to child has not been documented in the United States. Hepatitis D is spread primarily through contaminated needles and exposure to blood products. Sexual transmission of hepatitis D is less efficient than for hepatitis B.

Symptoms Hepatitis D cannot be distinguished from other causes of hepatitis. The development of a new episode of acute hepatitis in a patient with known chronic hepatitis B infection should prompt a search for evidence of a new hepatitis D infection.

Treatment There is no reliable treatment for hepatitis D. Interferon-A is not as promising as hoped.

Prevention The hepatitis B vaccine can prevent hepatitis D, since hepatitis B infection is required for hepatitis D infection to occur.

herpes Any of a variety of inflammatory skin conditions characterized by spreading or creeping small clustered blisters caused by the herpes simplex virus. Forms of the virus cause COLD SORES and the sexually transmitted disease genital herpes (see HERPES, GENITAL) characterized by blisters on the sex organs. The virus also causes many other conditions affecting the skin.

More than 80 known viruses exist within the herpes family. Of these, eight are known to cause disease in humans, the most common being herpes simplex virus 1 and 2. HSV1 and HSV2 look identical under the microscope, and either type can infect the mouth or genitals. Usually, however, HSV1 occurs above the waist, and HSV2 below the waist. In children, HSV2 is usually associated with infections of babies who acquire the disease during birth. However, there is a certain amount of overlap between the two, and conditions usually caused by HSV2 may be caused by HSV1, and vice versa. Both types are highly infectious, spread by direct contact with the lesions or by the fluid inside the blisters.

Herpes simplex virus most commonly causes cold sores in infants and children, and genital herpes in adolescents. Herpes simplex virus is also responsible for eye infections in children and for lesions on the parts of fingers and at other sites.

Newborn Infection

A much greater concern is herpes simplex virus infection in newborn infants. The virus is most frequently transmitted to an infant from the mother during vaginal delivery or, sometimes, via ascending infection. Transmission is much more likely to occur during a vaginal birth in a mother who is having a first episode of genital herpes. In such cases, the rate of transmission may be 33 to 50 percent. Unfortunately, in most cases, infected neonates are born to women in whom neither the history nor the physical examination suggests active infection.

Herpes simplex infection in newborns can range from a local infection of the skin, eyes, and mouth to a generalized systemic infection or a localized infection of the central nervous system. Neonatal MENINGITIS is extremely rare.

Symptoms

Most children are eventually infected with HSV1. While the first infection with this virus may cause no symptoms at all, there may be a flu-like illness in addition to ulcers on the skin around the mouth; afterward, the virus remains in the nerve cells of the face. Many people experience recurrent reactivations of the virus, suffering with repeated attacks of cold sores, especially during a fever or prolonged sun exposure.

Sometimes the virus infects the finger, causing painful blisters called herpetic whitlows. In patients with a preexisting skin condition, such as DERMATITIS, the virus may cause an extensive rash of blisters called eczema herpeticum.

A child suffering an immunodeficiency disorder, such as AIDS, who is exposed to the virus may experience a severe generalized infection that can be fatal.

Other Herpes Viruses

Varicella-zoster virus (VZV)   A close cousin of the herpes simplex virus, the varicella-zoster virus is responsible for two other skin blistering disorders—first CHICKEN POX, and later SHINGLES (or "herpes zoster"), an acute inflammatory infection that produces painful blisters on the skin over the sites of nerves. Although shingles is most common in adults over age 50, it can occur in children who have already had chicken pox. Like the herpes simplex virus, the varicella-zoster virus can affect the eyes or the brain in addition to the skin.

Epstein-Barr virus (EBV)   This herpes virus is associated with acute infectious MONONUCLEOSIS and chronic fatigue syndrome. Mononucleosis, also known as the "kissing disease," is spread by saliva and nasal secretions. Initial symptoms last up to 10 days and include fatigue, lethargy, and slight fever. The acute phase of the illness lasts up to another 10 days and is marked by sore throat, high fever, enlarged lymph nodes in the neck, enlarged spleen and, oftentimes, a faint, pink rash over the body. The fatigue and lethargy can last longer than other symptoms.

Cytomegalovirus (CMV)   This herpes virus causes many diseases in humans, particularly in infants. Symptoms of a cytomegalovirus (CMV) infection include swollen glands, fever, and fatigue and may take the form of HEPATITIS, mild mononucleosis or, in newborns, JAUNDICE and low birth weight. In severe cases of infected infants, CMV may cause brain damage, deafness, blindness, and death.

Herpes virus 6   This virus causes ROSEOLA infantum (a fever and pale pink body rash), most common in children between ages six months and three years. Most cases trigger a fever but no rash. In older children the virus can cause mononucleosis-like symptoms. The virus and its effects on humans are still being studied.

Herpes viruses 7 and 8   These viruses and their effects on humans are still being studied.

Treatment

The most dramatic results of the use of antiviral therapy in healthy children have been seen with the use of acyclovir in the treatment of herpes. A recent survey of all causes of neonatal meningitis in England and Wales during the years 1975 to 1991 found only 10 cases that were due to herpes simplex virus among 26,090 reported cases. For this reason, the American Academy of Pediatrics does not recommend treatment of infants born to mothers with active primary or recurrent genital herpes infections unless cultures are positive or obvious symptoms of herpes simplex virus infection occur.

Infants with documented herpes simplex virus infections should be treated with acyclovir for at least 14 days and up to 21 days. Treatment varies according to the type of virus, its site, and severity. The antiviral drug acyclovir (taken internally or applied topically to the blisters) is effective in shortening the symptoms during a primary attack, and there is some indication that the drug taken prophylactically may lessen future attacks.

herpes, genital   Until AIDS appeared, genital herpes was the most common sexually transmitted disease in the country. Despite popular hysteria, the medical community has always considered genital herpes to be more of a discomfort rather than a dangerous or life-threatening situation.

Cause

Herpes simplex virus type II causes 85 percent of genital herpes cases. Type I, which causes most herpes infections above the waist, is responsible for the other 15 percent. The infection is spread by contact with the genital secretions of a person with an active lesion. It is possible, however, for a person with no active lesion to shed virus and infect a sex partner.

The virus can infect any skin or mucous membrane surface on the body. For example, a person with a cold sore who engages in oral sex can transmit genital herpes to a partner.

"Neonatal herpes" is the term for a herpes infection in newborns that is acquired from an infected mother during birth.

Symptoms

Only about 40 percent of patients with herpes ever have symptoms. When they do, the first appearance of herpes lesions is the worst, with many painful lesions lasting up to 10 days; it may take two to three weeks to completely recover from this first attack. When the sores fade away, the virus remains behind. The virus is now *latent*. During the first attack, some people have a generalized sick feeling, with swollen glands in the pelvic area and fever, fatigue, headache, muscle ache, and nausea. People with no antibodies to herpes type I (cold sores) usually will be sicker during a first attack. Girls usually have lesions on the cervix or vulva, with recurrences on the vulva, the skin between vagina and anus, upper thighs, anal area, or buttocks. Boys have lesions on the head or shaft of the penis and the anus.

Most people have a recurrence within six months of their first attack that begins with a tingling, itching, or prickling sensation in the area where the virus entered the body. This is followed in a few days by a raised cluster of small painful blisters; there may be several groups of blisters. Eventually, the sores will crust over and dry up. Most people do not have the generalized sick feeling with recurrent infections.

Patients are infectious until the sores heal completely, usually up to 12 days; recurrent infections usually remain infectious for up to a week. Recent studies have shown that it is quite possible to shed virus without symptoms, which is how it is possible to infect a partner when no sores are present.

Neonatal herpes can take many different forms. About one-third of affected babies will have skin, eyes, or mouth lesions before any other symptoms; another third will have a brain infection (ENCEPHALITIS), PNEUMONIA, or infection of other organs; and the final third will have symptoms of both types. Respiratory distress, fever, skin lesions, or convulsions are common herpes symptoms in newborns.

Diagnosis

Doctors may diagnose genital herpes by symptoms alone, but there are also several lab tests that can confirm the infection. A specimen from the base of a lesion can identify the type of cell. Herpes also grows rapidly in tissue culture; specimens from a new lesion can be identified within 48 hours in the lab. Blood tests can look for antibodies to herpes; the newest blood tests can tell the difference between type I and II.

Treatment

The antiviral drug acyclovir (Zovirax) became available in the 1980s to treat herpes, but it is not a cure, since it does not kill the virus. However, it can significantly reduce the severity of symptoms. Available in ointment, capsule, liquid, and intravenous (IV) forms, capsules are usually used to treat primary genital herpes or a severe recurrence, or to suppress a frequent recurrence. Taking acyclovir at the first sign of a recurrence—that is, during the tingling phase before lesions begin—can shorten the healing time from four or five days to one day.

People with more than six recurrences in a year can take daily acyclovir to prevent recurrence. Most patients do not take acyclovir for more than three years. Very few people report side effects with this drug.

Intravenous acyclovir is given for severe primary herpes for hospitalized patients, and for babies born with or exposed to herpes during birth.

Symptoms can be eased with frequent sitz baths in lukewarm water. A small amount of petroleum jelly on the sores can reduce the irritation during urination. Very painful sores may be eased with an anesthetic ointment. While sores are present, girls should wear loose cotton underwear, avoiding pantyhose and tight pants.

Complications

Rarely, herpes MENINGITIS (infection in the lining of the brain or spinal cord) or herpes encephalitis (infection in the brain) follows an initial infection. In the past, it was believed that there could be a link between herpes and cancer of the cervix; new studies show that genital herpes probably has no role in cervical cancer.

herpes encephalitis   See ENCEPHALITIS.

herpes zoster   See SHINGLES.

hiccups   Hiccups happen when the muscles of the diaphragm tighten. The diaphragm lies on top of the stomach, a thin shelf-like muscle separating the lungs and heart from the stomach and intestines. The intercostal muscles controlling the diaphragm lie between the ribs. When these muscles function normally, they help a child breathe, speak, sing, and cough. But sometimes the nerves controlling these muscles do not work right, usually in a younger child.

Hiccups can be quite common in infants and are noted by mothers before their babies are born. Babies usually get hiccups because they swallow air when feeding; as the stomach gets bigger, it squeezes the diaphragm, which is why burping a baby can help hiccups. In newborns the lack of muscle tone at this age makes hiccups appear to control the baby's whole body, but they do not hurt children and usually will stop on their own after a brief period. Overstimulation can trigger hiccuping in infants as well.

Sucking hard or eating too much can make hiccups worse. Older children get hiccups from drinking too much soda pop or eating too much too fast. An upset or full stomach can lead to hiccups. Hiccups can hurt, but they are usually harmless, and children tend to outgrow them by late adolescence.

Treatment

Several home remedies can be effective. A child with hiccups can swallow one teaspoon of sugar fast, three or more times (once every two minutes) if the hiccups do not stop right away. Babies can be given a swallow of water. Lying down may help.

Call the Doctor

Consult a physician if

- hiccups last longer than 20 to 30 minutes
- hiccups occur in association with a prolonged cough, muscle weakness on one side of the body, or severe vomiting

high blood pressure   While high blood pressure is primarily a problem among older Americans, it can occur in children—even newborns. About 1 percent of American children have high blood pressure.

Blood pressure is the measure of two forces—the force as the heart pumps blood into the arteries and through the circulation system, and the force from the arteries as they resist this flow. High blood pressure, known medically as hypertension, occurs when the blood pressure rises significantly above normal. This can have devastating effects on the body, because the higher pressure forces the heart to work harder.

Blood pressure is always measured using two numbers—the first number (systolic) measures the pressure while the heart beats, and the second number (diastolic) measures the blood's pressure when the heart is resting between beats. In an adult, a blood pressure of 120/70 is considered very healthy; hypertension is considered to be 130/85.

Normal blood pressure readings are lower for younger children and rise with age, varying according to age, gender, and height of a child. An occasional high reading does not necessarily indicate hypertension, but consistent high readings could indicate a problem.

Cause

High blood pressure in childhood can usually be traced to a specific cause. Hypertension in a newborn may indicate congenital heart disease, such as a constriction in the aorta. If this constriction is strong enough, the baby's heart could fail unless it is surgically repaired.

Between 80 percent and 85 percent of cases are due to kidney diseases. Less than 5 percent of high blood pressure cases are caused by hormonal disorders or tumors. Heart disease makes up less than 3 percent; rare cases of meningitis, encephalitis, and brain tumors are other known causes.

If a parent has high blood pressure, a child is twice as likely to develop the condition as someone with no family history. Children who are overweight usually have higher blood pressure than those who are not. In fact, most children have hypertension for the same reasons as adults: family history, obesity, and lack of regular exercise.

Symptoms

The most common symptoms are headaches, dizziness, and light-headedness, but these are often so mild that the child ignores them. Many children with high blood pressure have no symptoms at all. Irritability, excessive crying, failure to gain weight, poor feeding, and low-grade fever are the only symptoms in children younger than two or three years.

In severe cases, symptoms of encephalopathy, cardiac failure, blindness, or kidney failure occur and require hospitalization.

Diagnosis

The only reliable way of diagnosing hypertension is with regular blood pressure measurements. The most important thing is for parents to have their child's blood pressure checked regularly by the pediatrician. An occasional high reading may only be due to nervousness while at the doctor's office. On the other hand, consistently high readings taken over a period of time (three separate readings a week apart) are more likely to be caused by true high blood pressure.

A child with high blood pressure should then be checked further as part of a focused physical examination looking for evidence of damage. A test called an echocardiogram uses sound waves to assess the child's heart and its function.

Treatment

Most doctors prefer not to prescribe medication to treat children who have mild hypertension. Instead, the doctor may try to lower blood pressure through weight loss, cutting down on salt, behavior modification (such as relaxation techniques), and exercise.

Staying fit is important in weight and blood pressure control. A minimum of 30 minutes of aerobic exercise three to four times a week may help.

When the cause of hypertension is treated, blood pressure usually returns to normal. A child with high blood pressure is not doomed to struggle with hypertension as an adult, but a child who remains overweight, has high blood pressure readings, and has a family history of hypertension is at higher risk.

histoplasmosis An uncommon infection caused by inhaling fungus spores that infect the lungs. Spontaneous recovery is typical, although small calcifications remain in the lungs and affected lymph glands. While anyone can get histoplasmosis, it is found most often among those with an impaired immune system, such as AIDS patients.

Infection confers immunity. The disease is most common in the Mississippi and Ohio River Valleys.

Cause

Histoplasmosis is caused by the organism *Histoplasma capsulatum,* which is a single budding yeast at body temperature, and a mold at room temperature. The fungus is spread by airborne spores from soil contaminated with bird droppings and is commonly found in the Mississippi River Valley.

The fungal infection enters the body when a child breathes in spores of the fungus from dried bird droppings. In addition to the lungs, the fungus may occasionally invade other parts of the body. Birds (especially chickens), bats, dogs, cats, rats, skunks, opossums, foxes, and other animals also can get the disease and may play a role in spreading it. Outbreaks may occur in groups with common exposure to bird or bat droppings, or recently disturbed soil in chicken coops, caves, or elsewhere. Person-to-person spread of the disease does not occur. Past infection with histoplasmosis usually reduces chances of getting the disease again, but permanent immunity does not occur.

Symptoms

Most infected children do not have any symptoms. Those who do will experience mild to severe fever, malaise, cough, and swollen lymph nodes between five and 18 days after exposure. Progressive histoplasmosis is a sometimes-fatal generalized form of the disease, characterized by ulcers in the mouth and nose, enlarged spleen, liver, and lymph nodes, and serious lung infection.

Diagnosis

Examination and blood test will confirm the disease.

Treatment

Progressive histoplasmosis is treated with amphotericin B; less severe cases may be treated with ketoconazole. (See also FUNGAL INFECTIONS.)

HIV See HUMAN IMMUNODEFICIENCY VIRUS.

hives Raised, red blotchy welts of various sizes that can appear and disappear randomly on the surface of the skin. This reaction is known medically as *urticaria* (from the Latin word *urtica* for "nettle").

About one in five children experiences hives at some point in their lives, which are physically uncomfortable but generally harmless. Eventually, hives will disappear on their own without leaving any marks or scars.

Cause

While the cause of the reaction is often unknown, hives appear when a child is exposed to a trigger, prompting certain cells in the body to release histamine, a chemical released during allergic reactions. Hives appear when histamine causes blood plasma to leak from the small blood vessels under the skin.

A wide variety of triggers have been known to cause hives, including food, pollen, animal dander, drugs, insect bites, infections, illness, cold, heat, light, or stress. Foods that have been linked with hives include shellfish, fish, berries, nuts, eggs, and milk. Penicillin and aspirin are two types of drugs that may also trigger hives in susceptible patients.

In rare cases, hives can swell significantly and affect deeper layers of the skin and other parts of the body. This condition is called angioedema. In some children, there may be a genetic component to the angioedema. Termed "hereditary angioedema," this condition is characterized by nonitchy swellings lasting three or four days that may be triggered by trauma or may appear spontaneously. With angioedema, the hands, feet, eye-

lids, lips, and even breathing passages can swell. Treatment for these is the same as for common hives.

Diagnosis

The pediatrician may be able to determine the cause of hives with a detailed medical history, including a detailed diary of exposure to foods, chemicals, new products, and possible irritants over a period of two weeks to a month before onset. However, because hives may be triggered by such a wide variety of irritants, it may never be possible to find out the exact cause.

Treatment

In many cases, hives will disappear or fade away on their own without any treatment. More persistent cases will respond to antihistamines, but other drugs also may be prescribed by the pediatrician, including adrenaline or epinephrine, terbutaline, oral corticosteroids, or cimetidine.

home alone The age at which a child can legally be left alone at home varies from state to state, although many laws stipulate age 11 as a minimum. The age at which a child is emotionally, mentally, and physically able to stay at home varies from child to child. Most children and young teens feel more comfortable if a sibling or friend stays home with them.

A child who is home alone should be instructed never to tell anyone he is alone and not answer the door. Children should have phone numbers not just for a parent, but for the police and a close neighbor as well. An extra key left with a neighbor or relative is a good idea.

Hong Kong flu See INFLUENZA.

hookworm A small, round, bloodsucking worm that penetrates the skin, causing a red, itchy rash on the feet. In the United States, children can become infested when the common hookworm is passed through a dog's feces and is deposited into the soil.

Once inside the body, hookworms travel to the lungs and then inside the small intestine, where they attach themselves and drain blood for nourishment. Heavy hookworm infestation can cause considerable damage to the intestinal wall. While one hookworm extracts only a fraction of a teaspoon of blood from the circulation every day, more severe infestations can be more serious. Since children cannot replace lost blood quickly, this may cause an iron deficiency and malnutrition. Chronic infestation with worms can lead to slowed growth and impaired behavioral, cognitive, and motor development. Occasionally hookworm infestation can be fatal (especially in infants). Since transmission of hookworm infection requires development of the larvae in soil, hookworm cannot be spread person to person.

Symptoms

There may be no symptoms in a minor infestation; in more severe cases, the worms can cause abdominal pain, anemia, cough, diarrhea, mental slowness, and pneumonia, in addition to an itchy rash.

Treatment

In the United States, hookworm infections are generally treated for one to three days with medication such as mebendazole to kill the worms. The drugs are effective and appear to have few side effects. For children under the age of two, the decision to treat should be made by a pediatrician.

Another stool exam should be repeated one to two weeks after therapy. If the infection is still present, treatment will be given again. Iron supplements will be ordered if the patient has anemia.

Prevention

The best prevention is to improve sanitation so that transmission cannot occur, which is how hookworm infestations were eradicated from the southeastern United States. Children should not walk barefoot or contact the soil with bare hands in areas where hookworm is common, or where there is likely to be feces in the soil or sand.

hordeolum See STYE.

hospice, children's A system of comprehensive services for children that provides coordinated home care and inpatient care through an interdisciplinary team coordinated by a physician and nurse.

The team provides medical, nursing, psychosocial, and spiritual care as core services, along with trained volunteer and other services as appropriate. Hospice care for children is also attentive to needs related to loss and grieving for all concerned both prior to and following a death. Nursing services are available 24 hours a day as needed in any setting in which care is provided. Services are systematically evaluated for appropriateness and effectiveness.

Hospice care for children incorporates both a concept for caring and a system of comprehensive, interdisciplinary services. These complementary aspects address the unique needs and issues of care for children and adolescents with life-threatening conditions, and for those family members or significant others who provide the child's immediate support.

Children's hospice encourages day-to-day communication so that the family can look back and treasure the time spent together, enabling the family to cope with life more effectively. With children's hospice support, families are strengthened and can return to positive, productive lives. The primary focus of hospice for children is to maintain a good quality of life for the dying child while watching out for the ongoing, strengthened life of the family.

As a concept, hospice care for children incorporates specific principles and values for the care of children and their families. Its goal is enhancement of quality of life for the child and family. Hospice includes the child and family in the decision-making process about services and treatment choices. It addresses, in a comprehensive and consistent way, the physical, developmental, psychological, social, and spiritual needs and issues of children and families through an individualized plan of care. It ensures continuity and consistency of care in all settings where services are provided.

hospitalization A hospital stay can mean new and sometimes frightening experiences for a child. While each child is unique and reacts differently to hospitalization, helping a child understand what to expect may help make the hospital experience less stressful.

The best way to prepare a child for a hospital stay is to talk about what will happen before admission in words the child can understand. How parents describe the event can affect a child's attitude during the hospital stay. Parent and child can pack together for the hospital stay and include a favorite toy; the entire family should be included in a pre-hospital discussion. It is a good idea for parents to borrow a library book that describes a hospital stay and read it with the child.

A child's questions should always be answered simply and honestly. When to bring up the subject of hospitalization varies according to the age of the child. For example, a youngster under age three should be told just a few days before admission, whereas teens should have at least a week's notice.

If the child does not talk about the upcoming hospitalization, the parent should start casual conversations about the event, especially if the child does not ask specific questions. This gives the child a chance to express feelings about being hospitalized. It is important to explain clearly to a child the need for the hospitalization honestly. In addition, the child needs to know that there will be doctors and nurses at the hospital, and that the parent will make regular visits and spend the night whenever possible. (Many hospitals allow parents to stay overnight.)

It is important that children understand what to expect ahead of time. With guidance from the child's doctor, parents can explain how things will feel, whether there will be pain, how long it will last, and that crying is a healthy way to express feelings.

Parents should clearly discuss any potential changes in the child's appearance, such as a scar or cast. Because the child's friends may not know what to say, the child should explain to them what happened. When a discharge date is given, the parent and child can discuss what they will do together afterward. No matter how tempting, parents should avoid telling a child things that are not true. If procedures will hurt, parents should say so.

If surgery is planned, parents should discuss how the child can expect to feel after an operation, emphasizing that the hospital stay is only temporary.

Younger Than Age Three

At this age, a child's greatest worry is usually being away from parents. Being with a child as much as possible during the hospital stay will make the child feel more secure. Younger children (especially those under age three) often think of hospitalization as a punishment for misbehavior. Parents should encourage a child to express fears and concerns and explain clearly why the hospital stay is necessary.

Ages Four to Six

Children in this age group fear damage to their bodies, so parents need to be careful when explaining what will take place, avoiding phrases that a child may misconstrue. For example, parents should never describe anesthesia as "being put to sleep," especially if a child may associate being put to sleep with an experience with a pet, assuming it means death. Instead, parents should tell children that the doctors will help a child take a nap for a few hours. When talking about surgery, parents should use terms such as "make an opening" instead of "cut."

Ages Six to 12

Children older than six will worry about losing control as well as the potential damage to their bodies. Older children may also worry about doing or saying embarrassing things while under anesthesia. Parents should not deny that there will be pain after an operation, if this is the case, but explain that the pain will be temporary and the child will be made to feel as comfortable as possible.

Teenagers

Parents should not assume a teenager can handle hospitalization just like an adult. Teens are often reluctant to ask questions, leading parents to believe that they understand more than they actually do. Parents should encourage teens to ask the doctors and nurses questions and include the child in discussions about their care plan to help them feel in control.

hot tub safety   Young children should not use a hot tub or spa because of the dangers of extremely warm water and the potential for drowning. In fact, the main hazard from hot tubs and spas is the same as that from pools—drowning. Since 1980 there have been more than 700 reported accidental deaths in spas and hot tubs; about a third of those were children under age five. For this reason, consumers should keep a locked safety cover on the spa whenever it is not in use and keep children away unless there is constant adult supervision.

The design of older spas and tubs caused numerous drownings by entangling hair in drains or entrapping body parts in the equipment. The U.S. Consumer Product Safety Commission (CPSC) helped develop standards to prevent hair entanglement and body part entrapment in spas, hot tubs, and whirlpools. These standards should help prevent deaths and injuries. Consumers should fix their old spas, hot tubs, and whirlpools with new, safer drain covers.

Hair Entanglements

There have been 49 incidents and 13 deaths since 1978 caused by having a person's hair sucked into the suction fitting of a spa, hot tub, or whirlpool, holding the victim's head under water. Hair entanglement occurs when a bather's hair becomes entangled in a drain cover as the water and hair are drawn through the drain. In some incidents, children were playing a "hold your breath the longest" game, which allowed their long hair to be sucked into the drain.

The CPSC helped develop a voluntary standard for drain covers that helps reduce the risk of hair entrapment, and consumers should be sure they have new drain covers that meet this standard. If there is any doubt, a pool or spa professional can check the spa. A child should never be allowed to play in a way that could permit the child's hair to come near the drain cover. If a drain cover is missing or broken, the spa should be shut down until the cover is replaced.

Body Entrapment

Since 1980 there have been 18 incidents in which parts of the body have been entrapped by the strong suction of the drain of pools, wading pools, spas, and hot tubs. Of these, 10 people were disemboweled and five others died.

The CPSC helped develop a standard requiring dome-shaped drain outlets and two outlets for each pump, which reduces the powerful suction if one drain is blocked. Consumers with older spas should have new drain covers installed and may want to consider getting a spa with two drains.

Hot Tub Temperatures

There have been several reported deaths from extremely hot water (about 110°F) in a spa, which can cause drowsiness and unconsciousness. In addition, high body temperature can lead to heat stroke and death.

As a result, in 1987 new laws required temperature controls to make sure that spa water temperatures never exceed 104°F. Pregnant women and young children should not use a spa before consulting a physician.

Skin Infections

Skin infections can be spread by contaminated hot tub and spa water. Because hot tubs and spas have warmer water than pools, chlorine or other disinfectant levels evaporate faster. For that reason, it is important that chlorine or disinfectant levels in hot tubs and spas be checked even more regularly than in swimming pools.

Safety Precautions

The following safety precautions are recommended when anyone uses a hot tub, spa, or whirlpool:

- A locked safety cover should always be used; young children should be kept away from spas or hot tubs unless there is constant adult supervision.

- The spa must have dual drains and drain covers as required by current safety standards.

- A professional should check the spa or hot tub on a regular basis and make sure it is in good, safe working condition, and that drain covers are in place and not cracked or missing.

- Homeowners should know where the cutoff switch is located for the spa pump so it can be turned off in an emergency.

- No one should use the spa while drinking alcohol.

- The water temperature in the spa should be at 104°F or below.

human granulocytic ehrlichiosis (HGE)   See EHRLICHIOSIS, HUMAN GRANULOCYTIC.

Human Growth Foundation   A nonprofit, volunteer organization dedicated to helping children and adults with disorders of growth and growth hormone through research, education, support, and advocacy. The Human Growth Foundation (HGF) includes concerned parents and friends of children with growth problems and interested health professionals.

The foundation was established in 1965 by five families of children with growth disorders. Their primary purpose was to identify other parents and children with similar problems, and to seek support for research and treatment, principally for growth hormone deficiency.

Today, with the advent of synthetic growth hormone for humans, the foundation has broadened its goals to encompass many other growth disorders. The foundation has more than 1,000 members in 30 chapters and publishes a quarterly newsletter and multiple booklets. HGF also sponsors "starter grants" to encourage research in both physical and psychosocial areas of growth disorders. HGF also sponsors internet support lists and a chat room for parents of children, and adults, with growth disorders; and a Parent-to-Parent Program for parents who desire one-on-one contact with other parents outside of the context of the chapters. (For contact information, see Appendix I.)

human immunodeficiency virus (HIV)   The retrovirus that causes acquired immune deficiency syndrome (AIDS) via transmission through contact with infected person's blood, semen, cervical secretions, or cerebrospinal fluid. AIDS is a condition in which an acquired immune deficiency, which lowers the body's resistance to disease, results in infections, some forms of cancer, and the degeneration of the nervous system.

It is possible to be infected with HIV and not have AIDS; some children are infected for years before they get sick. HIV infection leading to AIDS has been a major cause of illness and death among children.

Nationally, HIV infection leading to AIDS was the seventh leading cause of death in 1992 among children one to four years of age. By 1995 the Centers for Disease Control and Prevention (CDC) had received reports of about 5,500 children who had acquired HIV infection at birth.

During the 1990s nearly 90 percent of existing AIDS cases reported among children and virtually all new HIV infections among children in the United States could be attributed to transmission of the HIV virus at birth. An increasing proportion of AIDS cases were reported in children whose mothers were infected with HIV before the child was conceived through heterosexual contact with an infected partner whose infection status and risk factors were not known by the mother.

Cause

Infants   Nearly all HIV infections in U.S. children under age 13 are from infection while in the mother's womb or while passing through the birth canal, although not every child born to an infected mother will have the virus. Between 6,000 and 7,000 children are born to HIV-infected mothers each year in the United States.

Between 1992 and 1997 the number of infants who became HIV positive when born to an infected mother plummeted by 50 percent as a result of new antiretroviral medications now given to the mother during delivery.

Because transmission often occurs during delivery, cesarean section may be indicated for some women. The virus also has been detected in breast milk, so infected mothers should not breast-feed.

Children   Before 1985 a small group of children were infected with the virus by contaminated blood products. Since then, blood products have been screened for the virus and risk of infection from this route has been virtually eliminated.

Teens   In adolescents HIV is most commonly spread by sexual contact with an infected partner. The virus enters the body through the lining of the vagina, vulva, penis, rectum, or mouth through sexual activity. Teens between the ages of 13 and 19 represent one of the fastest growing HIV-positive groups. HIV is also spread by sharing needles, syringes, or drug use equipment with someone who is infected with the virus.

In general, HIV infection is not very contagious from one child to another. Across the country there have been only a few reported transmissions, all of which involved direct blood contact in a family setting. Despite widespread concerns, there are no reported transmissions of the HIV virus within a school or child-care setting.

Since the largest danger is direct blood contact, those in schools and child-care programs should routinely use gloves when in contact with blood. As children with HIV become older and the latency period stretches longer, counseling and education are imperative to prevent sexual transmission of the virus.

Diagnosis

Early HIV infection often causes no symptoms and must be detected by testing a child's blood for the presence of disease-fighting proteins called antibodies. HIV antibodies usually do not reach levels high enough to detect by standard blood tests until one to six weeks after infection, and it may take as long as six months. Children exposed to HIV should be tested for HIV infection as soon as they are likely to develop antibodies to the virus. When a child is highly likely to be infected with HIV and yet antibody tests are negative, a test for the presence of HIV itself in the blood is used. Repeat antibody testing at a later date, when antibodies to HIV are more likely to have developed, is often recommended.

When a new baby is born to an HIV-infected mother, however, an antibody test is almost guaranteed to be positive, since babies have their HIV-infected mother's antibodies for up to 18 months after birth. Uninfected infants will gradually lose their mother's antibodies during this time, whereas infected infants generally remain antibody positive. Instead, a diagnosis can be made in early infancy by using a viral culture (PCR—polymerase chain reaction), or a p24 antigen test.

According to the U.S. Public Health Service, HIV-infected women should be encouraged to obtain HIV testing for any of their children born after they became infected or, if they do not know when they became infected, for children born after 1977. Children over age 12 should be tested with proper consent. Women should be informed that the lack of signs and symptoms suggestive of HIV infection in older children may not mean that the child is not infected.

Symptoms

Although there are no immediate physical signs of HIV infection at birth, children born with HIV can develop the opportunistic infection *Pneumocystis carinii* pneumonia (PCP) in the first months of life. Opportunistic infections like PCP take advantage of an HIV-infected child's weakened immune system. In the past 10 percent to 20 percent of children infected at birth rapidly developed this progressive disease and died by two years of age. However, in more recent years all babies born to mothers with HIV or AIDS are suspected of having the virus and

are routinely treated, so as a result, fatalities have been greatly reduced.

Other possible symptoms of babies born with HIV infection include low birth weight. Within two to three months, the infected child also may experience poor weight gain, THRUSH, enlarged lymph nodes, enlarged liver and/or spleen, neurological problems, bacterial infections, and pneumonia.

In children with HIV, the following opportunistic conditions can frequently occur:

- *Pneumocystis carinii* pneumonia (PCP)—pneumonia caused by a microorganism that cannot be fought off due to a weakened immune system
- lymphoid interstitial pneumonia (LIP)—walking pneumonia that becomes chronic and is sometimes characterized by coughing and shortness of breath
- bacterial, viral, and yeast infections
- meningitis
- fungal infections
- esophagitis—inflammation of the esophagus
- shingles (zoster)
- parasitic infections

Unlike adult cases, malignancies are rare in children with HIV. The two most difficult conditions among children infected with HIV or who have AIDS are wasting syndrome (the inability to maintain body weight due to lack of appetite), and HIV encephalopathy or AIDS dementia (infection of the brain that can cause brain swelling or atrophy). Wasting syndrome can sometimes be helped with nutritional counseling, while encephalopathy remains extremely difficult to treat.

Treatment

There is no known cure for AIDS. While current treatment advances can slow the progression of the disease and improve quality of life, life expectancy is still reduced significantly. Although all children with HIV will eventually become sick, recent advances in treatment have prolonged the onset of this inevitability.

A major factor in reducing the number of deaths from HIV and AIDS in this country has been highly active antiretroviral therapy (HAART). HAART is a treatment regimen that combines reverse transcriptase inhibitors and protease inhibitors to treat patients who are newly infected with HIV. However, researchers have shown that HAART cannot eradicate HIV entirely from the body.

There are a number of drugs to help treat opportunistic infections to which children with HIV are especially prone, including foscarnet and ganciclovir to treat CYTOMEGALOVIRUS eye infections, fluconazole to treat yeast and other FUNGAL INFECTIONS, and trimethoprim/sulfamethoxazole (TMP/SMX) or pentamidine to treat *Pneumocystis carinii* PNEUMONIA (PCP).

Children can receive PCP preventive therapy when certain T-cell counts drop to levels considered below normal for their age group. Regardless of their cell counts, however, HIV-infected children who have survived an episode of PCP take drugs for the rest of their lives to prevent a recurrence of the pneumonia.

HIV-infected children who develop cancers can be treated with radiation, chemotherapy, or injections of alpha interferon, a genetically engineered naturally occurring protein.

Prevention

Infants can contract HIV during a natural delivery, and cesarean delivery can decrease the likelihood that this will occur. However, a C-section is by no means a routine option when the mother is infected with HIV or has AIDS. The more invasive nature of the C-section can create risks for mother and child, additional costs, and danger to health workers exposed to the mother's infected blood.

Fortunately, medications can safely be given to mother and child that prevent HIV transmission. To prohibit transmission of the virus, mothers are given intravenous zidovudine (AZT) during their second and third trimesters. Infants are then given a six-week course of AZT by mouth. This intensive treatment has greatly reduced transmission of the disease. Multidrug regimens have also been used to treat pregnant women with even more promising results.

There are three classes of medications currently available for treatment:

- *nucleoside antiretrovirals:* zidovudine (AZT), DDI, DDC, D4T, 3TC

- *protease inhibitors:* indinavir, nelfinavir, ritonavir, saquinavir

- *non-nucleoside reverse transcriptase inhibitors (NNRTIs):* nevirapine, delavirdine, efavirenz

Because these medications work in different ways, doctors generally prescribe a "combination cocktail" of these drugs. Most of these treatments have been studied in children. While a number of drugs are available to treat HIV infection and slow the onset of AIDS, unless they are taken and administered properly, the virus quickly becomes resistant to the particular mix of medications. This means that if a treatment plan is not followed precisely, a new regimen will need to be established with different drugs.

If this is not followed, the virus will in turn become resistant to it. Because the number of drugs in each class is still limited, the very real danger is that children can quickly use up all the potential treatments, especially if they resist taking their medication. In addition to the difficulty of getting young children to take their medication on a timed schedule, the medications also have unpleasant side effects, such as a bad flavor, while others are only available in pill form, which may be difficult for children to swallow.

humidifiers The use of a humidifier in a child's bedroom during the winter can help keep mucous membranes moist and healthy—but poorly maintained humidifiers can be the source of infection.

The nose, throat, and lungs work best when the air has a relative humidity of about 40 percent. If the air during the winter falls below that level, moisture will be absorbed into the heated air from the mucous membranes. Since dried mucous membranes cannot clean themselves, they become more vulnerable to invasion from cold viruses. A well-maintained humidifier can keep the air humid and nose and throat moist.

However, it is important that the device be used correctly. If the air becomes too humid, or the machine is not properly cleaned, mold and dust mites can multiply. To keep the risk of infection from molds or bacteria to a minimum, the humidity should not be allowed to rise above 40 percent. In addition, the water reservoir in the humidifier should be cleaned daily with a vinegar solution.

hydrocephalus An excess of cerebrospinal fluid within the skull, also known as "water on the brain." This condition is often present at birth in association with other abnormalities, especially SPINA BIFIDA. Untreated, the condition will progress to extreme sleepiness, seizures, and severe brain damage, and it may be fatal in a few weeks.

Cause

Hydrocephalus is caused by the excessive formation of spinal fluid, by a blockage of this fluid, or both. It may be present at birth or develop after a severe head injury, brain hemorrhage, infection (such as MENINGITIS), or brain tumor.

Symptoms

If the condition is present at birth, the symptoms include an enlarged head that continues to grow at an excessively fast rate, because the baby's skull bones are not rigid, and they expand to accommodate the fluid. Other symptoms may include leg rigidity, EPILEPSY, irritability, lethargy, vomiting, and absence of reflexes.

If the condition occurs later in childhood, the skull cannot swell and the symptoms will be caused by a rising pressure within the skull characterized by HEADACHE, vomiting, loss of coordination, and deteriorating mental function.

Diagnosis

The condition is diagnosed with computerized axial tomography (CAT) or magnetic resonance imaging (MRI) brain scans, which can reveal the location and nature of the problem.

Treatment

Excess fluid can usually be drained away by using a shunt from the brain to another part of the body (such as the lining of the abdomen), where it can be absorbed by the body. The shunt is inserted into the brain through a hole in the skull; sometimes, the device will be left in place indefinitely.

In older children, treatment may be aimed at resolving the underlying condition (head injury, brain hemorrhage, infection, or tumor).

hyperactivity Constant and excessive movement and activity. A child with hyperactivity may not be able to stop an action when directed to, or to sit still for any period of time. Hyperactivity often occurs with inattentiveness and impulsivity. An affected child might have trouble sitting still, fidget excessively, and move about excessively even during sleep. Onset occurs before age seven. Behaviors are chronic (present throughout the child's life), present throughout the child's day, and are not due to other factors such as anxiety or depression.

In older children, symptoms of hyperactivity may be more subtle, displaying themselves in restlessness, fidgeting, a tendency to interrupt in class, or in conflict-seeking behaviors with peers and family members. (See also ATTENTION DEFICIT HYPERACTIVITY DISORDER.)

hypertension See HIGH BLOOD PRESSURE.

hypoglycemia A condition of low levels of sugar in the blood that causes muscle weakness, uncoordination, mental confusion, and sweating. Hypoglycemia is a very serious condition that must be treated immediately. If untreated, it can progress to a coma. Hypoglycemia can occur in any infant or child who takes insulin injections for diabetes, or in people with type 2 diabetes taking certain medications. Almost every child who takes insulin will have low blood sugar at one time or another.

Cause

When blood sugars drop too low, the brain cannot get the glucose it needs to function properly. The level at which low blood sugar gets serious depends on the child's age, health, and whether or not the child has had hypoglycemia before.

Symptoms

The symptoms of low blood sugar range from mild to severe. Mild symptoms include hunger, sweating, headache, rapid heartbeat, and pallor. Moderate signs include irritability, poor coordination, lethargy, and confusion. Severe signs include losing consciousness or having seizures.

While severe symptoms are easy to spot, mild to moderate low blood sugar is not always easy to recognize. Some of the same symptoms might simply indicate a tired or sick child. The only way to tell for sure is to check the blood sugar levels. If for some reason a test is not possible, it is safer to assume that the cause of the child's behavior is low blood sugar and treat the suspected low with carbohydrates. It is safer to treat a child for low blood sugar when levels are normal, than to ignore a situation in which the blood sugar is actually low.

Symptoms that a child may have low blood sugar at night include nightmares or bad dreams, stomachache or headache in the morning, ketones in the urine, and/or high or low blood glucose levels when the child wakes up. If these symptoms appear, blood sugar should be checked around midnight and again at 3 A.M. If a child is having lows during the night, the nighttime insulin dosage, type, or timing of the insulin injections may need to be adjusted. A meeting with the child's diabetes treatment team is necessary.

The more lows a child has, the greater the risk for lows that go unrecognized in the future, because fewer warning signs actually appear. This is called "hypoglycemia unawareness." On the other hand, symptoms of hypoglycemia can increase if the number of lows is decreased. A child who is having too many episodes of low blood sugar on a regular basis (such as every day) needs to have an adjustment in the diabetes regimen.

Treatment

To treat low blood sugar during the day, the child should immediately take 15 grams of glucose or a sugar source such as three or four glucose tablets, four ounces (half a cup) of 100-percent fruit juice, four ounces (half a cup) of regular (not diet) soda, or one tablespoon of sugar or honey.

If the symptoms do not go away in 10 to 15 minutes, the blood sugar test should be repeated. If the reading is still less than 70 mg/dl, the child should repeat the sugar treatment.

To treat low blood sugars at night, if blood sugar is below 70 mg/dl to 100 mg/dl at bedtime, the child should have one-and-a-half snacks. The blood sugar reading needs to rise to 120 mg/dl before the child goes to bed. The child's blood sugar should be rechecked during the night, at about 3 A.M.

In the case of severe low blood sugar reading, the child should be given glucagon as prescribed. Although glucagon is rarely needed, it is vital to keep it on hand and to know how to use it if the blood sugar drops so low that the child cannot eat or drink. Glucagon is a very serious intervention.

Signs that it is needed include lethargy, unconsciousness, or the inability to swallow normally. A glucagon kit usually contains a syringe with liquid, and a bottle with glucagon powder.

Prevention

It is possible to prevent hypoglycemia. Children should not skip meals or snacks, but if a child does not eat appropriately or eats less than usual during the day, blood glucose should be checked more often than usual during the rest of the day. If the blood glucose reading is too low (usually around 70 mg/dl), treatment should be given. A middle-of-the-night blood glucose reading should be done if a child has eaten less than usual during the day.

While exercise is important, extra physical activity can cause blood glucose levels to drop lower than usual, either during the exercises or much later (particularly during the night). When a child exercises more than usual, more carbohydrates (such as peanut butter and crackers) should be given.

To help prevent nighttime lows, a child's blood sugar should be checked at bedtime and then followed with a snack. If the reading is below 100 mg/dl, it should be checked again in the middle of the night.

It is also important that everyone who cares for a child with diabetes (even school bus drivers) should know that the child has diabetes and takes insulin. They must also understand what hypoglycemia is, how to lessen the risk, and how to recognize and treat the problem. It is important to emphasize at school that a child who might be having a hypoglycemic episode should not be sent to the nurse's office alone, even for a blood sugar check. A responsible person carrying a sugar source should accompany the child. Teachers should also understand that low blood sugar can be triggered by an altered mealtime, a skipped meal or snack, or extra physical activity. Low blood sugar can also occur at any time without an obvious reason.

hypoxia Lack of oxygen to the brain, which may occur during DROWNING, childbirth, or choking. Hypoxia during birth is one of the primary causes of CEREBRAL PALSY and may be related to LEARNING DISABILITIES.

ibuprofen, pediatric An over-the-counter anti-inflammatory drug that can be bought without a prescription and used instead of aspirin to reduce fever or treat minor aches and pains or headaches and reduce swelling, stiffness, and joint pain.

Children who are allergic to aspirin should not use ibuprofen. In addition, pediatric ibuprofen should not be taken with ACETAMINOPHEN or pain reliever/fever reducer unless directed by a doctor. Pediatric ibuprofen should not be given to a child who is dehydrated because of vomiting, diarrhea, or lack of fluids.

Ibuprofen can be taken with or without food, but if the child gets an upset stomach after a dose, it should thereafter be given with food. Ibuprofen should only be given using the dropper or medicine cup that came with the medicine, not a kitchen spoon. Spoons are different sizes and are not good measuring tools. It is also available as a chewable tablet. Ibuprofen should not be given to infants under six months of age.

Side Effects
Side effects include nausea, heartburn, stomachache, cramps, diarrhea, gas, vomiting, constipation, or feelings of dizziness, fatigue, or confusion.

Call the Doctor
A doctor should be called at once if a child experiences:

- blood in the stool or vomit, or coughing up blood
- blue skin color
- bruising or bleeding
- chest tightness
- cough
- diarrhea
- fever
- hives
- rash
- ringing in the ears
- swelling in the face, lips, tongue, or throat
- vision changes
- vomiting
- wheezing

ichthyosis A family of at least 20 rare skin disorders characterized by dry, thickened rough, scaling, darkened skin triggered by too much keratin (the main protein component of skin). This group of genetic diseases ranges from mild generalized dry skin (ichthyosis vulgaris) to severe widespread thickened scaly dry skin (lamellar ichthyosis). The disorder's name is derived from the Greek word *ichthus* meaning "fish" because the appearance and condition of the skin resemble fish scales. It affects more than one million Americans.

Symptoms
Ichthyosis vulgaris, which affects the thighs, arms, and backs of the hands, usually appears at or shortly after birth and improves as the child grows up. However, in severe conditions, the infant may be stillborn, encased in skin as hard as armor plate. It is not contagious and is not caused by germs.

Treatment
There is no cure for any of the ichthyoses, which are lifelong diseases, but lubricants and ointments may help the skin dryness, and bath oils can moisten the skin. Ichthyosis improves in a warm, humid climate and worsens in cold weather. Washing with soap aggravates the condition.

imaginary friends   Imaginary playmates are a perfectly normal part of childhood that can offer youngsters a feeling of control in their lives. These invisible friends are not an indication of a mental health problem but are a common fact of life in many well-adjusted, creative children. Many children develop imaginary playmates between the ages of three and five, when they begin to form their own identities and to test the boundaries between fantasy and reality.

Imaginary friends enable children to try out different roles and allow children to explore issues of control and power without worrying about interactions with real authority figures. An imaginary friend can help a child work out difficult emotions and handle anxieties associated with major changes in the child's life. Parents can monitor their child's relationship with an imaginary friend to gain insights into how the child is coping.

While it is perfectly acceptable for parents to support the child's belief, they should not get too involved in the playacting so that the children feel they have lost control of the game. Parents should not belittle the relationship nor let the imaginary playmate take the blame for the child's mistakes. Children who see their parents taking the imaginary friend too seriously may worry that the adults don't know what is real and what is make believe.

An imaginary friend should become of concern only when the child avoids meaningful interaction with other children in favor of playing exclusively with an invented friend. Most children abandon their imaginary friends once kindergarten begins. A child who continues to focus intently on an imaginary playmate beyond that time may benefit from a professional consultation to explore any hidden worries.

immune system   An intricate combination of organs and cells that helps a child's body protects itself against invasion from a wide variety of infectious diseases. This network works most efficiently when the child is well rested, eats a healthy diet, and is not under too much stress. Genetics also play a part; some children are born with a stronger immune system than others.

When a germ enters the body, the immune system triggers the white blood cells (lymphocytes) to attack. White blood cells move throughout the body via the organs of the immune system, including bone marrow, lymph nodes, tonsils, adenoids, blood, and lymphatic vessels.

Both types of white blood cells—B cells and T cells—produce antibodies that destroy bacteria and viruses. A third type of white blood cell (the large phagocytes) surrounds invading microbes and swallows them.

This immune response is often the source of all of the symptoms children experience during an infection—chills, fever, aches, appetite loss, fatigue, inflammation, and rash.

Children whose immune systems are not working well, such as youngsters with AIDS, have more trouble fighting off invading germs. That is why anyone with an impaired immune system gets sick more often and more seriously, with illnesses that might not even harm a child whose immune system is working properly.

Vaccinations during the first year of life are important because a young baby's immune system is often not strong enough to fight off potentially fatal diseases such as measles and meningitis. This is why babies currently receive four shots at age two months. Receiving combination vaccines means that a child can get protection from these diseases in fewer shots. Vaccines are made of weakened or inactivated viruses or bacteria that are designed to stimulate the production of antibodies without infecting the body and provoking an immune system attack. This is how vaccines give a child immunity without causing illness.

Until four to six months of age infants generally receive some level of immunity from their mother's antibodies, which cross the placenta during the third trimester.

immunization   A method of producing immunity to disease via vaccination. When a naturally occurring disease-causing germ infects the body, the immune system produces special proteins called antibodies to destroy the invader. If the same germ is encountered a second time, the immune system recognizes it and produces antibodies much more quickly, killing the germ before the disease can develop. This is why a person who had a disease such as measles as a child is immune from the disease if ever exposed again.

Vaccines work by the same principle. Vaccines are made from tiny amounts of bacteria or viruses (antigens) that are weakened or killed so that they are harmless to the body. When they are introduced into the body, the immune system still makes antibodies against the vaccine's altered germs—so when the body later encounters the actual invading germ, it can fight off the disease. This is why a child who received a measles vaccine also would be immune to the disease if exposed later in life. A few vaccines produce immunity from a disease with just one dose, but most require two or more doses. For some vaccines (such as TETANUS), periodic booster shots are required to maintain lifelong immunity.

Immunity can be strong or weak and short- or long-lived, depending on the type of antigen, the amount of antigen, and the route by which it enters the body. When faced with the same antigen, some people's immune systems will respond forcefully, others feebly, and some not at all.

One hundred years ago about half of all children born in the United States died by the age of five, many of them of diseases that today can be prevented with vaccination. By 1979 SMALLPOX had been wiped out entirely, thanks to a worldwide vaccination effort. Vaccination has eliminated POLIO in the Western Hemisphere, and it has nearly eliminated MEASLES in the United States. Current guidelines call for children to receive a total of 24 doses of seven different vaccines protecting against 11 diseases, most of the doses given in the first two years of life.

Preschoolers are the most vulnerable to communicable disease, which is why infants soon after birth are started on a U.S. government-required series of immunizations. While at present there are a series of shots that must be given to protect against childhood diseases, scientists are working on a "mega vaccine" involving just one shot that can protect against six childhood diseases.

Although the terms vaccinate (vaccination) and immunize (immunization) often are used interchangeably, they are not strictly the same thing. To immunize means "to render immune." One way to do this is to vaccinate (to give a vaccine to produce immunity). Vaccination is considered active when the body responds to the vaccine by making antibodies against the pathogen, but immunity against infectious diseases also can be produced in other ways, such as being given preformed antibodies (immunoglobulin) against a particular disease (passive immunization) or by developing natural long-term immunity when personally exposed to that disease.

Controversy

Immunization is not straightforward. As infectious diseases continue to decline, some people have become less interested in the consequences of preventable illnesses like diphtheria and tetanus. Instead, they have become increasingly concerned about the risks associated with vaccines. Some vaccines are perceived by the public as carrying a risk, especially the pertussis part of the DPT (diphtheria-pertussis-tetanus) vaccine, which had been linked to seizures and other serious side effects. In response to these concerns, a safer acellular version of the pertussis vaccine is now in use DTaP.

Other concerns focused on the preservative thimerosal, a mercury compound, which used to be included in many vaccinations and which some parents believe has been linked to autism. A review by the Food and Drug Administration found no evidence of harm caused by doses of thimerosal in vaccines, except for minor local reactions. Nevertheless, in July 1999 the Public Health Service agencies, the AMERICAN ACADEMY OF PEDIATRICS, and vaccine manufacturers agreed that thimerosal levels in vaccines should be reduced or eliminated as a precautionary measure. Today almost all vaccines for children are thimerosal free.

Medical experts argue that a vaccine is not licensed unless it is considered safe and its benefits far outweigh perceived risks. For a vaccine to be included on the annual Recommended Childhood Immunization Schedule for the United States, it must first be approved by the Advisory Committee on Immunization Practices from the Centers for Disease Control and Prevention, the American Academy of Pediatrics, and the American Academy of Family Physicians. Scientists and physicians in these organizations carefully weigh the risks and

Recommended Childhood and Adolescent Immunization Schedule—United States, January–June 2004

Legend
Range of Recommended Ages
Catch-up Immunization
Preadolescent Assessment

Vaccine ▼ / Age ▶	Birth	1 mo	2 mo	4 mo	6 mo	12 mo	15 mo	18 mo	24 mo	4-6 y	11-12 y	13-18 y
Hepatitis B[1]	HepB #1	only if mother HBsAg (–) — HepB #2			HepB #3						HepB series	
Diphtheria, Tetanus, Pertussis[2]			DTaP	DTaP	DTaP			DTaP		DTaP	Td	Td
Haemophilus influenzae Type b[3]			Hib	Hib	Hib[3]	Hib						
Inactivated Poliovirus			IPV	IPV	IPV		IPV			PV		
Measles, Mumps, Rubella[4]						MMR #1				MMR #2	MMR #2	
Varicella[5]						Varicella				Varicella		
Pneumococcal[6]			PCV	PCV	PCV	PCV	PCV		PCV	PPV		
Hepatitis A[7]									Hepatitis A series			
Influenza[8]						Influenza (yearly)						

Vaccines below this line are for selected populations

This schedule indicates the recommended ages for routine administration of currently licensed childhood vaccines, as of December 1, 2003, for children through age 18 years. Any dose not given at the recommended age should be given at any subsequent visit when indicated and feasible. ▨ Indicates age groups that warrant special effort to administer those vaccines not previously given. Additional vaccines may be licensed and recommended during the year. Licensed combination vaccines may be used whenever any components of the combination are indicated and the vaccine's other components are not contraindicated. Providers should consult the manufacturers' package inserts for detailed recommendations. Clinically significant adverse events that follow immunization should be reported to the Vaccine Adverse Event Reporting System (VAERS). Guidance about how to obtain and complete a VAERS form can be found on the Internet: http://www.vaers.org/ or by calling 1-800-822-7967.

1. Hepatitis B (HepB) vaccine. All infants should receive the first dose of hepatitis B vaccine soon after birth and before hospital discharge; the first dose may also be given by age 2 months if the infant's mother is hepatitis B surface antigen (HBsAg) negative. Only monovalent HepB can be used for the birth dose. Monovalent or combination vaccine containing HepB may be used to complete the series. Four doses of vaccine may be administered when a birth dose is given. The second dose should be given at least 4 weeks after the first dose, except for combination vaccines which cannot be administered before age 6 weeks. The third dose should be given at least 16 weeks after the first dose and at least 8 weeks after the second dose. The last dose in the vaccination series (third or fourth dose) should not be administered before age 24 weeks.

Infants born to HBsAg-positive mothers should receive HepB and 0.5 mL of Hepatitis B Immune Globulin (HBIG) within 12 hours of birth at separate sites. The second dose is recommended at age 1 to 2 months. The last dose in the immunization series should not be administered before age 24 weeks. These infants should be tested for HBsAg and antibody to HBsAg (anti-HBs) at age 9 to 15 months.

Infants born to mothers whose HBsAg status is unknown should receive the first dose of the HepB series within 12 hours of birth. Maternal blood should be drawn as soon as possible to determine the mother's HBsAg status; if the HBsAg test is positive, the infant should receive HBIG as soon as possible (no later than age 1 week). The second dose is recommended at age 1 to 2 months. The last dose in the immunization series should not be administered before age 24 weeks.

2. Diphtheria and tetanus toxoids and acellular pertussis (DTaP) vaccine. The fourth dose of DTaP may be administered as early as age 12 months, provided 6 months have elapsed since the third dose and the child is unlikely to return at age 15 to 18 months. The final dose in the series should be given at age ≥4 years. **Tetanus and diphtheria toxoids (Td)** is recommended at age 11 to 12 years if at least 5 years have elapsed since the last dose of tetanus and diphtheria toxoid-containing vaccine. Subsequent routine Td boosters are recommended every 10 years.

3. Haemophilus influenzae type b (Hib) conjugate vaccine. Three Hib conjugate vaccines are licensed for infant use. If PRP-OMP (PedvaxHIB or ComVax [Merck]) is administered at ages 2 and 4 months, a dose at age 6 months is not required. DTaP/Hib combination products should not be used for primary immunization in infants at ages 2, 4 or 6 months but can be used as boosters following any Hib vaccine. The final dose in the series should be given at age ≥12 months.

4. Measles, mumps, and rubella vaccine (MMR). The second dose of MMR is recommended routinely at age 4 to 6 years but may be administered during any visit, provided at least 4 weeks have elapsed since the first dose and both doses are administered beginning at or after age 12 months. Those who have not previously received the second dose should complete the schedule by the 11- to 12-year-old visit.

5. Varicella vaccine. Varicella vaccine is recommended at any visit at or after age 12 months for susceptible children (i.e., those who lack a reliable history of chickenpox). Susceptible persons age ≥13 years should receive 2 doses, given at least 4 weeks apart.

6. Pneumococcal vaccine. The heptavalent **pneumococcal conjugate vaccine (PCV)** is recommended for all children age 2 to 23 months. It is also recommended for certain children age 24 to 59 months. The final dose in the series should be given at age ≥12 months. **Pneumococcal polysaccharide vaccine (PPV)** is recommended in addition to PCV for certain high-risk groups. See MMWR 2000;49(RR-9):1-38.

7. Hepatitis A vaccine. Hepatitis A vaccine is recommended for children and adolescents in selected states and regions and for certain high-risk groups; consult your local public health authority. Children and adolescents in these states, regions, and high-risk groups who have not been immunized against hepatitis A can begin the hepatitis A immunization series during any visit. The 2 doses in the series should be administered at least 6 months apart. See MMWR 1999;48(RR-12):1-37.

8. Influenza vaccine. Influenza vaccine is recommended annually for children age ≥6 months with certain risk factors (including but not limited to children with asthma, cardiac disease, sickle cell disease, human immunodeficiency virus infection, and diabetes; and household members of persons in high-risk groups [see MMWR 2003;52(RR-8):1-36]) and can be administered to all others wishing to obtain immunity. In addition, healthy children age 6 to 23 months are encouraged to receive influenza vaccine if feasible, because children in this age group are at substantially increased risk of influenza-related hospitalizations. For healthy persons age 5 to 49 years, the intranasally administered live-attenuated influenza vaccine (LAIV) is an acceptable alternative to the intramuscular trivalent inactivated influenza vaccine (TIV). See MMWR 2003;52(RR-13):1-8. Children receiving TIV should be administered a dosage appropriate for their age (0.25 mL if age 6 to 35 months or 0.5 mL if age ≥3 years). Children age ≤8 years who are receiving influenza vaccine for the first time should receive 2 doses (separated by at least 4 weeks for TIV and at least 6 weeks for LAIV).

For additional information about vaccines, including precautions and contraindications for immunization and vaccine shortages, please visit the National Immunization Program Web site at www.cdc.gov/nip/ or call the National Immunization Information Hotline at 800-232-2522 (English) or 800-232-0233 (Spanish).

Approved by the Advisory Committee on Immunization Practices (www.cdc.gov/nip/acip), the American Academy of Pediatrics (www.aap.org), and the American Academy of Family Physicians (www.aafp.org).

benefits of newly developed vaccines, monitor the safety and effectiveness of existing vaccines, and track cases of vaccine-preventable diseases.

The topic of vaccine safety became prominent during the mid-1970s as lawsuits were filed on behalf of those presumably injured by the diphtheria, pertussis, tetanus (DPT) vaccine. In order to reduce liability and respond to public health concerns, Congress passed the NATIONAL CHILDHOOD VACCINE INJURY ACT (NCVIA) in 1986. Designed for citizens injured or killed by vaccines, this system provided a no-fault compensation alternative to suing vaccine manufacturers and providers. The act also created safety provisions to help educate the public about vaccine benefits and risks, and to require doctors to report adverse events after vaccination as well as keep records on vaccines administered and health problems which occur following vaccination. The act also created incentives for the production of safer vaccines.

Reports from health departments across the country estimate that less than half of American children are properly immunized by age two; in the inner city, the rate drops to less than a third. Since 1991 most insurance companies cover children's immunizations, and some health departments offer free shots.

While a serious illness precludes a vaccination, minor colds with low fevers do not interfere with immunization. Slight soreness and swelling at the injection site are normal and are not an indication that the child should not finish the series of shots. Antibiotics prescribed for another illness also will not interfere with the vaccination (except for the oral typhoid vaccine). In that case, Tylenol may be given.

A child should not be vaccinated if there has been a serious allergic reaction to a previous shot. Anyone who has a severe allergy to eggs should not receive the MMR (measles-mumps-rubella), INFLUENZA, or YELLOW FEVER vaccines.

impetigo   A superficial skin infection, most commonly found in childhood, that is caused by streptococcal or staphlococcal bacteria. Impetigo should be treated as soon as possible to avoid spreading the infection to other children and to prevent a rare complication—a form of kidney disease called acute glomerulonephritis.

Cause

Impetigo is spread by touching and usually is found on exposed body areas such as the legs, face, and arms. Because impetigo is spread quickly through play groups and day care, children with the infection should be kept away from playmates and out of school until the sores disappear.

Symptoms

The condition starts as tiny, almost imperceptible blisters on a child's skin, usually at the site of a skin abrasion, scratch, or insect bite. Most lesions occur on exposed areas, such as the face, scalp, and extremities. The red and itchy sores blister briefly, then begin to ooze for the next few days, leaving a sticky crust. Untreated, the infection will last from two to three weeks. Impetigo is most common during hot, humid weather.

Treatment

Children with impetigo need immediate medical care to avoid spreading the infection to others. Medication includes dicloxacillin, cephalosporin, or erythromycin for 10 days, together with topical application of mupirocin ointment.

Complications

Rarely, impetigo can lead to possible kidney disease known as acute glomerulonephritis.

Prevention

Cleanliness and prompt attention to skin injuries can help prevent impetigo. Children with the condition and their families should bathe regularly with antibacterial soaps and apply topical antibiotics to insect bites, cuts, abrasions, and infected lesions immediately. Impetigo in infants is especially contagious and serious. To prevent spreading, pillowcases, towels, and washcloths should not be shared and should be boiled after each use.

impetigo, bullous   Also called "staphylococcal impetigo," this is a superficial skin infection caused by *Staphylococcus aureus* bacteria that requires immediate attention. This disease has been more frequently diagnosed since the 1970s.

Symptoms

Thin-walled, flaccid blisters that rupture easily and contain fluid ranging from clear to pus. After rupture, the base quickly dries to a shiny veneer, which looks different than the thicker crust found in common IMPETIGO. Lesions are usually found grouped in one area.

Treatment

As with common impetigo, bullous impetigo is treated with dicloxacillin, cephalosporin, or erythromycin. Topical treatment is not necessary and could cause more harm than good. Septic complications are rare.

inborn errors of metabolism A group of more than 200 inherited disorders in which the body cannot metabolize food components normally. These disorders are usually caused by gene defects that cause a particular enzyme to be defective or missing. Enzymes are proteins that help the body use food, produce energy, and do work. The particular enzyme involved determines what the body cannot do and what the resulting problem may be. The likelihood of having an inborn error of metabolism is about one in 5,000 live births. Some of the more common inborn errors of metabolism are cystic fibrosis, hypothyroidism, SICKLE-CELL DISEASE, PHENYLKETONURIA (PKU), and TAY-SACHS DISEASE. Other inborn errors of metabolism include fructose intolerance, which causes a problem in the breakdown of the carbohydrate fructose; galactosemia, which causes a problem in breaking down galactose to glucose; and maple sugar urine disease, in which there is a problem with the breakdown of certain amino acids.

Symptoms

The symptoms of inborn errors of metabolism vary a great deal. A baby's symptoms may indicate a problem by showing signs of FAILURE TO THRIVE (not gaining weight, not eating well, or having developmental delays). Vomiting and diarrhea are among other symptoms that may prompt the doctor to test for an inborn error of metabolism. Several inborn errors of metabolism cause MENTAL RETARDATION if not controlled.

Cause

The enzyme defects are caused by abnormal genes. In most cases, the child must inherit an abnormal gene from each parent in order to have the problem. Defects have been observed in almost all bio-logical reactions, and the responsible genes are scattered among the chromosomes. The enzyme defects that lead to the inborn errors of metabolism are caused by genetic abnormalities present from the time of conception.

Parents who have had one child with an inborn error of metabolism are at risk to have other affected children. One in four pregnancies of such parents can be expected to result in an affected child.

Some inborn errors of metabolism are more often found in certain racial and ethnic groups. For example, sickle-cell anemia occurs among those of African descent, Tay-Sachs occurs more often among Ashkenazi Jewish populations, and those of northern European heritage are more likely to pass on defective genes for cystic fibrosis.

Diagnosis

Physical features such as malformations of the skeleton usually make a diagnosis obvious. A diagnosis can be confirmed by checking the blood or urine for one or more of the compounds involved. Tests for urine amino acids can be helpful. There may be too much of a compound, not enough of another, or abnormalities among others. The compounds may also be studied in tissue from biopsies. DNA tests may also confirm the diagnosis.

Treatment

Many of the inborn errors of metabolism can be treated effectively, depending on the missing or defective enzyme and how easily the compounds involved can be eliminated or replaced. Inborn errors of metabolism often require diet changes, the type and extent of which depend on the specific metabolic error.

The diseases caused by the inborn errors may be preventable if the missing enzyme can be supplemented or a harmful buildup eliminated. For example, the disease phenylketonuria involves phenylalanine building up in the body, causing problems. When phenylalanine is eliminated from the diet, the child's body will function normally.

Prevention

Screening programs of potential carriers of certain IEM, such as Tay-Sachs—or amniocentesis—can be performed in cases with two partners who are both carriers.

indigestion Another name for an upset stomach that usually results when a child eats too much food, or eats too quickly. Also known as dyspepsia, only very rarely does indigestion mean a person may have a more serious digestive problem or an ulcer in the digestive tract. Stress and not enough sleep may make indigestion worse. Obesity also tends to promote indigestion.

Symptoms
Indigestion causes pain or burning in the middle of the belly, nausea, bloating, uncontrolled burping, and heartburn.

Prevention
The best way to prevent indigestion is to avoid foods that seem to cause it. Children with the tendency toward indigestion should eat healthy, smaller meals throughout the day, avoiding junk food, fatty foods, too much chocolate, and too many citrus fruits. Eating slowly and avoiding stress can also help. In addition, children should never exercise with a full stomach.

Indigestion is fairly common, but usually it only happens occasionally. A child who gets indigestion despite a healthy diet, plenty of exercise, and enough sleep should see a pediatrician for an examination or stomach X-rays and tests to make sure indigestion is not the sign of another problem in the digestive tract.

infant botulism See BOTULISM, INFANT.

infectious parotitis See MUMPS.

inflammatory bowel disease (IBD) The general name for diseases that cause inflammation of the bowels, including ulcerative colitis and Crohn's disease. Although these two diseases are similar, there are also some important distinctions.

Ulcerative colitis is an inflammatory disease of the inner lining of the large intestine, which becomes inflamed and ulcerates. Ulcerative colitis is often most severe in the rectal area and can cause frequent bloody diarrhea. Crohn's disease, on the other hand, affects the last part of the small intestine, although it can also affect any part of the digestive tract. Moreover, Crohn's disease tends to involve the entire bowel wall, whereas ulcerative colitis affects only the lining.

Inflammatory bowel disease (IBD) occurs most often among people aged 15 to 30, but it can affect younger children. There are significantly more reported cases in western Europe and North America than in other parts of the world.

Cause
Scientists do not yet know what causes inflammatory bowel disease, although they suspect that a number of factors may be involved, including the environment, diet, and heredity. Smoking appears to increase the likelihood of developing Crohn's disease. A new theory suggests that Crohn's disease may be caused by infection (similar to CAT SCRATCH DISEASE).

Symptoms
The most common symptoms of both ulcerative colitis and Crohn's disease are mild to severe diarrhea and abdominal pain. Pain is usually caused by abdominal cramps caused by irritation of the nerves and muscles controlling intestinal contractions. Severe diarrhea can lead to dehydration, rapid heartbeat, and low blood pressure, and continued loss of small amounts of blood in the stool can lead to anemia. Sometimes children with Crohn's disease may experience constipation if the intestines become partially obstructed. In ulcerative colitis, constipation may be a symptom of inflammation of the rectum.

Fever, fatigue, and weight loss may also occur in IBD as may malnutrition because of the loss of fluid and nutrients due to diarrhea and chronic inflammation of the bowel.

Children with IBD may experience a slowdown in growth and a delay in the onset of puberty.

Diagnosis
IBD can be difficult to diagnose because there may be no symptoms despite years of increasing bowel damage, or symptoms may mimic other conditions. Blood tests can reveal inflammation or abnormalities in the digestive tract. Increased white blood cell counts and sedimentation rates along with lower levels of albumin, zinc, and magnesium in the blood suggest IBD.

However, an accurate diagnosis of ulcerative colitis may require an examination of the colon by inserting a colonoscope, which allows doctors to see the degree of damage. A biopsy of the colon may help confirm the diagnosis. To diagnose Crohn's disease, barium X rays can reveal characteristic signs of inflammation in the lining of the intestine. An upper gastrointestinal endoscopy and colonoscopy may be performed to check for evidence of bowel damage caused by inflammation.

Treatment

Medication is the primary method for treating symptoms of IBD. Steroids, cyclosporin, azathioprine, and anti-TNF antibodies restrain the immune system from attacking the body's own tissues and causing further inflammation. Anti-inflammatory drugs are also used.

If a child with IBD does not respond to these medicines, surgery may be considered, although the recurrent nature of Crohn's disease makes surgery a last-ditch effort. An aggressive surgical approach to Crohn's disease also can cause other complications, such as short bowel syndrome (which reduces the ability to absorb nutrients and also may cause growth failure).

Children with ulcerative colitis may need to have the large intestine removed, along with a surgical procedure in which doctors form a pouch from the small bowel to collect stool in the pelvis. After another surgery to reconnect the bowel, feces can pass through the anus.

influenza   A contagious respiratory infection that often occurs in epidemics from November to March. While the disease is not dangerous in itself, it can lead to PNEUMONIA, a potentially fatal complication. Every year as winter begins, the flu spreads across the globe. In the United States, up to 50 million people may be infected. Field studies indicate the flu may affect children the most—up to 36 percent of children from ages one to 18 will get sick during an epidemic. While most deaths from flu occur among the elderly, children under age five are also at higher risk for complications. Some children who have chronic medical conditions may become sicker with the flu and may

require hospitalization, and flu in a newborn also can be hazardous.

In the past, because there were far more serious diseases to worry about, the flu did not attract much medical attention until the great Spanish flu pandemic of 1918, which killed 550,000 Americans. Worldwide, this pandemic left about 21 million dead out of about one billion cases before it vanished; scientists still do not know where it went, and they worry that another outbreak could occur. Since World War II, vaccines have helped cut the death rate.

Cause

The influenza virus today occurs in any of three types, known as influenza A, B, and C. However, strains A and B mutate quickly; several strains of each of these types now exist. The three basic flu types have variants that are designated according to where they first strike, such as New Jersey (A), Bangkok (A), and so on. The 1957 and 1968 Asian flu pandemics were caused by strains of type A.

The highly contagious virus is spread by direct contact, or via droplets and dust in the air over short distances away from patients who are coughing or sneezing. The virus also can survive for hours in dried mucus, so dirty tissues should be carefully thrown away.

Anyone can catch the flu, regardless of age, sex, or race, but certain groups are more likely to develop complications. The contagious period varies, but it probably starts the day before symptoms appear and extends for about a week.

An infection will confer immunity to the specific flu strain only. Because the viruses that cause flu are always changing, people who have been infected or who have gotten a flu shot in other years may still become infected with a new strain.

Avian Flu

One reason why authorities watch worldwide outbreaks of flu is the concern that the germs can mutate so quickly and jump from one species to another with deadly consequences. In May 2001 Hong Kong authorities ordered the slaughter of virtually all poultry in the territory to prevent the further spread of a virulent outbreak of bird flu. Imports of poultry from the rest of China were also suspended, and as many as 1.2 million birds were slaughtered. However, this virus does not affect people and was different from a 1997 strain that killed six people. What worried authorities was the fact that the 2001 infection was a new and highly virulent strain of avian flu that killed almost 800 chickens in cages in three separate markets during its first 24 hours. To prevent a possible jump to humans, all the chickens, ducks, geese, and quail in the territory's markets, along with all mature poultry on its farms, were slaughtered.

The appearance of the avian virus in Hong Kong in humans in 1997 prompted fears of a worldwide epidemic, since a study showed similarities between the virus and Spanish flu, an outbreak of which killed between 20 and 40 million people in 1918. A less serious strain infected two children in 1999, and there were unconfirmed reports of further cases in China's southern provinces. Most bird flu viruses do not replicate efficiently in humans.

Symptoms

About one or two days after exposure, symptoms of flu develop suddenly, with fever, headache, and body aches. Intestinal symptoms are uncommon. The throat is sore, dry, and red. A cough appears on the second or third day, followed by a drop in fever with drenching sweats by the third to fifth day. As the fever drops, the child becomes highly susceptible to secondary bacterial infection. Fatigue and depression may last for weeks afterward. Although most children are sick for only a few days, some have much more serious illness (such as pneumonia) and may need to be hospitalized.

Diagnosis

There is no easy way to diagnose influenza. While the virus can be isolated from the throat, and antibodies can be found in the blood, these tests are expensive and slow. Diagnosis is usually made on the basis of symptoms and the occurrence of other cases in the area.

Treatment

There is no specific cure for the flu. No known antibiotic has any effect on any type or strain of any virus, although antibiotics may be used to treat secondary bacterial infections. Treatment is usually aimed at reducing fever and alleviating symptoms. Rest and liquids usually help.

Two oral prescription drugs—amantadine (Symmetrel) and rimantadine (Flumadine)—may prevent or reduce the severity of influenza A, but they are not effective against type B (which accounts for 30 percent of flu cases). However, they are 70 to 90 percent effective in preventing illness caused by A viruses, and their onset of protection is quicker than vaccination, making them a useful alternative, especially during type A influenza epidemics. Rimantadine produces fewer side effects.

Amantadine and rimantadine are approved for preventing type A influenza in children over age one. These medications may be given to children who have received the flu vaccine for the first time, since adequate antibody levels take six weeks to develop. The drugs do not affect the development of antibodies in response to the vaccine.

Amantadine, but not rimantadine, is also labeled for the *treatment* of type A influenza in children. The drug is designed to shorten illness by preventing the flu virus from reproducing, and so it works best if taken as soon as the flu strikes. Prompt treatment within 48 hours of the onset of symptoms reduces the severity and shortens the duration of illness. However, the effect of treatment on the development of complications is not known.

Amantadine causes more side effects than does rimantadine, but both can cause nausea and loss of appetite. Central nervous system side effects can range from nervousness and light-headedness to delirium, hallucinations, and seizures. These adverse effects are dose-related.

Two new medicines, oseltamivir and zanamivir, have not yet been approved for children under age 12.

Prevention

Routine vaccination against the flu is the most important way to control the disease, but in the past experts have not recommended that children be vaccinated. However, the vaccine experts now recommend annually for all children over six months of age—especially those who have certain risk factors, including ASTHMA, heart disease, SICKLE-CELL DISEASE, HIV, MUSCULAR DYSTROPHY, cystic fibrosis, or diabetes. Children under age nine who are receiving the vaccine for the first time should receive two doses separated by at least four weeks. Every child should be vaccinated against the flu every year, because the viral strains from the previous year's vaccine will not fully protect against the next year's viral strains. However, research has shown that even in years when new strains emerge, people in high-risk groups who get yearly flu shots tend to have milder illnesses and are less likely to be hospitalized with complications.

Each year scientists at the U.S. Centers for Disease Control and the World Health Organization (WHO) make an educated guess about which kind of flu will predominate during the next winter season. These two groups maintain a global network that collects data required to select strains for the coming flu season's vaccine. A similar process is undertaken in Europe by the WHO and various national authorities there.

How it works   The vaccine, which is usually offered between September and mid-November (but may be given at other times of the year), creates immunity to the flu through an injection of relatively harmless microorganisms that come from or are similar to the viruses that cause the flu. Flu season is from November to April, with most cases occurring between late December and early March. The shots are up to 80 percent effective in preventing disease. Because the vaccine is made from a killed virus, it is not possible to get the flu from the shot.

After getting a flu shot, a child's body will create antibodies to fight the virus if exposed. Antibodies against flu develop and provide protection within one or two weeks after vaccination. For children under seven who are getting a flu shot for the first time, the vaccine is given in two separate shots a month apart.

Although it is still possible for an immunized child to get the flu, symptoms usually are fewer and milder. Because the flu vaccine prevents infection with only a few of the viruses that can cause flu-like symptoms, getting the vaccine is not a guarantee that a child will not get sick during the season.

Who should get the shot   All children should get vaccinated, but it is especially critical for:

- those older than six months who are on long-term aspirin therapy and may be at risk for REYE'S SYNDROME if they catch the flu

- children who were born prematurely and are at increased risk of developing lung problems if they get influenza

- children who have chronic heart or lung disorders, including asthma

- children who in the past year saw a doctor regularly or were hospitalized for chronic diseases such as diabetes mellitus, KIDNEY PROBLEMS, severe anemia, or immune deficiency (including HIV/AIDS and immunosuppression caused by drugs)

- children who live with someone in the high-risk group

Who should not get a shot   Children who are severely allergic to eggs and egg products should not get the flu vaccine. Although inhaled flu vaccine (Flumist) is available for healthy children over age five, the American Academy of Pediatrics does not recommend it for children. Children allergic to thimersal should request the thimersal-free shot.

Side effects   Most children do not experience any side effects from the flu shot. The few who do may experience soreness or swelling at the site of the shot, and about 10 percent have mild side effects such as headache or low-grade fever that last about 24 hours after vaccination. Side effects are most likely to occur in children who have not been exposed to the flu before.

Children with these symptoms should not be given aspirin unless a pediatrician requests it because of its link to Reye's syndrome. Instead, a warm compress can ease soreness or swelling at the injection site and acetaminophen (Tylenol) or ibuprofen (Advil or Motrin) can treat headache or low-grade fever.

The most serious side effect from a flu shot is an allergic reaction in a person allergic to eggs or egg products. People who have a serious reaction—hives or breathing difficulty—should get medical attention immediately.

See also SEVERE ACUTE RESPIRATORY SYNDROME (SARS).

information processing disorders   Problems in any of the ways a child processes information, such as visual discrimination or understanding spatial relationships. A child's senses of sight, smell, hearing, taste, and touch are constantly providing information, which is stored in short- and long-term memory. For each of the hundreds of things children do each day, they need to quickly decide what information to use to complete the task. Managing all of the stored information and using it effectively is called "information processing."

A child with an information processing disorder may have trouble with one or more of the information processing skills, which interferes with using information efficiently, solving problems, or completing tasks. The inability to process information efficiently often causes frustration and learning failure.

Visual Discrimination

The ability to visually compare the features of different items to distinguish one from another. Children with problems in visual discrimination may find it hard to notice the small differences between some letters and numbers, certain colors, or between similar shapes and patterns.

Visual Figure-Ground Discrimination

The ability to separate a shape or printed character from its background. Children with problems in this area may find it hard to find the specific bit of information they need from a printed page or computer screen filled with words and numbers.

Visual Memory

Long-term visual memory is the ability to recall something seen a long time ago, while short-term visual memory is the ability to remember something seen very recently. Visual memory often depends upon the nature of the information being processed. For example, most people find it easier to remember what an object looked like four weeks ago if the object is associated with a special event. Children with problems in this area may find it hard to describe a place they have visited, remember the spelling of a familiar but irregularly spelled word, dial a telephone number without looking carefully at each of the numbers and letters on the telephone, or use a calculator, typewriter, or computer keyboard with speed and accuracy.

Visual Motor Processing

The kind of thinking needed to use feedback from the eyes to coordinate the movement of other parts of the body is called "visual motor processing." For example, eyes and hands need to work together if the child is going to write well with a pen or pencil. Children who have problems in this area may find it hard to write neatly or stay within the margins or on the lines of a page, use scissors, sew, move around without bumping into things, place objects on surfaces so they will not fall off, or participate in sports that require well-timed and precise movements in space.

Visual Closure

Visual closure is the ability to know what an object is when only parts of it are visible. Children with problems in this area may find it hard to recognize a picture of a familiar object missing some parts, or identify a word when a letter is missing.

Spatial Relationships

Spatial relationships refer to the way objects are positioned in space. Children use their ability to recognize and understand spatial relationships as they interact with their surroundings and also when they look at objects on paper. The ability to recognize and understand spatial relationships helps them understand whether objects are near or far, on the left or right, or over/under other objects. This skill is needed to learn to read, write, count, and think about numbers. Children with problems in this area may find it hard to find their way from one place to another, or write intelligibly, or do math.

Auditory Discrimination

The ability to notice, compare, and distinguish the distinct and separate sounds in words is called "auditory discrimination." In order to read efficiently, students must be able to isolate sounds, especially those that match letters in the alphabet. Children with problems in this area may find it hard to learn to read or understand spoken language, follow directions, and remember details.

Auditory Figure-Ground Discrimination

Auditory figure-ground discrimination refers to the ability to pick out important sounds from a noisy background. Children with problems in this area may find it hard to separate meaningful sounds from background noise.

Auditory Memory

There are two kinds of auditory memory: Long-term auditory memory is the ability to recall something heard long ago, whereas short-term auditory memory is the ability to remember something heard very recently. Children with problems in this area may find it difficult to remember people's names, memorize and recall telephone numbers, follow multistep spoken directions, recall stories they have been told, or remember lines from songs.

Treatment

There are things that can be done to help a child make it easier to process information. These include:

- simplify directions
- maintain eye contact while speaking
- speak slowly, especially when providing new information
- ask the child to repeat the information

Children with LEARNING DISABILITIES often have strong preferences for one type of information processing over another, which are sometimes called "learning or working styles." Something as simple as giving instructions both orally and in writing can be of enormous help to some children with learning disabilities.

intelligence   As commonly used, intelligence refers to the level of intellectual functioning and capacity of an individual—the ability to learn or understand.

Recently some experts have suggested that intelligence is not a single phenomenon, but that there exist "multiple intelligences," a number of discrete "intelligences," and that an individual will possess a unique pattern of strengths and abilities across this range of intellectual functions.

In the context of LEARNING DISABILITIES, the concept of intelligence is important for two reasons. First, there can often be significant discrepancies between intellectual ability and academic performance. Second, learning disabilities have often been misunderstood as a sign of lower intelligence despite extensive research and the achievement of many notable individuals with learning disabilities

such as Albert Einstein, Thomas Edison, and Nelson Rockefeller.

Intelligence is measured by intelligence tests, which provide an INTELLIGENCE QUOTIENT (IQ), a measure of intellectual development that is the ratio of a child's mental age to his chronological age, multiplied by 100.

intelligence quotient (IQ)   A measurement of intelligence based on performance on intelligence tests. Use of intelligence testing remains controversial because of the limitations of testing for specific abilities and knowledge, and because of possible cultural bias in the design of tests.

Nonetheless, intelligence quotient (IQ) is used in educational and psychological settings in combination with other types of tests in order to evaluate a child's mental capacity and to recommend appropriate remediation or treatment.

For children with learning disabilities, IQ scores can demonstrate superior intelligence despite weak language skills or poor academic performance. Conversely, poor performance on intelligence tests can inaccurately reflect true ability and potential, with many capable individuals outperforming the level of achievement their IQ scores might have predicted.

IQ is generally based on a mean of 100, with scores ranging in classification from "mentally retarded" at the low end to "very superior" at the high end.

The concept of intelligence has existed for centuries, but it was not until this century that scientists began testing it and debating whether or not they should. Intelligence testing was developed in the late 19th century as France's Alfred Binet began work on tests of individual differences, which led him to study "subnormal" children in Paris schools. Several years later Binet and Paris physician Theodore Simon recommended that an accurate diagnosis of intelligence be established for schoolchildren. The result was the Simon-Binet test of intelligence, which first appeared in 1905 and was revised in 1908.

Binet thought of the test as a tool for selecting students who needed special remedial teaching, not as a measure of absolute innate ability. The test was translated into English for the American audience in 1908 by Henry H. Goddard and revised several times, but it was not until 1916 that the test was standardized with the revision by Lewis M. Terman in the form still known as the Stanford-Binet test.

In 1911 William Stern developed the idea of relating mental age to chronological age with his formulation of Intelligence Quotient. This simple formulation of IQ= MA/CA × 100 gave a number that would stand for the performance of the child. This allowed the IQ to be manipulated within statistical tests and to be used for prediction of later performance.

During World War I the first massive use of psychological tests of intelligence was begun with the testing of military recruits. Hundreds of psychologists and graduate students in psychology were recruited to administer the tests to recruits. After the war critics were outraged to find that the Army test suggested that southern and eastern Europeans were inferior to northern Europeans, and that blacks were inferior to whites. Some believe it was these test results that prompted restrictive emigration policies in America in 1924 and fanned the flames of racial prejudice against blacks and other minorities.

David Wechsler developed his tests in response to many of the criticisms of the Binet tests. In 1939 he introduced his Wechsler Adult Intelligence Scale (WAIS), the first of a stable of tests still much in use.

Since that time there have been many intelligence tests produced, some specifically aimed at reducing cultural and background effects on pencil-and-paper tests. In 1969 the debate about the inherent versus the environmental bases of intelligence exploded with an article by psychologist Arthur Jensen in which he argued for the inheritance of racial differences in intelligence. The debate continued into the last decade of the 20th century in response to further controversial work on intelligence and class structure in American life. In recent years influential books by psychologist Howard Gardner and others have supported the idea of multiple intelligences over a single global factor in intelligence.

International Academy for Child Brain Development A group of professionals from a variety of disciplines including physicians, psy-

chologists, and anthropologists who are interested in the physical and psychological processes involved in child brain development. The group seeks to gain recognition of the study of child brain development and establish criteria for child brain developmentalists. The group conducts research, offers courses in child brain development, and bestows awards.

Founded in 1985, the group sponsors an annual convention during the last week in November and publishes *Journal for Child Brain Development.*

International League Against Epilepsy A group of national organizations united to encourage scientific research on EPILEPSY and to promote optimal treatment and rehabilitation. The league fosters the development of and cooperation among associations with common interests. Founded in 1909, the group publishes a bimonthly journal.

International Rett Syndrome Association A support group for parents of children with RETT SYNDROME, professionals, and others interested in Rett syndrome, a disorder affecting girls who seem normal up until ages seven months to 18 months, when autistic-like withdrawal sets in. Although this symptom eases in time, higher brain functions continue to deteriorate, leading to severe MENTAL RETARDATION.

The association provides support to parents, encourages research, collects and disseminates information, helps identify Rett syndrome patients, and conducts activities aimed at the prevention, treatment, and eventual eradication of the condition.

Founded in 1985, the association has 1,500 members and publishes a quarterly newsletter and informational brochures. (For contact information, see Appendix I.)

intussusception A problem with the intestine in which one portion of the bowel slips into the next like a collapsible tube, blocking the intestine so that the walls of the bowel press against one another. This can lead to inflammation, swelling, and loss of blood to the intestines. The condition can occur in children between three months and six years of age, although most cases happen between five months and nine months. It affects between one and four infants out of 1,000 and is two to three times more common in boys.

Causes

In infants the causes of intussusception are unknown. Some experts believe that the problem is caused by the aftereffects of a viral intestinal infection. Viral infections can cause swelling of the infection-fighting lymph tissue that normally lines the intestine. Because intussusception is seen most often in spring and fall, this seems to suggest a possible connection to the kinds of viruses children catch at these times.

When an older child or adult develops intussusception, it is often the result of a tumor or polyp in the intestine.

Symptoms

Intussusception usually triggers loud, anguished crying from the intense pain, as the baby draws the knees to the chest. Other common symptoms include vomiting, fever, irritability, lethargy, abdominal swelling, shallow breathing or grunting, and constipation. There may be some blood and mucus mixed with the stools.

In some babies with intussusception the pain may come and go, and in between pains the infant may stop crying. However, the pain always returns. Over time, an infant can become weak and suffer from severe dehydration or shock.

Diagnosis

A detailed patient and symptom history, together with a physical exam on the baby, may reveal a sausage-shaped mass in the abdomen, which suggests intussusception. Additional tests may help diagnose intussusception, including an abdominal X ray. If the diagnosis is certain and the child seems to be very sick or is losing blood, the pediatric surgeon may decide to operate right away to correct the bowel obstruction. If the diagnosis is still uncertain after regular X rays and a surgical examination and the baby is not seriously ill, a barium or air enema may be prescribed. A barium enema is a special X ray in which a substance called barium is put in the baby's rectum, and several X rays are taken. Barium can outline a telescoping intestine, and the obstruction may be cured by the pres-

sure from placing the enema in the bowel. A rectal air enema can be used together with X rays to make the final diagnosis, but not many hospitals use them on children.

Treatment

Treatment often depends on the severity of the problem, but if the child is treated early enough, the enema will correct the problem and relieve the obstruction without surgery. Both procedures are very safe and usually well tolerated by the child, although there is a very small risk of infection or bowel perforation.

If these procedures do not cure the intussusception, or if the infant is too sick to have the enema, surgery will be required to fix the obstruction and save the bowel. If there is any dying or infected bowel, that part of the tissue will be removed. Most infants who are treated within the first 24 hours recover completely.

Complications

If left untreated, intussusception can cause many severe complications, including death of bowel tissue, perforation of the bowel, infection, and death.

Call the Doctor

Call a doctor immediately if a child exhibits symptoms. Intussusception is a medical emergency, but with early treatment most infants recover completely. In many cases, early diagnosis means surgery can be avoided.

ipecac, syrup of   An emetic derived from the dried roots of a poisonous shrub found in Europe and the Americas, used to treat accidental poisoning.

However, ipecac syrup should no longer be used routinely as a poison treatment intervention in the home, according to new guidelines issued in November 2003 by the American Academy of Pediatrics (AAP). The AAP, reversing its long-standing guidelines, said the new recommendations are based on a lack of clear evidence of ipecac's benefit and the risk of people abusing the product. Instead, in case of possible poisoning, parents should contact the national Poison Control Hotline at 1-800-222-1222, or contact a pediatrician.

For decades, doctors have recommended that parents keep a bottle of ipecac on hand to induce vomiting when children ingest something poisonous. The antidote, made from roots of the tropical ipecac plant, induces vomiting. In the past, recommendations for using ipecac had been based more on intuition rather on than any hard evidence that home use is effective. Although earlier recommendations advised parents to call a doctor or poison control center before using the syrup, parents have not always heeded that advice. Too often, parents used ipecac inappropriately.

Scientific advisers to the U.S. Food and Drug Administration (FDA) recommended in June 2003 that the agency end over-the-counter sales of ipecac. A final FDA decision was expected in 2004.

Poison-control centers have been phasing out ipecac because it sometimes caused prolonged vomiting and lethargy similar to drowsiness that could have been caused by an overdose of sedative pills. Those symptoms can complicate diagnosis and treatment. It also may not totally empty the stomach of poison, or may linger and cause a child to vomit up other antidotes.

Another study found that home use did not reduce emergency room visits and did not improve outcomes. It is based on an analysis of data from the American Association of Poison Control Centers, which also is preparing new ipecac guidelines.

Ipecac syrup that has not expired does not need to be thrown out, but parents should not use ipecac before consulting a physician. Alternative home treatments for poisoning, such as activated charcoal or natural products, have not been shown to be effective, and in some cases are not safe or feasible to administer. Because of this, the American Academy of Pediatrics does not recommend using these products at home.

In any case, charcoal is harder for parents to administer than ipecac, because children object to the tasteless, gritty solution. For this reason, many experts believe there is still a place for syrup of ipecac in the home, although it must always be given with poison control center guidance.

While the correct dosage should be prescribed by a doctor or poison control center, a typical dose for a child over age one is two tablespoons followed by at least two to three glasses of water—*not milk*. If the child has not vomited within 20 minutes, the dose may be repeated. If the child still does not vomit, the poison control center should be called for further instructions.

If possible, the child should vomit into a container so that the material can be identified by medical experts at a hospital. Vomiting is effective only if it occurs within four hours of ingestion of a solid substance, or within two hours of ingestion of a liquid.

iron Dietary supplements containing iron (ferrous sulfate, ferrous gluconate, ferrous fumarate) are commonly given to children as part of a daily vitamin, but it is an often-overlooked potential source of poison to youngsters.

An accidental overdose of iron can damage the stomach, liver, and small intestine, affect blood circulation, and lead to shock and even death. Young children have been seriously injured by swallowing doses of 200 mg to 400 mg of iron, equivalent to 14 to 27 children's vitamin-and-mineral supplements with iron—or just four to seven tablets of a typical adult iron supplement.

More than 2,000 people are poisoned each year with iron, and a large number of those poisonings are fatal. Mortality may be as high as 50 percent.

In 1997 the U.S. Food and Drug Administration ruled that packages of all preparations that contain iron must now display a warning that accidental overdose of these products is a leading cause of fatal poisoning in children under age six. In addition, products containing 30 mg or more of iron per unit must be packaged as individual doses that will limit the number of pills or capsules a small child could swallow.

Despite resistant packaging, accidental overdose of iron remains a leading cause of poisoning deaths in children under age six. Since 1986 more than 11,000 incidents of children ingesting iron have been reported, and 35 children have died. Most of the serious injuries have occurred with products having more than 30 mg of iron per dosage unit. This includes most prenatal iron products, which are likely to be found in households with young children.

The exact mechanism behind iron poisoning is not known, nor is it understood how death results—whether from shock, systemic effects, or from the metabolic effects of absorbed iron, which causes respiratory collapse.

Symptoms

Within 30 minutes of overdose the first symptoms appear: lethargy, vomiting, fast weak pulse, low blood pressure, shock, pallor, blue-tinged skin, clotting problems, and coma. Then the child may seem to improve, but a few days later the patient goes into shock with pulmonary edema, collapse, coma, and death within 12 to 48 hours.

Treatment

Iron poisoning is a medical emergency that should be treated in the hospital with stomach pumping and chelating agents. Dialysis or an exchange transfusion may be needed.

irritable bowel syndrome   A condition in which there is abnormally rapid movement of the small and large intestine often linked to emotional stress or diet, which produces diarrhea and pain.

Irritable bowel syndrome (IBS) can affect children (especially girls), giving them a puzzling set of digestive complaints. Sometimes it is cramps, gas, and diarrhea; sometimes it is bloating and constipation; and sometimes it is alternating bouts of both. Children with IBS may sometimes pass mucus with their bowel movements, but they have no rectal bleeding or fever. IBS often troubles children during times of stress—family problems, divorce, moving, taking exams, even going on vacations, but IBS is not a psychological problem; it has a physical cause.

Cause

People with IBS have bowels that go into spasms more easily than those who do not, but scientists do not yet know why. What they do know that certain types of foods (milk, chocolate, caffeine) can trigger IBS in children.

Treatment

Not surprisingly, IBS symptoms often improve when trigger foods are limited. Increasing fiber in the diet and using techniques to relieve stress also seem to help. If necessary, the child's doctor may prescribe medicines to relieve symptoms.

isotretinoin (Accutane)   A synthetic oral form of vitamin A, isotretinoin has been used since the late 1970s to mitigate severe cystic ACNE that has not responded to other treatment. Isotretinoin is the only known cure for acne. It works by decreasing formation of oily plugs of sebum, reducing the formation of keratin (the tough outer layer of skin) and shrinking the oil-producing sebaceous glands. It works so well that it can cause unpleasant side effects, such as skin dryness and nosebleeds.

Isotretinoin cures or greatly reduces severe disfiguring acne in up to 80 percent of cases. However, because it can cause severe birth defects, pregnancy must be avoided during treatment and for at least two months after treatment has ended.

Currently, initial treatment with isotretinoin is given for four to six months. After treatment has stopped, the skin condition may continue to improve for at least two more months and sometimes for as long as a year, although the sebum production gradually returns to its original levels. More than 60 percent of patients with severe acne never again require treatment. If a second course is needed, it should be given only after a six-month hiatus. This second course may require higher doses.

Adverse Effects

Isotretinoin is an extremely effective anti-acne preparation, but in a small number of patients (less than 1 percent) it may be associated with symptoms of a major depressive episode. In these cases, symptoms resolve rapidly (within two to seven days) after stopping the medicine. After a period off medication, treatment can begin again at a lower dose.

In a "Dear Doctor" letter to 210,000 dermatologists, family doctors, and psychiatrists, the maker of the drug (Roche) wrote that the strengthened depression warning on its boxes was tied to uncommon adverse reactions. But the "potential consequences" led to label changes, warning physicians that isotretinoin may cause "depression, psychosis, and rarely, suicidal ideation, suicide attempts, and suicide." Stopping the drug may not be enough to ease the depression, the label warns.

Although the link between depression and isotretinoin has not been scientifically proven (the manufacturer insists there is no link), several people who have taken it claim they experienced depression, mood swings, and even suicidal thoughts. Both the FDA and the drug company said depression is common among acne patients, whether or not they take isotretinoin. It appears that patients who are prone to depression may be at higher risk for developing depression while taking isotretinoin.

Other side effects may include thinning hair, itching, dry and flaky skin, occasional aching muscles, and, rarely, liver damage.

itching That familiar tickling sensation on the skin is the most prominent symptom in many skin diseases and allergies. Skin that is too dry and scaly commonly causes itching as well, and many drug reactions result in itching (especially reactions to codeine and some antibiotics). Some types of rough clothing, soap, and detergents can trigger an itching response in some sensitive children.

In addition, a wide range of disorders produce itching, including HIVES, ECZEMA, FUNGAL INFECTIONS, and PSORIASIS. Itching all over the body may be caused by diabetes mellitus, kidney failure, JAUNDICE, thyroid problems, or blood disorders. Anal itching in children is usually caused by worms, although it also may be caused by an anal fissure or persistent diarrhea, or by too-rough cleansing after defecation. Infestations of LICE or SCABIES, or insect bites, can cause severe itching. Itching around the vulva may be caused by a yeast infection or hormonal changes at puberty.

Treatment

Specific treatment of itching depends on the underlying cause, but in general cooling lotions such as calamine can ease the itch and irritation of the skin. Emollients can reduce skin drying and ease itching for those with dry skin. Soothing lukewarm baths in colloidal oatmeal or Aveeno bath can ease the itch caused by hives or skin rashes such as CHICKEN POX or POISON IVY.

Because soap can irritate itchy skin, especially if the skin is dry or has a rash, it should be used only when really necessary. Mild cleansing solutions or water alone may be enough to keep itchy skin clean.

While scratching can temporarily ease an itch, it can actually make itching worse over time by over-stimulation. The urge to scratch can be suppressed by using lotions or salves or by applying cool wet compresses to the affected area. Systemic medications such as antihistamines also can be effective.

jaundice   Yellow discoloration of the skin caused by the accumulation in the blood of the yellow-brown bile pigment called bilirubin. Jaundice is a primary symptom of many different disorders of the liver and biliary systems.

Bilirubin is formed from hemoglobin as old red blood cells break down. The pigment is absorbed from the blood by the liver, where it is dissolved in water and excreted in bile. The process can be disrupted in one of three ways, causing one of the three types of jaundice—hemolytic, hepatocellular, and obstructive.

Jaundice in a newborn is often caused by hemolytic jaundice, in which the body breaks down too many red blood cells, producing too much bilirubin. This occurs in newborns when the liver has not yet developed the capacity to break down bilirubin, and where bilirubin is concentrated.

In hepatocellular jaundice, the transfer of bilirubin from liver cells to bile is prevented, causing a buildup of bilirubin. This is usually the result of acute hepatitis or liver failure.

Obstructive jaundice is caused by a block of the bile ducts, which prevents the bile from flowing out of the liver. Obstructive jaundice can also occur if the bile ducts are missing or have been destroyed. As a result, bile cannot pass out of the liver, and bilirubin is forced back into the blood.

JC virus   A virus that infects about 65 percent of all children by the age of 14, and that may play a role in the development of medulloblastoma—the most common type of malignant brain tumor found in the young. This type of cancer is diagnosed annually in about one out of every 200,000 children under the age of 15. Very aggressive, this cancer is difficult to treat and is often fatal.

Proteins from the JC virus were found in 20 specimens of brain tumors taken from children,

according to researchers at Temple University. The presence of the virus suggests it may play a role in the development of these tumors.

The name of the virus comes from the initials of a patient, John Cunningham, from whom the virus was first isolated in the 1970s. Earlier studies have shown that JC virus causes cancer in rats and mice, and that it can cause brain tumors in certain monkeys. JC virus, a type of neutropic polyomavirus, typically infects the upper respiratory system in the same way as the common cold. The virus causes no disease unless a patient's immune system is weakened or destroyed. In addition to the brain tumors, the JC virus can cause a fatal brain disease known as progressive multifocal leukoencephalopathy (PML). About four percent of all AIDS patients develop PML.

If scientists can conclusively prove that JC virus does play a role in the brain cancer, it may be possible to develop a vaccine that could help in treating the tumor or preventing its spread.

jealousy   See SIBLING RIVALRY.

jellyfish stings   The jellyfish family includes about 200 species that drift along the shoreline, dragging tentacles capable of stinging when touched. While most stings from jellyfish may cause little harm, some jellyfish can inflict severe stings, causing a child to panic and drown. In the water the shock of the sting often causes the child to jerk away, which only stimulates the tentacles to release more poison. If stung by a jellyfish on dry land, more poison is released if the child tries to rip off the sticky threads of the tentacles.

Symptoms

Stings can cause a severe burning pain with a red welt or row of lesions at the sting site. There also may be more general symptoms, including headache, nausea, vomiting, muscle cramps, diarrhea, convulsions, and breathing problems. The wound site becomes red and blistered and can leave permanent scars. One or two weeks after the sting, the child may experience a recurrence of the lesions at the site.

The sting of the Portuguese man-of-war is rarely fatal but causes hives, numbness, and severe chest, abdominal, and extremity pain. Death is usually the result of panic and drowning.

Treatment

Because tentacles continue to discharge their stinging cells as long as they remain on the skin, the most important first aid intervention is to remove all of the tentacles. Alcohol, ammonia, or vinegar and salt water (not freshwater) can be poured over the sting site to deactivate the tentacles, which should then be scraped off with a towel. Tentacles must not be removed by hand. Instead, they should be pulled (not rubbed) away. Baking soda in a paste can be applied to the sting to relieve pain; after an hour, it should be scraped off with an object (such as a credit card) to remove any remaining stinging cells. Calamine lotion will ease the burning sensation, and painkillers may help with the stinging pain.

Antivenin is effective against more dangerous species, but it must be given immediately. Jellyfish stings also may cause an allergic reaction, which can be treated with Benadryl or corticosteroids. A severe reaction to the sting may require hospitalization.

jock itch The common term for tinea cruris, a common fungal infection of the genital area. It is most common in the tropics and among boys.

Cause

The infection is caused by certain fungi of the genera *Trichophyton, Microsporum,* or *Epidermophyton floccosum*. These fungi live on dead body tissue such as hair, the outer layer of skin, and nails. The fungi are transmitted from boy to boy by sharing towels, benches, or shower stalls in locker rooms. Since fungi grow best in warm, moist environments, they thrive in hot, humid weather and among boys who wear tight clothing or who are obese.

Symptoms

Jock itch is a mild but annoying infection characterized by reddened, itchy scaly areas spreading from the genitals outward to the inner thighs. The rash may be dry, crusted, bumpy, or moist; the scrotum is not usually affected. Some people are prone to jock itch and are often reinfected.

Diagnosis

A fungal culture from skin scrapings will provide a definite diagnosis. However, it may be difficult to differentiate jock itch from other yeast infections in the groin. It is important to have the condition correctly diagnosed.

Treatment

The area should be bathed well with soap and water, removing all scabs and crusts, followed by application of antifungal cream on all lesions. Antifungal drugs (such as miconazole and clotrimazole) are often prescribed as a lotion, cream, or ointment to ease the itchy rash.

To prevent recurrence, treatment should be continued for some time after the symptoms have passed to make sure the fungi have been eliminated. Mild infections on the skin surface may require treatment for up to six weeks.

In very severe cases or if there is no improvement with the cream after a few days, some people require oral medication; griseofulvin is used only for these severe, resistant cases. Scratching the rash can lead to additional skin infection.

Juvenile Diabetes Foundation (JDF) The world's leading nonprofit, nongovernmental supporter of diabetes research, the only major diabetes organization focused exclusively on research. The foundation was founded in 1970 by the parents of children with juvenile diabetes—a disease that strikes children suddenly, makes them insulin-dependent for life, and carries the constant threat of devastating complications.

Volunteers help define research priorities, select research grant recipients, lead advocacy efforts, and provide guidance to overall operations. The Juvenile Diabetes Research Foundation (JDRF) has 93 chapters and affiliates worldwide, which have helped to raise more than $500 million for diabetes research. Volunteers help raise funds through a "Walk to Cure Diabetes," galas and golf tourna-ments, community activities, advocacy, and private donations. JDRF receives no federal funding. (For contact information, see Appendix I.)

juvenile rheumatoid arthritis   See ARTHRITIS, JUVENILE RHEUMATOID.

Kawasaki disease A childhood disease primarily characterized by inflammation of the blood vessels, affecting children under age five. Kawasaki disease is the most common cause of acquired heart disease in children. If not detected and treated immediately, it can result in heart damage and death.

Known medically as "mucocutaneous lymph node syndrome," it was first described in Japan in 1967. The acute illness itself is self-limited, but 15 percent to 25 percent of untreated children will suffer damage to the coronary arteries resulting in dilation or aneurysms. Although damage can occur in any medium-sized muscular artery, the vessels most often affected are the coronary arteries.

Kawasaki disease was first described in the United States in the early 1970s. Although Japanese children have the highest risk of this illness, Kawasaki disease occurs in all races. Black children have the second highest rate of occurrence, followed by whites.

Almost 85 percent of cases occur in children under age five years, with the greatest likelihood of occurrence in the toddler age group (one- to two-year-olds). Infants often experience atypical symptoms, but infant males have the highest risk of developing severe coronary artery disease. Recent research has also documented a higher incidence of coronary artery aneurysms in children older than age six years. Boys are affected more often than girls.

Although experts do not know how many children in the United States develop Kawasaki disease each year, estimates based upon hospital discharge summaries suggest that at least 2,000 to 3,000 cases occur annually.

Cause
Little is known about how the syndrome is spread or how a person contracts it, although it does not appear to be transmitted from one person to another. Experts suspect the disease is related to an infectious agent for a number of reasons:

- The disease almost exclusively affects children, which suggests that people develop passive immunity by adulthood.
- Geographic outbreaks occur with more cases in the late winter and early spring.
- The symptoms of Kawasaki disease look very much like other infectious diseases, such as SCARLET FEVER.

Genetic susceptibility may play a role in Kawasaki disease, since children of Japanese origin, no matter where in the world they live, are more likely to acquire Kawasaki disease, and siblings of children with the disease are more likely than other neighborhood children to develop the illness at a later time. Finally, Kawasaki disease has been reported in the children of parents who themselves had been affected in childhood.

Interestingly, epidemiological studies have found associations between the occurrence of Kawasaki disease and recent exposure to carpet cleaning and living near a body of stagnant water.

Symptoms
Most children experience a high fever that does not respond to antibiotics and lasts more than five days. There also may be red eyes and lips, strawberry tongue, a rash, and swollen lymph nodes. The rash may cover the entire body and may be followed by peeling of the skin on hands and fingers.

The course of the illness can be divided into three stages: acute, subacute, and convalescent phases. The acute phase begins with the abrupt onset of fever, which lasts for at least five days but averages 11 days without treatment. Often one symptom appears as another disappears, making the diagnosis challenging, especially for children who see different doctors during the early days of their illness. Arthritis in fingers and toes appears in about a third of patients. Although unusual, cardiac rhythm (electrical) disturbances may occur.

The subacute phase begins as the fever drops. During this stage, the skin of the palms and soles starts to peel off, beginning under the fingertips and toes. Arthritis, if present, generally affects the larger weight-bearing joints in this phase. In those patients who develop coronary artery abnormalities, an echocardiogram will reveal dilation or aneurysms in this phase.

The third stage is a convalescent phase, during which the child continues to recover and laboratory values return to normal. Unfortunately, although the child is usually feeling better at this time, coronary aneurysms may continue to enlarge, reaching their maximum dimension four to six weeks from the first day of fever.

Diagnosis

There are no tests for this disease. Physicians must diagnose Kawasaki disease by the symptoms alone. Echocardiography is performed at the time of diagnosis to evaluate cardiac function and establish a baseline for evaluation of coronary artery size and shape.

Treatment

Most patients are treated in the hospital where they can be watched and given aspirin and immunoglobulins. Intravenous gamma globulin is highly effective if administered immediately.

Complications

The most common complication is a ballooning of the vessels of the heart (called a coronary artery aneurysm). Among children who do not receive intravenous immunoglobulins (IVIG) treatment in the acute phase, 15 percent to 25 percent will develop damage to the coronary arteries. The longer the fever persists, the greater the risk of the development of coronary aneurysms.

Coronary artery abnormalities often are not detected until the second week after the onset of fever; however, they have been detected as early as seven days into the illness. The affected vessels can continue to enlarge through the fourth week of illness, at which time they have generally reached their maximum dimension.

Kawasaki Disease Foundation The only non-profit organization dedicated exclusively to addressing issues related to KAWASAKI DISEASE, established in 2000 by a group of parents and professionals. The foundation strives to unite the personal insight of families with the expertise of medical professionals. The group tries to raise awareness among the medical community, child-care providers, and the general public and also provide support among families to help them cope with this uncommon illness and the potentially devastating effects of heart damage. The group also raises money for research. (For contact information, see Appendix I.)

kerion An inflamed area of the skin that develops as an immune reaction to a fungus, usually RINGWORM of the scalp.

Symptoms

A kerion is characterized by a red swelling that lasts up to two months and may leave a scar and permanent loss of hair from the affected area.

Treatment

While the swelling may heal without treatment, applications of ichthamnol paste and antifungal agents are used.

kidney problems The kidneys play a critical role in filtering out harmful minerals and chemicals from the blood so that waste products do not build up in the blood and damage the body. Children can develop several different problems with the kidneys, including birth defects, urinary tract blockages, and disease of the kidney itself.

Birth Defects

The most common kidney diseases in children are birth defects such as:

- *Posterior urethral valve obstruction* A narrowing or obstruction of the urethra
- *Fetal hydronephrosis* Dilatation or enlargement of one or both of the fetal kidneys due to a problem in the developing urinary tract
- *Hydronephrosis* Swelling of parts of the kidney that can occur in infancy or childhood due to a blocked urinary tract or vesicoureteral reflux (VUR), which is caused by a problem in the function of the mechanism that prevents urine from backing up from the bladder to the kidneys.
- *Cystic kidney diseases* These are usually present at birth. One type is polycystic kidney disease (PKD), in which many fluid-filled cysts in the kidneys take up most of the space in the kidneys, leading to kidney failure. Some forms of PKD are inherited. Multicystic kidney disease is another type of cystic kidney problem in which a developmentally abnormal kidney grows large cysts and eventually stops functioning. Although PKD always affects both kidneys, multicystic kidney disease frequently affects only one.

Diseases of the Kidney

While many kidney problems are present at birth, others do not appear until later in childhood. Some of these kidney diseases include:

- *Renal tubular acidosis* In this condition, the kidneys do not properly regulate the amount of acid in the body.
- *Wilms' tumor* A type of CHILDHOOD CANCER of the kidney
- *Nephritis* An inflammation or infection of the filtering unit of the kidney (nephron) that may be inherited or may be the result of an infection; more often, the cause is unknown.
- *Nephrosis* A change in the nephron that is not inflammatory
- *Nephrotic syndrome* This condition occurs when large amounts of protein are lost from the body through the urine.
- *Infection* Repeated kidney and urinary tract infections can cause kidney damage.

- *Other diseases* SICKLE-CELL DISEASE, LUPUS, HIGH BLOOD PRESSURE, and diabetes also can cause kidney damage.
- *Accidents* A serious injury such a car accident or a major fall could potentially damage a child's kidneys.
- Kidney stones

Symptoms

The signs and symptoms of kidney disease can vary quite a bit from one child to the next. Children with chronic kidney failure may not have symptoms until 80 percent of their kidney function is lost. If symptoms do appear, they may include:

- fever
- swelling around the eyes, feet, and ankles
- burning or pain during urination
- significant increase in the frequency of urination
- problems in controlling urination in children who are toilet trained
- recurrence of nighttime bed-wetting in children who have been dry for several months
- bloody urine
- high blood pressure
- fatigue
- nausea and vomiting
- concentration problems

Diagnosis

Kidney disease can be diagnosed by either the child's pediatrician or a nephrologist (kidney specialist) using urine tests, blood tests, imaging studies, or a biopsy.

Urinalysis A urinalysis can quickly reveal problems such as too many red or white blood cells that may signal inflammation or irritation in the urinary tract. Urinalysis also can reveal the presence of casts (cylindrical structures made up of cells or protein that form in the presence of some kidney diseases). While a lack of casts does not rule out the possibility of a kidney disease, their presence suggests it.

Blood tests Some blood tests reveal how well the kidneys filter waste products and balance the bloodstream's chemical makeup. Creatinine and blood urea nitrogen (BUN) are two common blood level tests that doctors use to monitor kidney function.

Blood pressure/growth Two other important diagnostic tools a doctor may use during an initial physical exam are blood pressure and growth measurements. The heart is not the only important organ in regulating blood pressure—the kidneys also play a vital role. High blood pressure in a child, which is quite unusual, is an important sign that the kidneys need to be evaluated. Accurate growth measurements can provide a clue in diagnosing some kidney diseases because children with chronic kidney disease often grow poorly.

Biopsy A pediatrician may recommend a kidney biopsy to evaluate a child's kidney function. During a biopsy, a small piece of kidney tissue is removed with a needle while a child is under anesthesia. This simple procedure can help make an accurate diagnosis of the kidney problem in about nine out of 10 cases. It is especially helpful in the diagnosis of nephritis and nephrosis.

Scans In addition to standard X rays, a doctor may use computerized tomography (CT) scans or ultrasound to help diagnose kidney diseases. Of all the different types of scans, ultrasound is used most often because it is painless and requires no X-ray exposure or special preparation. A kidney ultrasound shows details of the anatomy of the kidneys and bladder and can be used to rule out or diagnose obstructions, developmental abnormalities, tumors, and stones in the kidneys and urinary tract.

A CT scan is often helpful in revealing the anatomy of the kidneys or bladder and, in some cases, is better than ultrasound for finding kidney stones. It can show if the kidneys have developed properly or if the flow of urine is blocked by a stone or a developmental abnormality.

With a renal nuclear scan, the doctor injects a radioactive material into a vein to compare the kidneys to each other in size, shape, and function. It also can detect scarring or other evidence of recurrent or chronic kidney infection.

Treatment

The first and simplest way to treat kidney diseases is by modifying the diet and taking medicine, such as vitamins, calcium, bicarbonate, and blood pressure pills. Newer injectable medicines are available for treating anemia and growth failure in some children with chronic kidney disease. Erythropoetin can increase the red blood cell count, which often improves the energy and activity levels of a child with kidney failure. Recent studies have shown that many children with chronic kidney disease will grow more normally with the help of human growth hormone injections.

Nearly all children with end-stage kidney disease eventually receive transplants. If a living related donor cannot be found, dialysis may be required until a donor kidney is found.

A child with chronic kidney disease may have several needs to address, including diet changes. Ensuring that your child takes in adequate calories and proper amounts of various nutrients can be a challenge for both you and your child. Supplementing your child's diet with extra carbohydrates and fats may help to increase calorie intake. As kidney failure develops, it produces a taste in the mouth that leads to an aversion to certain foods, especially proteins.

Dairy products have to be restricted because they contain large amounts of phosphorus, but if they are eliminated, it can be hard to provide enough calcium in a child's diet to maintain bones and support other body needs, particularly in a growing child. In children with more severe degrees of kidney failure, reducing the intake of dairy products and other protein-rich foods (such as meat, fish, or eggs) can make the filtering work of the kidneys easier and can sometimes put off the need for dialysis. It is important to remember that children do need enough protein for growth, and strict protein restriction (the kind that is recommended for adults) should not be used.

Many foods (including fruits and vegetables) contain potassium, but too much of it can be dangerous for children with kidney failure. Foods that are high in potassium include orange juice, bananas, tomato sauces, raisins, and melons.

It is also important to monitor fluid intake, because if the child's ability to produce urine is declining, fluid intake needs to be limited. Some children with kidney disease, particularly those with high blood pressure, may need to restrict their intake of sodium. The advice of a child's doctor or a dietitian may be valuable in learning about the sodium content of various foods. A child's nephrologist can discuss an appropriate diet that meets a child's need for calories and nutrients while minimizing damage to kidneys and avoiding other complications.

knock-knees Many children show a moderate tendency toward knock-knees between the ages of four and six as the body goes through a natural shift of alignment during the first years of life. After this period, the body tends to straighten. Many perfectly normal children are bowlegged and then become knock-kneed during normal development. Special shoes or wedges make no difference. Only when an inward turning of the knees is severe and associated with other problems is further evaluation or treatment necessary.

Most pediatricians can recognize when the condition is severe enough to warrant special care, but parents may want to seek a specialist's opinion if they believe their child's feet or legs are not developing normally. BOWED LEGS, FLATFEET, knock-knees, PIGEON TOE, and TOE-WALKING are all examples of normal variations of the human anatomy that rarely require treatment.

labial adhesion   A very common condition in infant girls in which the labia (the folds of tissues covering the genitals) stick together. Labial adhesions are almost always unnoticed by parents and occasionally by doctors, but between 25 percent to 40 percent of infant girls have some degree of adhesions. The tissue may cover part or all of the hymen (opening to the vagina) and the urethra (the opening to the bladder) and sometimes extend up to the clitoris.

Symptoms

This tissue usually breaks apart spontaneously before it is ever noticed or causes problems. Most of the time, adhesions do not cause any symptoms and naturally disappear with the hormonal changes of puberty. A physician will notice the condition during an infant's physical exam.

Treatment

The adhesions should not be forcefully separated because the area is very sensitive, and small tears in the tissue may be more likely to reattach themselves and become scarred. Thin adhesions may break apart on their own without special treatment.

If they do not, a pediatrician may prescribe hormonal creams, especially if the adhesions are thickened, recurrent, or causing symptoms. Because the estrogen in the cream is absorbed and will cause breast development and darkening of the labia skin when used for an extended time, the therapy is usually given for a short term and closely monitored.

Prevention

Once the tissues separate, daily baths, good hygiene, and lubrication of the tissues with a diaper ointment are recommended to prevent the tissues from sticking together again. Once the child is out of diapers, the problem should not recur.

Complications

If the adhesion is thick and large, sometimes the child will develop discomfort or burning during urination if the urine is trapped behind the adhesion. Urinary tract infections are also a rare complication of this problem.

La Crosse encephalitis   See ENCEPHALITIS, LA CROSSE.

lactose intolerance   The inability to digest milk sugar (lactose) because of a lack of the digestive enzyme lactase normally produced in the cells lining the small intestine. Lactase breaks down milk sugar into simpler forms that can then be absorbed into the bloodstream. When there is not enough lactase to digest the amount of lactose consumed, the results are gas, bloating, and abdominal pain. It is more common in African Americans than Caucasians.

While not all children deficient in lactase have symptoms, those who do are considered to be lactose intolerant. Even though lactose intolerance is widespread, it need not pose a serious threat to good health. Children who have trouble digesting lactose can learn which dairy products and other foods they can eat without discomfort and which ones they should avoid. Many will be able to enjoy milk, ice cream, and other such products if eaten in small amounts or eaten with other food. Lactase liquid or tablets may also help digest the lactose.

Even growing children who must avoid milk and foods made with milk can meet most of their special dietary needs by eating greens, fish, and other calcium-rich foods that are free of lactose. A carefully chosen diet, with calcium supplements if the doctor or dietitian recommends them, is the key to reducing symptoms and protecting future health.

Symptoms

Common symptoms include nausea, cramps, bloating, gas, and diarrhea, which begin about 30 minutes to two hours after eating or drinking foods containing lactose. The severity of symptoms varies depending on the amount of lactose each child can tolerate.

In rare cases, children are born without the ability to produce lactase. For most children, however, lactase deficiency is a condition that develops naturally over time. After about the age of two, the body begins to produce less lactase, but many people may not experience symptoms until they are much older.

Diagnosis

The most common tests used to measure the absorption of lactose in the digestive system are the lactose tolerance test, the hydrogen breath test, and the stool acidity test. These tests are performed on an outpatient basis.

The lactose tolerance test begins with the child fasting before the test and then drinking a liquid that contains lactose. Several blood samples are taken over a two-hour period to measure the child's blood sugar level, which indicates how well the body is able to digest lactose. Normally, when lactose reaches the digestive system, the lactase enzyme breaks down lactose into glucose and galactose. The liver then changes the galactose into glucose, which enters the bloodstream and raises the person's blood glucose level. If lactose is incompletely broken down, the blood glucose level does not rise and a diagnosis of lactose intolerance is confirmed.

The hydrogen breath test measures the amount of hydrogen in the breath. Normally, very little hydrogen is detectable in the breath, but undigested lactose in the colon is fermented by bacteria, and various gases (including hydrogen) are produced. The hydrogen is absorbed from the intestines, carried through the bloodstream to the lungs, and exhaled. In the test, the child drinks a lactose-loaded beverage, and the breath is analyzed at regular intervals. Raised levels of hydrogen in the breath indicate improper digestion of lactose. Certain foods and medications can affect the test's accuracy and should be avoided before the test is taken.

The lactose tolerance and hydrogen breath tests are not given to infants and very young children who are suspected of having lactose intolerance. A large lactose load may be dangerous for very young individuals because they are more prone to dehydration that can result from diarrhea caused by the lactose. If a baby or young child is experiencing symptoms of lactose intolerance, many pediatricians simply recommend changing from cow's milk to soy formula and waiting for symptoms to stop. If necessary a stool acidity test, which measures the amount of acid in the stool, may be given to infants and young children. Undigested lactose fermented by bacteria in the colon creates lactic acid and other fatty acids that can be detected in a stool sample. In addition, glucose may be present in the sample as a result of unabsorbed lactose in the colon.

Treatment

Fortunately, lactose intolerance is relatively easy to treat. Symptoms in young children can be controlled by diet in which foods containing lactose are eliminated. Most older children need not avoid lactose completely, although children differ in the amounts and types of foods they can eat. For example, one child may not be able to drink a small glass of milk without symptoms, while another can eat ice cream but not other dairy products. Each child will need to learn through trial and error how much lactose can be tolerated.

Children who react to very small amounts of lactose or who have trouble eliminating lactose can take lactase enzymes. One type of enzyme is available as a liquid which is added to a quart of milk; after 24 hours in the refrigerator, the lactose is reduced by 70 percent. The process works faster if the milk is first heated; adding a double dose of the enzyme produces milk that is 90 percent lactose free. Chewable lactase enzyme tablets also can help children digest solid foods that contain lactose. Lactose-reduced milk and other products are available at most supermarkets.

One concern for lactose intolerant children is whether they are getting enough calcium in their diet, which is contained in dairy products and which is essential for the growth and repair of bones throughout life. Research suggests that yogurt with active cultures may be a good source of calcium for children with lactose intolerance, because even though it contains a lot of lactose, the bacterial cultures in the yogurt produce some of the lactase enzyme required for proper digestion.

Foods to Avoid

Although dairy products are the only natural sources of lactose, it is often added to prepared foods such as bread and baked goods, processed breakfast cereals, instant potatoes, breakfast drinks, margarine, lunch meats, salad dressings, candies, and mixes for pancakes, biscuits, and cookies. Some products labeled "nondairy," such as powdered coffee creamer, also contain lactose because they include ingredients derived from milk.

Consumers need to check for foods made not only with milk and lactose but with ingredients including whey, curds, milk by-products, dry milk solids, and nonfat dry milk powder. In addition, lactose is used as the base for more than 20 percent of prescription drugs and about six percent of over-the-counter medicines.

language delay A lag in the development of communication skills, progressing more slowly than would be expected based on age, environment, or specific deprivation or disease. Children with LEARNING DISABILITY are likely to have language delays. Language delay includes the diagnostic subgroups of language disorder, language and learning disability, MENTAL RETARDATION, and AUTISM.

language disabilities A range of deficits in linguistics, whether related to expressive language, written or oral, or auditory processing, the processing of sounds and meaning.

language disorder A developmental disorder involving disabilities of reception, integration, recall, and/or production of language. Language disorders may be spoken, written, or both. (See also LEARNING DISABILITY.)

language processing disabilities The most common type of LEARNING DISABILITY, this problem may cause children to have trouble with any aspect of language, such as:

- hearing words correctly
- remembering verbal material
- understanding the meaning of words
- communicating clearly

The child with this problem has trouble with the spoken word, which usually interferes with reading and writing when the child first starts school. This learning problem may range from mild to extremely severe—so difficult that the child may find that coping with reading and writing is like learning a foreign language. They may be slow in learning to speak and speak in brief sentences, and their memory for verbal directions is poor.

Many children with this problem may speak in a garbled fashion because their brains may have trouble sorting out the right sounds; these children may pronounce "elephant" as "efelunt." They may have a poor grasp of grammar and trouble with word sequencing in a sentence and may confuse words that sound alike. These types of errors usually get worse if the children must speak in public or before an authority figure.

laryngitis An inflammation and swelling of the voice box (larynx) and the area around it, usually associated with hoarseness or loss of the voice. The problem is most common in late fall, winter, or early spring.

Cause

The voice box contains the vocal cords and is located at the top of the airway to the lungs. When the vocal cords become inflamed or infected, they swell, which can cause hoarseness and may even obstruct the child's airway.

The most common form of laryngitis is caused by a viral infection, although it also may be caused by a bacterial infection or the common cold, bronchitis, flu, or pneumonia. Common laryngitis is not normally associated with any breathing difficulty.

Several other forms of laryngitis in children—CROUP and EPIGLOTTITIS—can lead to fatal obstruction of the respiratory tract. Other causes of laryngitis include laryngeal polyps, laryngeal paralysis, precancerous changes of the throat, malignant tumors, allergies, and trauma.

Symptoms

Symptoms include a recent upper respiratory infection, fatigue, hoarseness, fever, and swollen lymph nodes or glands in the neck.

Treatment

Since most common laryngitis is viral, treatment with antibiotics is generally not necessary. Resting the voice helps to reduce inflammation of the vocal cords, and a humidifier may ease the raw feeling sometimes associated with laryngitis. Decongestants and painkillers may ease symptoms from the upper respiratory infection.

Call a Doctor

Rarely, severe respiratory distress may develop. A doctor should be consulted if the child has trouble breathing or swallowing, or if a small child is drooling. A doctor should be called if a child less than three months old is hoarse, or if an older child has been hoarse for more than a week.

Prevention

Avoiding upper respiratory infections during cold and flu season may help prevent laryngitis. This can be done by thorough hand-washing, avoiding others with infections, and wiping surfaces in the home when people are sick.

latex allergy Allergic responses to latex (rubber) products are fairly common among children and can range from mild irritation to life-threatening reaction. It is an extremely common compound found in many products, including underwear bands, rubber gloves, toys, elastic bandages, baby bottle nipples, pacifiers, and balloons. Anyone with a latex allergy should avoid exposure to all products that contain latex, but children most at risk are those with birth defects requiring multiple surgeries early in life. Between two and eight percent of the population are allergic to latex.

The first incidents of latex allergy in the United States were reported in 1988. Numbers had increased to at least 500,000 by 1992. Between 1990 and January 1991, nine children at a children's hospital in Milwaukee had anaphylactic reactions within 30 minutes after general anesthesia was started but before any surgical incisions had been made. The latex connection was the anesthe-

sia equipment and intravenous catheters. Eight of the children required intensive care.

Symptoms

Typical symptoms include watery eyes, wheezing, hives, rash, swelling, and, in severe cases, anaphylaxis. (In anaphylactic shock, a child can develop shortness of breath, swollen lips, and throat, heart, and breathing problems within minutes.) These responses can occur when items containing latex touch the skin, the mucous membranes (the mouth, genitals, bladder, or rectum), open areas, or bloodstream (especially during surgery). Lips and the face may swell after contact with latex balloons.

Cause

A latex allergy occurs when the immune system reacts to proteins found in latex, triggering a defensive reaction that can cause unpleasant and, in some cases, life-threatening symptoms. However, certain children are at greater risk of becoming allergic to latex. Those at higher risk include children who are frequently exposed to latex. As many as 65 percent of children with spina bifida have latex allergy. More than 25 percent of children with spinal injuries are allergic to latex, as are 33 percent of children with multiple congenital defects (especially urinary tract defects) and any child who has had three or more surgeries. It is the repeated exposure to latex (usually through catheterization) that sensitizes children to latex. This progressive allergy worsens with increased exposure.

Children who develop latex allergy also can be sensitive to food allergens. A number of fruits, vegetables, nuts, and cereals contain proteins that are similar to the proteins found in latex. A child's body can generalize an allergic reaction from one protein to another similar one (cross-reactivity). The following foods cross-react with latex: avocados, bananas, pineapples, apricots, grapes, kiwis, tomatoes, papayas, passion fruit, cherries, figs, peaches, nectarines, plums, celery, raw potatoes, hazelnuts, and chestnuts.

Diagnosis

A sensitivity to latex can be diagnosed from a review of past medical history, a physical exam, and blood tests for latex-specific IgE antibodies. Test results define the presence of sensitivity, but once a sensitivity is present, IgE antibodies cannot be used to predict how severe a reaction will occur.

Treatment

There is no cure for a latex allergy. Children at high risk can prevent the development of latex allergy by avoiding latex products in all areas. If a child has already developed latex allergy, avoidance may lessen the response. In order to protect themselves, students with latex allergies should carry nonlatex gloves at all times for health-care professionals to use during both routine examinations and emergency procedures. School nurses should have a supply of nonlatex gloves available for use. Highly allergic children also should wear a Medic Alert bracelet and carry an emergency epinephrine kit (Epipen) in case they are accidentally exposed to latex and go into anaphylactic shock. The school nurse, playground aides, and classroom teacher should be aware of what to do in case of an allergic reaction. The physical education instructor should also be familiar with the student's allergy because equipment is often made from rubber-based products. Cafeteria workers may need to adjust their food preparation practices to address the student's sensitivity.

lawn mower safety The power lawn mower is one of the most dangerous tools around the home, especially for children. In 1990 about 10,000 children younger than 15 years were seen in emergency rooms with lawn mower injuries. More than seven percent of pediatric mower-related injuries require hospitalization, which is about twice the hospitalization rate for consumer product-related injuries overall.

Older children and teens were most often hurt while cutting lawns, but younger ones were most often injured by riding on lawn mowers with a parent. Lawn mower injuries include deep cuts, loss of fingers and toes, broken and dislocated bones, burns, and eye and other injuries.

To prevent lawn mower injuries to children, the American Academy of Pediatrics recommends:

- Parents should only use a power mower with a control that stops the mower if the handle is let go. This control should never be disconnected.

- Children under age 16 should not use ride-on mowers, and children under age 12 should not use walk-behind mowers. Children should not operate lawn mowers until they have displayed appropriate levels of judgment, strength, coordination, and maturity necessary for their safe operation

- Children should always wear sturdy shoes (not sandals or sneakers) while mowing.

- Objects such as stones or toys should be picked up from the lawn before mowing to prevent injuries from flying debris. A collection bag for grass clippings or a plate that covers the opening where cut grass is released should be used.

- Anyone using a mower should wear protective eyewear.

- While the lawn is being mowed, children younger than six years should be kept indoors.

- Mowers should be started and refueled outdoors, not in a garage or shed. Mowers should be refueled with the motor turned off and cool.

- Blade settings should only be done by an adult, with the mower off and the spark plug removed or disconnected.

- Children must not be allowed to ride as passengers on mowers or to be towed behind mowers in carts or trailers. They should not be permitted to play on or around the mower when it is in use or in storage.

- Children should receive a period of operational training, safety instruction, and supervision by an adult before they are allowed to operate a mower by themselves.

lazy eye The common term for amblyopia, in which a child's reduced vision is not caused by any eye disease and is not correctable by glasses or contact lenses. Instead, the problem is caused by the brain's refusal to acknowledge the images seen by the lazy eye, causing reduced vision. This almost always affects only one eye, although vision may be reduced in both. It is estimated that three percent of children under six have some form of amblyopia. If not detected and treated early in life, amblyopia can cause a permanent loss of vision. Detection and correction before the age of two is the best way to restore normal vision. Between 2 and 3 percent of all children have lazy eye.

Cause

All babies are born with poor eyesight, but as they grow, their eyesight improves. Good eyesight needs a clear, focused image that is the same in both eyes. If the image is not clear in one eye, or if it is not the same in both eyes, the vision pathways will not develop correctly, or may get worse.

Amblyopia usually is caused by either a misalignment of a child's eyes (such as crossed eyes) or a difference in image quality between the two eyes (one eye focusing better than the other). In both cases, one eye becomes stronger, suppressing the image of the other eye. If this condition persists, the weaker eye may become useless. Anything that interferes with clear vision in either eye during the critical period from birth to six years of age will cause amblyopia.

Amblyopia vs. Strabismus

Although many people call strabismus (crossed eyes) "lazy eye," in fact they are two different conditions; strabismus is one cause of amblyopia. Amblyopia can result from a constant strabismus in which the right or left eye turns all of the time, but alternating strabismus in which an eye only sometimes turns rarely causes amblyopia.

Diagnosis

Since amblyopia usually occurs in only one eye, children may not notice the condition, and because many parents do not have their infants or toddlers take a comprehensive vision exam, many children go undiagnosed until they have their eyes examined later. The most important diagnostic tools are special visual acuity tests.

Treatment

The earlier the treatment, the better the opportunity to reverse the vision loss. Amblyopia can be treated between the ages of two and six, but the success rate decreases with age. The best results from treatment occur between six months and two years.

Glasses are commonly prescribed to improve focusing or misalignment of the eyes. Surgery may be performed on the eye muscles to straighten the eyes if other means have not been successful.

Eye exercises may be recommended either before or after surgery to correct faulty visual habits associated with strabismus and to teach comfortable use of the eyes. The correction may be followed by patching or covering one eye for a few weeks to as long as a year. The better-seeing eye is patched, forcing the "lazy" one to work, thereby strengthening its vision.

Eye drops or ointment may be used to blur the vision of the good eye in order to force the weaker one to work, although this is generally a less successful approach than eye patching.

Although true amblyopia cannot be cured after the age of six, treatment for older children still can usually improve vision. Treatment of amblyopia after the age of six requires more effort and includes vision therapy. If not treated early enough, an amblyopic eye may never develop good vision and may even become functionally blind.

lead poisoning   Lead poisoning is one of the most common and preventable childhood health problems today, affecting more than one million children under age six. More than one-fifth of African-American children living in housing built before 1946 have elevated blood lead levels. Alarmingly, even very small exposures can produce subtle but dangerous health effects in young children.

Lead is a neurotoxin, which means that it will impair both physical and mental function and development. For many years, people assumed that children would have to ingest large amounts of lead before being harmed, but today experts believe even small exposures (such as raising and lowering a window painted with lead paint in the presence of a child) can result in subtle developmental and intellectual delays.

Youngsters ingest lead by licking or eating flakes of old paint containing lead, or by drinking water flowing through pipes contaminated with lead, solder, or brass fittings. Babies who drink reconstituted formula made with water flowing through lead pipes can ingest an alarming percentage of tainted water.

Lead poisoning causes most damage to the brain, nerves, red blood cells, and digestive system. A cumulative poison, it remains in the kidneys for seven years and in the bones for more than 30 years. Several studies have also shown that high levels of lead in the blood can interfere with a child's growth; poisoning during critical periods of bone and brain cell growth can seriously interfere with a child's development.

Lead poisoning in children is particularly serious because it does not take much to harm a child—and the potential damage to the child's developing neurological system is much more serious. Furthermore, the danger of lead poisoning is especially great with young children, who tend to put everything into their mouths, including contaminated lead dust and flecks from old lead paint. Worst of all, there may be no symptoms of lead poisoning for a very long time until the damage has already been done. Because its effects vary wildly from one child to another, it is almost impossible to predict how an individual child will fare.

Lead Prevention

The most effective way to protect children from lead poisoning is to prevent lead from building up in blood, tissues, and bones. The Centers for Disease Control and Prevention (CDC) recommends testing every child at 12 months of age, and if resources allow, at 24 months. Screening should start at six months if the child is at risk of lead exposure (for example, if the child lives in an older home built before 1960 which has peeling or chipping paint). Decisions about further testing should be based on previous blood lead test results, and the child's risk of lead exposure. In some states, more frequent lead screening is required by law. The CDC in 1991 identified a number of reasons for testing a child for lead poisoning, including:

- child lives or regularly visits a house built before 1960 being renovated or that has peeling, chipped paint
- sibling or classmate is being treated for lead poisoning
- child lives with someone whose hobby includes exposure to lead, such as making pottery or stained glass, working in auto repair or bridge or highway construction
- child lives near industry likely to release lead

- child received treatment for foreign object in ear, nose, or stomach
- child often swallows nonfood items
- any child under six with unexplained developmental delays, hearing problem, irritability, severe attention deficit, violent tantrums, or unexplained anemia

The test will identify how many micrograms of lead are found in one deciliter of the child's blood. Based on what is known today, children should have under 10 micrograms per deciliter (10 mcg/dl) of blood lead concentration. If higher levels are found, there are certain steps that can be taken.

At 10–19 mcg/dl, a child has mild lead poisoning and should be retested in a few months. The home and all the places where the child spends time should be checked for lead sources, and identified lead hazards should be controlled. Frequent wet cleaning and hand-washing will help reduce lead dust. Good nutrition can help the child fight lead.

A blood lead level between 20 and 44 means the child has moderate lead poisoning. Sources of lead in the child's environment must be removed, and the child may need chelation therapy to remove lead from the body. Chelation therapy means the child is given a drug capable of binding lead and reducing its acute toxicity. All drugs have potential side effects and must be used with caution.

A blood lead concentration of 45–69 is severe lead poisoning. A child with this concentration needs both medical treatment and lead removed from the environment.

A blood lead level over 70 is an acute medical emergency. The child may stay in the hospital for treatment and not be released until he or she can return to a lead-free safe home.

While many products contain lead, it is most often associated with paint; until about 1960, *all* house paint contained some. Lead was added to paint because it helped the paint dry quicker and gave it a shiny, hard finish. In fact, the more lead in a can of paint, the better and more expensive the product—some paints were as much as 50 percent lead.

By the late 1970s the government began to regulate the amount of lead in paint, but nothing was done about the lead-filled paint already on the walls in millions of older homes throughout the United States. It is this lead-based paint (often found in inner-city homes) that causes most of the lead poisoning in children. More than three-fourths of American homes built before 1980 still contain lead paint, and 14 million housing units have high levels of lead in dust or chipping paint—3.8 million housing young children. If a house was built before 1950, it is almost guaranteed that its paint contains the toxic substance; if it was built between 1950 and 1978, there is a 50 percent chance of lead paint.

The average blood lead level in the general population has been gradually dropping over the past 20 years since lead was eliminated from gasoline, but an estimated seven million tons of lead remain in the soil.

Symptoms

Lead poisoning is usually a chronic problem, building up in the body over a period of time. When a child eats lead, the body absorbs about 10 to 15 percent of the metal, and the rest is slowly excreted. Most of the absorbed lead is stored in the child's bones, with smaller amounts deposited in bone marrow, soft tissues, and red blood cells. If the lead poisoning continues, it will accumulate to toxic levels.

Lead is excreted very slowly from the body, so it builds up in tissues and bones and may not even produce detectable physical effects, although it can still cause mental impairment. If they do appear, early symptoms include listlessness, irritability, loss of appetite and weight, constipation, and a bluish line in the gums, followed by clumsiness, vomiting and stomach cramps, and a general "wasting."

If untreated, the toxic lead levels in a child's body can lead to serious cognitive complications as well, including mental retardation. Babies exposed to high levels of lead before birth reveal impaired attention span, hearing and language ability, and intelligence. After birth, the affected infants may be able to recover, but only if they are no longer exposed to lead. If lead exposure continues, their cognitive performance will continue to be affected for at least the first five years of life.

In addition, some researchers suggest that there may be an association between exposure to lead pre- and postnatally and HYPERACTIVITY, behavior disorders, and ATTENTION DEFICIT HYPERACTIVITY DISORDER.

While lead poisoning is almost always a chronic problem, it is possible—albeit extremely rare—to suffer from an acute case of lead poisoning, when a large amount of lead is taken in by the body over a short period of time. Acute poisoning symptoms include metallic taste in the mouth, abdominal pain, vomiting, diarrhea, collapse, and coma. Large amounts directly affect the nervous system and cause headache, convulsions, coma and, sometimes, death.

Treatment

According to the CDC, unless widespread screening has revealed no lead problems, a baby should be tested at 12 months of age and again at two years, *even without symptoms*. This is because symptoms may be subtle or nonexistent.

Lead screening includes a simple blood test that determines the level of lead in the blood. A child with elevated blood lead levels, or enough absorbed lead in the body to show symptoms, will probably require hospitalization. Treatment usually includes the administration of medicines (called chelating agents) to help the body rid itself of lead. In mild cases, the chelating agent penicillamine may be used alone; otherwise, it may be used in combination with edetate calcium disodium and dimercaprol. Chelation therapy has its risks, however, and must be properly monitored to avoid kidney damage. In acute cases, stomach pumping may be necessary.

What Else Parents Can Do

When renovating an older home, consumers should call an expert to ascertain whether or not there is a lead problem and, if so, how to handle the situation. Because children who live near factories that melt metal may also have a lead poisoning problem, parents who live near a factory can find out if lead is being released from the stacks by checking the Environmental Protection Agency's (EPA) Toxics Release Inventory available at public libraries.

To temporarily reduce lead paint and dust, floors, windowsills, and window wells should be cleaned at least twice a week with a trisodium phosphate

LEAD POISONING GUIDE

The following recommendations have been provided by the U.S. Centers for Disease Control:

Lead Levels	Complications	Treatment
0–9 mcg/dl*	None	Annual checks until age six
10–14 mcg/dl	Borderline (possible test inaccuracy); risk for mild developmental delays	Nutrition, housecleaning
15–19 mcg/dl	Risk for IQ decrease; no symptoms usually noticed	Test for iron deficiency
20–44 mcg/dl	Risk of IQ impairment increases	Eliminate lead; drug treatment possible
45–69 mcg/dl	Colic, anemia, learning disabilities	Remove from home until lead is removed; drug treatment
70 mcg/dl	Vomiting, anemia, critical illness	Immediate hospitalization; lead removal

*mcg/dl = micrograms per deciliter of blood

detergent available at hardware stores. Sponges used for this purpose should not be used for anything else. Cribs and playpens should be moved away from chipped or peeling paint, mantels, windowsills, and doors. Baby furniture that may be decorated with lead paint should be stripped or removed. The child's hands, face, bottle nipples, and toys should be washed often. Children and pregnant women should not be in the area while removing lead paint. Because the seams of imported canned foods may be soldered with lead, which can leach into the contents, they should be avoided.

Children should be given calcium, iron, and protein, with plenty of milk, breads, low-fat foods, and green leafy vegetables, because these diminish lead's effects in the body. In addition, parents should limit the amount of dirt tracked in the home and avoid storing acidic food (such as orange juice and tomatoes) in ceramic or crystal containers that may contain lead glaze. Pregnant women should not drink out of ceramic mugs.

The home's water lead level should be tested; it should not exceed 15 parts per billion. Water should never be boiled to eliminate lead; boiling only concentrates lead. Cold water should be allowed to run only for a few minutes before using, and parents should never cook with hot water from the tap (especially when making baby food) since lead leaches more quickly into hot water. A water-treatment device to remove lead from tap water might be a good investment. If the soil tests high in lead, it should be covered with clean soil and seed or sod.

learning disability   A neurobiological disorder in which a child's brain works, or is structured, differently, affecting one or more of the basic processes involved in understanding or using spoken or written language. Such a disability may result in a problem with listening, thinking, speaking, reading, writing, spelling, or doing mathematical calculations. Experts believe that children with learning disabilities have a problem with the way the brain handles information that hinders the normal learning process.

Learning disabilities affect one in seven children and represent a national problem of enormous proportions. Every year 120,000 more students are diagnosed with learning disabilities, a diagnosis now shared by 2.4 million schoolchildren in the United States. Many thousands more are never properly diagnosed or treated, or they do not get treatment because they are not considered eligible for services.

All children learn in highly individual ways. Children with learning disabilities simply process information differently, but they are generally of normal or above-average intelligence. The most common learning disability is a problem with language and reading.

Sometimes overlooked, learning disabilities are often not easily recognized, accepted, or considered serious once detected. The impact of the disability, which can be hereditary, ranges from relatively mild to severe. Learning disabilities can affect many parts of a child's life: school or work, daily routines, friendships, and family life. Some children have many overlapping learning disabilities, while others may have a single, isolated learning problem that has little impact on other areas of their lives.

Learning disabilities are not the same as MENTAL RETARDATION, AUTISM, deafness, blindness, or behavioral disorders, nor are learning disabilities caused by poverty, environmental factors, or cultural differences. Learning disabilities are not curable, but individuals can learn to compensate for and even overcome areas of weakness. Attention deficits and hyperactivity sometimes appear with learning disabilities, but not always.

Common learning disabilities include:

- DYSLEXIA A language-based disability in which a person has trouble understanding words, sentences, or paragraphs
- *Dyscalculia* A mathematical disability in which a person has a very difficult time solving arithmetic problems and grasping math concepts
- *Dysgraphia* A writing disability in which a person finds it hard to form letters correctly or write within a defined space
- *Auditory and visual processing disabilities* Sensory disabilities in which a person has difficulty understanding language despite normal hearing and vision

More than one in six children will encounter a problem learning to read during the first three years in school, according to the U.S. Department of Education. Currently, more than 2.8 million school-age children receive special education services as students with learning disabilities, which represents about five percent of all children in public schools. However, these statistics do not include the thousands of students who attend private and religious schools, nor does it include the scores of students who may have serious problems with learning but who may not meet the criteria established by school districts to receive special education services.

Symptoms

The earlier a learning disability is detected, the better chance a child will have of succeeding in school and in life. Parents are encouraged to understand the warning signs of a learning disability from as early as preschool, since the first years in school are especially crucial for a young child.

There is no one indication of learning disabilities. Although most children have an occasional problem with learning or behavior, a consistent pattern of the following problems may suggest the need for further testing:

Preschool:

If the child has problems

- learning the alphabet
- rhyming words
- connecting sounds and letters
- counting or learning numbers
- being understood when speaking to a stranger
- using scissors, crayons, or paint
- reacting too much or too little to touch
- using words or using phrases
- pronunciation
- walking up and down stairs
- talking (identified as a "late talker")
- remembering names of colors
- dressing

Elementary School:

Does the child have trouble with:

- learning new vocabulary
- speaking in full sentences
- understanding conversation rules
- retelling stories
- remembering information
- playing with peers
- moving from one activity to another
- expressing thoughts
- holding a pencil
- handwriting
- handling math problems

- following directions
- self-esteem
- remembering routines
- learning
- reading comprehension
- drawing or copying shapes
- deciding what information presented in class is important
- modulating voice
- neatness and organization
- meeting deadlines
- playing age-appropriate board games

Adulthood:

Does the adult have trouble with:

- remembering new information
- organization
- reading comprehension
- getting along with peers or coworkers
- finding or keeping a job
- sense of direction
- understanding subtle jokes
- making appropriate remarks
- self-expression
- following directions
- reading, writing, spelling, and math
- self-esteem
- using proper grammar
- meeting deadlines

Symptoms may appear in only one skill area, such as reading or writing, in many people with learning disabilities. The following is a brief outline of warning signs for possible learning disabilities in specific skill areas:

Attention:

- has short attention span
- is impulsive
- has difficulty conforming to routines
- is easily distracted

Auditory:

- does not respond to sounds of spoken language
- consistently misunderstands what is being said
- is overly sensitive to sound
- has trouble differentiating simultaneous sounds

Language:

- can explain things orally but not in writing
- has trouble telling or understanding jokes or stories
- misinterprets language
- does not understand what is said
- responds in an inappropriate manner, unrelated to what is said
- responds only partially to what is said

Math:

- has problems with arithmetic, math language, and math concepts
- reverses numbers
- has problems with time, sequencing, or problem solving

Memory:

- learns information presented one way but not another
- has trouble memorizing information
- is unable to repeat what has just been said

Movement:

- performs similar tasks differently each day
- has trouble dialing phone numbers or holding a pencil
- has poor coordination, is clumsy; poor motor planning
- is unaware of physical surroundings
- has a tendency to self-injury

Organization:

- has trouble following a schedule
- is often late
- has trouble learning about time
- has difficulty organizing belongings

Reading:

- has poor reading ability or poor comprehension
- may misread information
- has problems with syntax or grammar
- confuses or reverses similar letters or numbers
- has problems reading addresses, small print, and/or columns

Social:

- has trouble with social skills
- misinterprets nonverbal social cues
- experiences social isolation
- does not use appropriate eye contact

Thinking Skills:

- acquires new skills slowly
- has trouble following directions
- confuses right/left, up/down, under/over, behind/between
- gets lost in large buildings
- seems unaware of time or sequence of events

Writing:

- has problems writing down ideas
- has problems organizing thoughts on paper
- reverses or omits letters, words, or phrases when writing
- has problems with sentence structure, writing mechanics
- may spell the same word differently in a single paper
- may read well but not write well (or vice versa)

What Is Not LD

It is also important to understand what is not included in the LD category. For example, while attention deficit disorder (ADD) and ATTENTION DEFICIT HYPERACTIVITY DISORDER (ADHD) are not learning disabilities themselves, there is a 20 percent probability that a child with ADD or ADHD also has one or more learning disabilities. Other conditions that are not considered to be learning disabilities themselves include AUTISM, blindness and deafness, emotional problems, hyperactivity, illiteracy, mental retardation, "slow learner," or physical disability.

Diagnosis

"Learning disabilities" is a broad term that covers a range of possible causes, symptoms, and treatments. Partly because learning disabilities can show up in so many forms, it is difficult to diagnose or to pinpoint the causes.

Not all learning problems are necessarily learning disabilities; many children are simply slow to develop certain skills. Because children show natural differences in their rate of development, sometimes what seems to be a learning disability may simply be a delay in maturation. To be diagnosed as a learning disability, problems must occur either in developmental speech and language disorders, academic skills disorders, or other coordination disorders and learning handicaps. Each of these categories includes a number of more specific disorders.

Developmental Speech and Language Disorders

Speech and language problems are often the earliest indicators of a learning disability. Children with developmental speech and language disorders have trouble producing speech sounds, using spoken language to communicate, or understanding what other people say. Depending on the problem, the specific diagnosis may be:

- Developmental articulation disorder
- Developmental expressive language disorder
- Developmental receptive language disorder

With a developmental articulation disorder, children may have trouble controlling their rate of speech, or they may lag behind their friends in learning to make speech sounds. These disorders are common, appearing in at least 10 percent of children younger than age eight. Fortunately, articulation disorders can often be outgrown or successfully treated with speech therapy.

Some children with developmental expressive language disorder have problems expressing themselves in speech, such as calling objects by the wrong names, speaking only in two-word phrases, or not being able to answer simple questions.

Some have trouble understanding certain aspects of speech; this is developmental receptive language disorder. This explains the toddler who does not respond to his name or the worker who consistently cannot follow simple directions. While hearing is normal, these individuals cannot make sense of certain sounds, words, or sentences. Because using and understanding speech are strongly related, many people with receptive language disorders also have an expressive language disability.

Of course, some misuse of sounds, words, or grammar is a normal part of learning to speak. It is only when these problems persist that there is any cause for concern.

Academic Skills Disorders

Students with academic skills disorders often lag far behind their classmates in developing reading, writing, or arithmetic skills. The diagnoses in this category include:

- developmental reading disorder
- developmental writing disorder
- developmental arithmetic disorder

Developmental reading disorder (also known as dyslexia) is quite widespread, affecting between 2 percent and 8 percent of elementary school children. The ability to read requires a rich, intact network of nerve cells that connect the brain's centers of vision, language, and memory. While a child can have problems in any of the tasks involved in reading, scientists have found that a significant number of children with dyslexia share an inability to distinguish or separate the sounds in spoken words. For example, a child might not be able to identify the word "cat" by sounding out the individual letters, c-a-t, or to play rhyming games. Fortunately, remedial reading specialists have developed techniques that can help many children with dyslexia acquire these skills. However, there is more to reading than recognizing words. If the brain cannot form images or relate new ideas to those stored in memory, the reader will not be able to understand or remember the new concepts. This is why other types of reading disabilities can appear in the upper grades when the focus of reading shifts from word identification to comprehension.

Writing, too, involves several brain areas and functions. The brain networks for vocabulary, grammar, hand movement, and memory must all work well if the child is to be able to write well. A *developmental writing disorder* may be caused by problems in any of these areas. A child with a writing disability, particularly an expressive language disorder, might be unable to compose complete, grammatical sentences.

Arithmetic involves recognizing numbers and symbols, memorizing facts such as the multiplication table, aligning numbers, and understanding abstract concepts like place value and fractions. Any of these may be difficult for children with *developmental arithmetic disorders.* Problems with numbers or basic concepts are likely to show up early, whereas problems that appear in the later grades are more often tied to problems in reasoning.

Many aspects of speaking, listening, reading, writing, and arithmetic overlap and build on the same brain capabilities, so it is not surprising that people can be diagnosed as having more than one area of learning disability. For example, the ability to understand language underlies the ability to learn to speak. Therefore, any disorder that interferes with the ability to understand language will also interfere with the development of speech, which in turn hinders learning to read and write. A single problem in the brain's operation can disrupt many types of activity.

"Other" Learning Disabilities

There are additional categories of learning disabilities, such as "motor skills disorders" and "specific developmental disorders not otherwise specified." These diagnoses include delays in acquiring language, academic, and motor skills that can affect the ability to learn but do not meet the criteria for a specific learning disability. Also included are coordination disorders that can lead to poor penmanship, as well as certain spelling and memory disorders.

Attention Disorders

Nearly four million school-age children have learning disabilities; of these, at least 20 percent have a type of disorder that leaves them unable to focus their attention. Some children who have attention disorders are easily distracted or appear to daydream constantly. Children with this problem may have a number of learning difficulties.

In a large proportion of affected children (mostly boys) the attention deficit is accompanied by hyperactivity, running into traffic or toppling desks. Hyperactive children cannot sit still: They blurt out answers, they interrupt, they cannot wait their turn. Because of their constant motion and explosive energy, hyperactive children often get into trouble with parents, teachers, and peers. By adolescence, physical hyperactivity usually subsides into fidgeting and restlessness, but the problems with attention and concentration often continue into adulthood.

At work, adults with ADHD often have trouble organizing tasks or completing their work. They do not seem to listen to or follow directions. Their work may be messy and appear careless.

While attention disorders (with or without hyperactivity) are not considered learning disabilities in themselves, because attention problems can seriously interfere with school performance, they often accompany academic skills disorders.

Causes

Experts do not know exactly what causes learning disabilities, but they are assumed to be disorders of the central nervous system triggered by many different factors. These may include heredity, problems during pregnancy or birth, and incidents after birth.

The fact that learning disabilities tend to run in families indicates that there may be a genetic link. For example, children who lack some of the skills needed for reading, such as hearing the separate sounds of words, are likely to have a parent with a related problem. However, a parent's learning disability may take a slightly different form in the child. A parent who has a writing disorder may have a child with an expressive language disorder. For this reason, it seems unlikely that specific learning disorders are inherited directly. Instead, what is inherited might be a subtle brain dysfunction that can lead to a learning disability.

There may be an alternative explanation for why LD might seem to run in families. Some learning difficulties may actually stem from the family environment. For example, parents who have expressive language disorders might talk less to their children, or the language they use may be distorted. In such cases, the child lacks a good model for acquiring language and therefore may seem to be learning disabled.

LD problems also may be caused by illness or injury during or before birth, or by the use of drugs and alcohol during pregnancy, untreated RH incompatibility with the mother, premature or prolonged labor, or lack of oxygen or low weight at birth.

Throughout pregnancy, the fetal brain develops from a few cells into a complex organ made of billions of specialized, interconnected nerve cells called neurons. During this process, things can go wrong that may alter how the neurons form or interconnect.

In the early stages of pregnancy, the brain stem forms, the part of the brain that controls basic functions such as breathing and digestion. Later, a deep ridge divides the cerebrum (the thinking part of the brain) into two halves, a right and left hemisphere. Finally, the areas involved with processing sight, sound, and other senses develop, as well as the areas associated with attention, thinking, and emotion.

As new cells form, they move into place to create various brain structures. Nerve cells rapidly grow to form networks with other parts of the brain. These networks allow information to be shared among various regions of the brain.

Throughout pregnancy, this brain development is vulnerable to disruptions. If the disruption occurs early, the fetus may die, or the infant may be born with widespread disabilities and possibly mental retardation. If the disruption occurs later, when the cells are becoming specialized and moving into place, it may leave errors in the cell makeup, location, or connections. Some scientists believe that these errors may later show up as learning disorders.

Scientists have found that mothers who smoke during pregnancy may be more likely to bear smaller babies, who tend to be at risk for a variety of problems, including learning disorders. Alcohol also may be dangerous to the fetus's developing brain, distorting the developing neurons. Heavy alcohol use during pregnancy has been linked to

FETAL ALCOHOL SYNDROME, a condition that can lead to low birth weight, intellectual impairment, HYPERACTIVITY, and certain physical defects. Any alcohol use during pregnancy may influence the child's development and lead to problems with learning, attention, memory, or problem solving. Drugs such as cocaine (especially crack cocaine) seem to affect the normal development of brain receptors that help to transmit incoming signals from skin, eyes, and ears. Because children with certain learning disabilities have trouble understanding speech sounds or letters, some researchers believe that learning disabilities (as well as ADHD) may be related to faulty receptors. Current research points to drug abuse as a possible cause of receptor damage.

After birth, learning disabilities may be caused by head injuries, nutritional deprivation, poisonous substances, or child abuse. New brain cells and neural networks continue to be produced for a year or so after the child is born, and these cells also are vulnerable to certain disruptions.

Some environmental toxins may lead to learning disabilities, possibly by disrupting childhood brain development or brain processes. Cadmium and lead, both prevalent in the environment, are becoming a leading focus of neurological research. Cadmium, used in making some steel products, can get into the soil, then into food. Lead was once common in paint and gasoline and is still present in some water pipes. A study of animals sponsored by the National Institutes of Health showed a connection between exposure to lead and learning difficulties. In the study, rats exposed to lead experienced changes in their brain waves, slowing their ability to learn. The learning problems lasted for weeks, long after the rats were no longer exposed to lead.

In addition, there is growing evidence that learning problems may develop in children with cancer who had been treated with chemotherapy or radiation at an early age. This seems particularly true of children with brain tumors who received radiation to the skull.

Diagnosis

By law, a learning disability is defined as a significant gap between a child's intelligence and the skills achieved at each age. This means that a severely retarded 10-year-old who speaks like a six-year-old probably does not have a language or speech disability, because he has mastered language up to the limits of his intelligence. On the other hand, a fifth grader with an IQ of 100 who cannot write a simple sentence probably does have LD.

Learning disorders may be informally flagged by observing significant delays in the child's skill development. A two-year delay in the elementary grades is usually considered significant, but for older students, such a delay is not as debilitating, so learning disabilities are not usually suspected at this age unless there is more than a two-year delay.

Parents and professionals should each gather information and discuss concerns about a child who is struggling with learning problems. The child's parents should arrange for a comprehensive educational evaluation, which can only take place with the parent's written consent. Evaluations can help identify the child's relative strengths and difficulties, and help determine whether the student is eligible for special assistance in school.

When parents and school staff agree, the public school system must provide an evaluation to determine if a student is entitled to special education services. Evaluations can be arranged for free through the school system, or through private clinics, private evaluators, hospital clinics, or university clinics. However, some school districts may not automatically accept test results from outside sources. Parents should check with their school district before seeking evaluation services from private facilities.

The actual diagnosis of learning disabilities is made using standardized tests that compare the child's level of ability to what is considered normal development for a person of that age and intelligence. Test outcomes depend not only on the child's actual abilities but on the reliability of the test and the child's ability to pay attention and understand the questions.

Each type of LD is diagnosed in slightly different ways. To diagnose speech and language disorders, a speech therapist tests the child's pronunciation, vocabulary, and grammar and compares them to the developmental abilities seen in most children that age. A psychologist tests the child's intelligence. A physician checks for any ear infections, and an audiologist may be consulted to rule out auditory problems. If the problem involves articulation, a doctor examines the child's vocal cords and throat.

In the case of academic skills disorders, academic development in reading, writing, and math is evaluated using standardized tests. In addition, vision and hearing are tested to be sure the student can see words clearly and can hear adequately. The specialist also checks if the child has missed much school. It is important to rule out these other possible factors because treatment for a learning disability is very different from the remedy for poor vision or missing school.

ADHD is diagnosed by checking for the long-term presence of specific behaviors, such as considerable fidgeting, losing things, interrupting, and talking excessively. Other signs include an inability to remain seated, stay on task, or take turns. A diagnosis of ADHD is made only if the child shows such behaviors substantially more than other children of the same age.

If the school fails to notice a learning delay, parents can request an outside evaluation. After confirming the diagnosis, the public school is obligated to provide the kind of instructional program the child needs.

Parents should stay abreast of each step of the school's evaluation, and they may appeal the school's decision if they disagree with the findings of the diagnostic team. Parents always have the option of getting a second opinion.

Treatment

Although a diagnosis is important, even more important is creating a plan for getting the right help. Schools typically provide special education programs either in a separate all-day classroom or as a special education class that the student attends for several hours each week. Some parents hire trained tutors to work with their child after school. If the problems are severe, some parents may choose to place their child in a special school for the learning disabled.

Planning a special education program begins with systematically identifying what the student can and cannot do. The specialist looks for patterns in the child's gaps, such as the failure to hear the separate sounds in words or other sound discrimination problems. Special education teachers also identify the types of tasks the child can do and the senses that function well. By using the senses that are intact and bypassing the disabilities, many children can develop needed skills. These strengths offer alternative ways the child can learn.

After assessing the child's strengths and weaknesses, the special education teacher designs an individualized education program (IEP). The IEP outlines the specific skills the child needs to develop as well as appropriate learning activities that build on the child's strengths. Many effective learning activities engage several skills and senses. For example, in learning to spell and recognize words, a student may be asked to see, say, write, and spell each new word. The student may also write the words in sand, which engages the sense of touch. Many experts believe that the more senses children use in learning a skill, the more likely they are to retain it.

An individualized, skill-based approach often succeeds in helping where regular classroom instruction fails. Therapy for speech and language disorders focuses on providing a stimulating but structured environment for hearing and practicing language patterns. For example, the therapist may help a child who has an articulation disorder to produce specific speech sounds. During an engaging activity, the therapist may talk about the toys, then encourage the child to use the same sounds or words. In addition, the child may watch the therapist make the sound, feel the vibration in the therapist's throat, then practice making the sounds before a mirror.

Assistive Technology

Learning disabilities cannot be cured, but with the help of certain tools a child with a learning disability can work around difficulties with reading, writing, numbers, spelling, organization, or memory. Complex, high-tech tools and devices, called assistive technology, can help people work around specific deficits.

Tools for people with learning disabilities can be as simple as highlighters, color coded files or drawers, books on tape, tape recorders, calculators, or a different paper color or background color on a computer screen. Sometimes standard technologies (such as voice recognition systems) can be adapted or designed to help people with learning disabilities perform everyday tasks. Complex assistive technology includes computers that talk to help people with reading and writing difficulties, speech recognition systems that translate oral language into written text, talking calculators that assist people with math difficulties, and software that predicts words for people with spelling difficulties.

Researchers are also investigating nonstandard teaching methods. Some create artificial learning conditions that may help the brain receive information in nonstandard ways. For example, in some language disorders, the brain seems abnormally slow to process verbal information. Scientists are testing whether computers that talk can help teach children to process spoken sounds more quickly. The computer starts slowly, pronouncing one sound at a time. As the child gets better at recognizing the sounds and hearing them as words, the sounds are gradually speeded up to a normal rate of speech.

Controversy

The term "learning disability" was coined by psychologist Samuel A. Kirk in 1963 to describe children who experience difficulty acquiring academic skills despite normal intelligence. He proposed this term because of his discomfort with the widespread use in an educational setting of medically oriented terms such as DYSLEXIA, congenital word blindness, and minimal brain dysfunction. Although the term has become widely accepted, there has been a great deal of controversy about the exact definition and methods of assessment and identification of the condition.

The term has provided a focal point for legislation and advocacy that has resulted in far-reaching changes in the nature of public and postsecondary education in the United States. At the same time, the term "learning disabilities," the range of potential learning problems that it includes, and the broad and rapidly changing field that it describes, continue to be controversial. In fact, there is still no consensus on the definition of learning disabilities or on what the category should include or exclude,

and the coming years are likely to see continuing debate on the fundamental issues of definition, classification, diagnosis, and treatment.

According to the National Joint Committee on Learning Disabilities, the term refers to a group of disorders marked by significant difficulties in listening, speaking, reading, writing, reasoning, or mathematical abilities. These disorders are presumed to be caused by central nervous system dysfunction and may occur at any time. Although learning disabilities may appear at the same time as other handicapping conditions (such as deafness, blindness, mental retardation, or serious emotional disturbance), they are not caused by these conditions.

The primary legal definition of a learning disability, according to Public Law 94-142 (as amended by Public Law 101-76), indicates a disorder in one or more of the basic psychological processes involved in understanding or in using spoken or written language. This may include an imperfect ability to listen, think, speak, read, write, spell, or do mathematical calculations. The term includes such conditions as perceptual handicaps, brain injury, minimal brain dysfunction, dyslexia, and developmental aphasia. The term does not include children who have problems primarily caused by visual, hearing, or motor disabilities, or mental retardation, emotional disturbance, or of environmental, cultural, or economic disadvantage.

Most definitions suggest that learning disabilities are permanent, affect a range of language and mathematics functions, and are caused at least in part from problems within the central nervous system. In addition, definitions of LD have generally focused on two key identifying factors: discrepancy and exclusion.

"Discrepancy" means that a child with a learning disability exhibits a significant gap between aptitude and performance. In many states, a diagnosis of a learning disability depends on a very strict statistical measurement of this discrepancy between achievement and aptitude.

"Exclusion" means that a learning disability is not caused by some other handicapping condition, such as physical impairment or social status. A child who struggles to learn because she cannot see, or because he comes from a background of poverty and disadvantage, is not considered to have a learning disability if these are the primary factors in the learning problems.

Both the discrepancy formulation for learning disabilities, and the role that exclusion of other conditions plays, have become subjects for increasing debate in recent years. Many researchers have proposed redefining the concept of learning disabilities to focus on specific language and thought processing problems that may be identified by appropriate testing, without necessarily involving the question of aptitude or intellectual potential. Some experts have argued that the exclusionary element in definitions of LD have led to the under-identification or misdiagnosis of individuals who come from poverty or from minority cultural, racial, or ethnic backgrounds. They argue that the difficulties such children have in learning are more likely to be ascribed to their backgrounds and upbringing than to a potential learning disability, and that approaches to diagnosis that depend on aptitude/achievement discrepancies are also likely to underrepresent such individuals.

The continuing controversy and debate that surround the concept of learning disabilities are complicated by different disciplines and theoretical perspectives, as well as the advocacy of parents, economic pressures on school districts, political, and legal developments. These controversies are likely to continue in the years to come.

Treatment for learning disabilities is extremely important if the child is to be successful. In fact, 35 percent of students with untreated learning disabilities do not finish high school. Most students with learning disabilities were not fully employed one year after graduating from high school. Adolescents with untreated learning disabilities are at higher risk for drug and alcohol abuse. One study showed that up to 60 percent of adolescents in treatment for substance abuse had learning disabilities.

Even though learning disabilities cannot be cured, there is still cause for hope. Because certain learning problems reflect delayed development, many children do eventually catch up.

Of the speech and language disorders, children who have an articulation or an expressive language disorder are the least likely to have long-term problems. Despite initial delays, most children do learn to speak. For people with dyslexia, the outlook is mixed. But an appropriate remedial reading program can help learners make great strides. With age, and appropriate help from parents and clinicians, children with ADHD become better able to suppress their hyperactivity and to channel it into more socially acceptable behaviors.

Consequences

Children with learning disabilities who have not been diagnosed or properly treated experience serious, lifelong negative consequences, including low self-esteem, delinquency, and illiteracy. Thirty-five percent of students identified with learning disabilities drop out of high school (this does not include students who drop out without being identified as having learning disabilities.) Fifty percent of young criminal offenders tested were found to have previously undetected learning disabilities; when offered educational services that addressed their learning disability, the recidivism rates of these young offenders dropped to below 2 percent.

Learning Disabilities Association (LDA) National nonprofit membership organization dedicated to enhancing the quality of life for children with LEARNING DISABILITIES and their families. It offers advocacy, education, research, and services. Formerly known as the Association for Children and Adults with Learning Disabilities, the Learning Disabilities Association was formed in 1964 by a group of concerned parents on behalf of children with learning disabilities. The LDA is the only national organization devoted to defining and finding solutions for the broad spectrum of these problems.

learning disorder A more specific term than LEARNING DISABILITY, without the same legal weight. A learning disorder may include any of a broad spectrum of dysfunctions in the ability to learn, including some syndromes and difficulties that are not generally grouped under the category of learning disabilities.

learning style A child's behavior, temperament, and attitude in a learning situation. Some of the best-known learning styles are visual, auditory, or kinesthetic. Some experts argue that is important to match a child's learning style with the style of instruction to make learning easier. For example, a child with a strong visual learning style should be taught to read with an emphasis on the shapes of words.

There are many different learning styles. Although a student may prefer one style over another, preferences develop like muscles: the more they are used, the stronger they become. Successful students have flexible and integrated learning styles. No one uses one of the styles exclusively, and there is usually significant overlap in learning styles.

Visual Learners

Children with this style relate most effectively to written information, notes, diagrams, and pictures. Typically they will be unhappy with a presentation where they cannot take detailed notes. To a degree, information does not exist for a visual learner unless it has been seen written down. This is why some visual learners take notes even when they have printed notes in front of them. Visual learners will tend to be most effective in written communication. They make up about 65 percent of the population.

Auditory Learners

Children with this style relate most effectively to the spoken word. They tend to listen to a lecture and then take notes afterward, or rely on printed notes. Because written information will often have little meaning until it is heard, it may help auditory learners to read written information out loud. Auditory learners may be sophisticated speakers and may specialize in subjects like law or politics. Auditory learners make up about 30 percent of the population.

Kinesthetic Learners

Children with this style learn best through touch, movement, and space, and they learn skills by imitation and practice. Kinesthetic learners can appear slow, because information is usually not presented in a style that suits their learning methods. Kinesthetic learners make up around 5 percent of the population.

left-handedness A child's preference for using the left hand for writing and other activities requiring coordination. Whether a child prefers the right or left hand (called "handedness" by scientists) is probably inborn. Four percent of children are left-handed and 96 percent are right-handed (percentages don't equal 100 because some are ambidextrous).

More than 90 percent of healthy children use the right hand for writing, and most (66 percent) favor the right hand for other activities requiring coordination. The rest are either left-handed or ambidextrous (able to use either hand). Handedness has no correlation to gender, and if the brain becomes damaged before age 12, it is possible to switch handedness without too much difficulty.

The propensity for using the left hand is related to the two hemispheres of the brain, each of which controls movement and sensation in the opposite side of the body. The dominant hemisphere in left-handed people is almost always the left, although a few left-handed children have a dominant right hemisphere. Others display no dominance at all.

Scientists suspect that some language disorders such as DYSLEXIA and STUTTERING are more common in left-handed children and may be related to a problem in developing cerebral dominance.

In earlier centuries, a left-handed child was considered to be unlucky at best, and evil at worst. (The word *sinister* comes from the Latin word for "left.") While this is no longer true today, so many people are right-handed that the pressure to conform is very high, especially in cultures that reserve the left hand for cleaning the anal area after defecating; in these cultures, the left hand is considered "unclean."

It is not clear whether left-handed children have special abilities. There is no evidence that more artists are left-handed, for example. In fact, about 60 percent of left-handed children, like right-handers, process speech in the left hemisphere, while the other 40 percent use both sides of the brain. This is one indication that each of the brain's hemispheres has the potential for processing any function.

leukemia Cancer of the blood cells that affects more than 2,000 children in the United States every year. Leukemia occurs when the body produces large numbers of abnormal blood cells—usually white blood cells, which help the body fight infection. The leukemia cells usually look different from normal blood cells, and they do not function properly.

There are several types of leukemia grouped by how quickly the disease develops and gets worse or by the type of blood cell that is affected. In acute leukemia, the abnormal blood cells remain very immature (called *blast cells*) and cannot carry out their normal functions; because the number of blast cells increases rapidly, the disease worsens quickly.

In chronic leukemia, on the other hand, while some blast cells are present, most cells are more mature and can carry out some of their normal functions. Also, the number of blasts increases more slowly than in acute leukemia, so chronic leukemia gets worse gradually.

Leukemia can occur in either of the two main types of white blood cells—lymphoid cells or myeloid cells. When leukemia affects lymphoid cells, it is called lymphocytic leukemia. When myeloid cells are affected, the disease is called myeloid or myelogenous leukemia.

Types of Leukemia

Acute lymphocytic leukemia (ALL) is the most common type of leukemia in young children. *Acute myeloid leukemia* (AML) occurs in both children and adults and is sometimes called acute nonlymphocytic leukemia (ANLL). *Chronic myeloid leukemia* (CML) affects only a very small number of children; it occurs mainly in adults.

Cause

Scientists know that leukemia affects more boys than girls, and more whites than blacks, but researchers cannot explain why one person gets leukemia and another does not. Scientists also know that certain genetic conditions can increase the risk for leukemia. In particular, children with DOWN SYNDROME are more likely to get leukemia than other children.

Some research suggests that exposure to electromagnetic fields (a type of low-energy radiation from power lines and electric appliances) is a possible risk factor for leukemia, but studies have not yet conclusively proven this link.

Symptoms

Leukemia cells are abnormal cells and cannot help the body fight infections. For this reason, children with leukemia often get infections and have fevers. Because children with leukemia often have fewer healthy red blood cells and platelets, there are not enough red blood cells to carry oxygen through the body. This causes anemia, making children look pale and feel weak and tired. When there are not enough platelets, children can bleed and bruise easily.

Depending on the number of abnormal cells and where these cells collect, children with leukemia may have a number of symptoms. In acute leukemia, symptoms appear and get worse quickly. In chronic leukemia, however, symptoms may not appear for a long time, and when they do appear, they seem mild at first and get worse gradually. Doctors often find chronic leukemia during a routine checkup before there are any symptoms.

Some of the common symptoms of leukemia include fever, chills, and other flu-like symptoms; weakness and fatigue; frequent infections; loss of appetite and/or weight; swollen or tender lymph nodes, liver, or spleen; easy bleeding or bruising; tiny red spots under the skin; swollen or bleeding gums; night sweats; and/or bone or joint pain.

In acute leukemia, the abnormal cells may collect in the brain or spinal cord and cause headaches, vomiting, confusion, loss of muscle control, and seizures. Leukemia cells also can collect in the testicles and cause swelling or cause sores in the eyes or on the skin. Leukemia also can affect the digestive tract, kidneys, lungs, or other parts of the body.

In chronic leukemia, the abnormal blood cells may gradually collect in various parts of the body. Chronic leukemia may affect the skin, central nervous system, digestive tract, kidneys, and testicles.

Diagnosis

A medical history and physical exam is the first step in diagnosing leukemia. In addition to checking general signs of health, the pediatrician will look for swelling in the liver, spleen, and the lymph nodes under the arms, in the groin, and in the neck. Although blood tests can help diagnose the condition, they may not show what type of leukemia it is. To check further for leukemia cells or to tell what type of leukemia a patient has, a doctor must examine a sample of bone marrow removed with a small needle. A bone marrow biopsy is performed with a larger needle and removes a small piece of bone and bone marrow.

If leukemia cells are found in the bone marrow sample, the doctor will order other tests to find out the extent of the disease. A spinal tap (lumbar puncture) checks for leukemia cells in the fluid that fills the spaces in and around the brain and spinal cord, and chest X rays can reveal signs of disease in the chest.

Treatment

Treatment is complex and depends on the type of leukemia and leukemia cells, the extent of the disease, and whether the leukemia has been treated before. It also depends on the child's age, symptoms, and general health.

Acute leukemia needs to be treated immediately; when there is no evidence of disease, more therapy may be given to prevent a relapse. Many children with acute leukemia can be cured.

Chronic leukemia patients who do not have symptoms may not require immediate treatment, but they should have frequent checkups so the doctor can see whether the disease is progressing. When treatment is needed, it can often control the disease and its symptoms, but chronic leukemia can seldom be cured.

Chemotherapy Most children with leukemia are treated with chemotherapy. Depending on the type of leukemia, they may take one drug or a combination of several, usually given intravenously. Because anticancer drugs often cannot cross the blood-brain barrier to reach cells in the central nervous system, doctors may inject them directly into the cerebrospinal fluid.

Chemotherapy is given in cycles of a treatment period followed by a recovery period, then another treatment period, and so on. In some cases, the patient has chemotherapy as an outpatient at the hospital, at the doctor's office, or at home. However, depending on which drugs are given and the patient's general health, a hospital stay may be necessary.

Radiation Some children may also may have radiation therapy together with chemotherapy for some kinds of leukemia. Radiation therapy uses high-energy rays to damage cancer cells and stop them from growing.

Bone marrow transplantation Some children may undergo this treatment for their leukemia, in which leukemia-producing bone marrow is destroyed by high doses of drugs and radiation and then replaced by healthy bone marrow. The healthy bone marrow may come from a donor, or it may be marrow that has been previously removed from the child. If the child's own bone marrow is used, it may first be treated outside the body to remove leukemia cells. A bone marrow transplant usually requires a hospital stay of several weeks. Until the transplanted bone marrow begins to produce enough white blood cells, children have to be carefully protected from infection.

Biological therapy Some children may be given substances such as interferon that affect the immune system's response to cancer.

Side effects Because leukemia patients get infections very easily, they may receive drugs to help protect them. Anemia and bleeding are other problems that often require supportive care. Leukemia and chemotherapy can make the mouth sensitive, easily infected, and likely to bleed. Because treatment also damages healthy cells and tissues, it causes side effects that depend on the type and extent of the treatment. Generally, anticancer drugs affect dividing cells, including healthy cells that divide often, such as blood cells, cells in hair roots, and cells in the digestive tract—all of which are likely to be damaged. This means the child's resistance to infection drops, they may have less energy and may bruise or bleed easily, they may lose their hair or have nausea, vomiting, and mouth sores. Most side effects go away gradually during the recovery periods between treatments or after treatment stops.

Some anticancer drugs can affect a patient's fertility, but most children treated for leukemia appear to have normal fertility when they grow up. However, depending on the drugs and doses used and on the age of the patient, some boys and girls may not be able to have children when they mature.

Radiation can cause reddened, irritated skin in addition to side effects similar to chemotherapy. Some side effects may be lasting. Children who receive radiation to the brain may develop subsequent problems with learning and coordination.

For this reason, doctors use the lowest possible doses of radiation and give this treatment only to children who cannot be treated successfully with chemotherapy alone. Radiation to the testicles is likely to affect both fertility and hormone production, and most boys who have this form of treatment are not able to have children later on. Some may need to take hormones.

Children who have a bone marrow transplant face an increased risk of infection, bleeding, and other side effects of the large doses of chemotherapy and radiation they receive. In addition, graft-versus-host disease (GVHD) may occur in children who receive bone marrow from a donor. This means that donated marrow reacts against the patient's tissues (most often the liver, the skin, and the digestive tract) at any time after the transplant (even years later). Drugs may be given to reduce the risk of GVHD and to treat the problem if it occurs.

Follow-Up Treatment

Regular exams are very important after treatment for leukemia to be sure the cancer has not returned, including exams of blood, bone marrow, and cerebrospinal fluid.

Leukemia and Lymphoma Society   A nonprofit health organization dedicated to finding the cure for LEUKEMIA, lymphoma, Hodgkin's disease, and myeloma, and to improve the quality of life of patients and their families. Since its founding in 1949 the society has provided more than $240 million for research specifically targeting blood-related cancers. The society was founded in 1949 by parents who lost their only son to leukemia and had recognized the need for the creation of a separate organization dedicated to finding cures for the disease through research. The society has grown to encompass 58 chapters throughout the country. (For contact information, see Appendix I.)

lice   Crawling insects that feed on human blood that are a common annoyance in elementary schools and day-care centers. Head lice live on and suck blood from the scalp, leaving red spots that itch intensely and can lead to skin inflammation and infection. The females lay a daily batch of pale eggs, called "nits," that attach to hairs close to the scalp. The nits hatch in about a week, and the adults can live for several weeks.

Head lice are found among people of all walks of life. About six million cases occur each year among U.S. schoolchildren between ages three and 12, even among those who shampoo daily. Children are most often infected via direct contact at school by sharing hats, brushes, combs, or headrests. Pets cannot get head lice.

Neighborhood parents and the child's school, camp, or child-care provider should be notified of the infestation. Children should be checked once a week for head lice.

Head lice lay eggs at the base of hairs growing on the head. While nits can be found anywhere on the hair, they are especially common behind the ears and at the back of the neck. Because lice move so quickly, it is usually the oval-shaped nits that are seen on the hair shaft. Nits are yellow when newly laid, turning to white once they hatch. They appear to be "glued" at an angle to the side of the hair shaft and hatch within eight days. The empty eggshells are carried outward as the hair grows.

Nits should not be confused with hair debris such as fat plugs or hair casts. Fat plugs are bright white irregularly shaped clumps of fat cells stuck to the hair shaft. Hair casts are long, thin cylinder-shaped segments of dandruff encircling the hair shaft; they are easily dislodged.

Head lice and nits also can be found on eyebrows and eyelashes. If one person in a family has head lice, all family members should be checked. However, only those who are infested should be treated with lice pesticide.

Diagnosis

Lice infestations are diagnosed by the presence of nits. By calculating the distance from the base of the hair to the farthest nits, it is possible to estimate how long the infestation has been.

Treatment

In order to get rid of head lice, all nits must be removed. Since no lice pesticide kills all nits, remaining nits left on the hair must be removed to eliminate the need for more treatments. Nits can be removed with a special nit removal comb, with baby safety scissors, or with the fingernails.

Drug treatment Lotions containing malathion or carbaryl kill lice quickly; the lotion should be washed off 12 hours after application, followed by combing the hair with a fine-toothed comb to remove dead lice and nits. Shampoos containing malathion or carbaryl are also effective if used repeatedly over several days. Combs and brushes should be plunged into very hot water to kill any attached eggs.

The National Pediculosis Association discouraged the use of lindane products (such as Kwell) because they appear to be potentially more toxic and no more effective than other treatments. Still, no product kills 100 percent of nits. Lice medications are not intended to be used on a routine or preventive basis.

All lice-killing medications are really pesticides and therefore should be used with caution. A health-care expert should be consulted before using or applying pesticides when the child has lice or nits in the eyebrows or eyelashes or has other health problems (such as allergies). Because head lice pesticides can be absorbed into the blood, they should not be used on open wounds on the scalp. These medications should not be used at all on infants and should be used with caution on children under age two. Instead, lice and nits can be removed by hand on very young children while wearing gloves.

The product should be used over a sink (not applied in a tub or shower) to minimize pesticide exposure to the rest of the body. The child's eyes should be kept covered while administering the pesticide.

Environmental treatments Bedding and recently worn clothing also should be washed in hot water and dried in a hot drier. Combs and brushes should be cleaned and then soaked in hot water for 10 minutes. Vacuuming is the best way to remove lice and attached nits from furniture, mattresses, rugs, stuffed toys, and car seats. According to the National Pediculosis Association, lice sprays should not be used.

Body Lice

Body lice live and lay eggs on clothing next to the skin, visiting the body only to feed. Body lice affect those who rarely change their clothes and are not a serious problem for American children. Body lice can be killed by placing infested clothing in a hot drier for five minutes, by washing clothes in very hot water, or by burning.

listeriosis A food-borne illness that may cause no symptoms in healthy children but is especially dangerous to newborns and very young children. Listeriosis occurs in about 7.5 cases for every one million people. Once thought to be exclusively a veterinary problem, it was identified as a human disease in 1981 when a Canadian outbreak was linked to tainted coleslaw made from cabbage grown in soil fertilized with *Listeria*-infected sheep manure. Four years later another outbreak was traced to Mexican-style soft cheese in California, which sickened 150 people, including many pregnant women, resulting in stillbirths.

From 1987 to 1992 the government recalled cooked products from 27 firms, including hot dogs, bologna, and other luncheon meat, chicken salad, ham salad, sausages, chicken, sliced turkey breast, and sliced roast beef. Cheese, dairy, sandwich, prepared salad, and smoked fish recalls from 1987 to 1992 included 516 different products from 105 firms.

Cause

Listeriosis is caused by one species in a group of bacteria called *Listeria monocytogenes* found in cow's milk, animal and human feces, soil, and leafy vegetables. In the past 10 years there have been several outbreaks that seem to have been linked to eating deli meats and soft cheeses such as feta, blue-veined cheeses, and some types of Mexican cheese. One recent study found that 2 percent of hot dogs tested contained the bacterium *L. monocytogenes*. Children with impaired immune systems also can catch the disease from undercooked chicken.

The bacteria is remarkably tough, resisting heat, salt, nitrite, and acidity much better than many other organisms. It can survive on cold surfaces and can multiply slowly at temperatures as low as 34°F. Freezing the food will stop the bacteria from multiplying, and commercial pasteurization will eliminate the organism in dairy products. *Listeria* does not change the taste or smell of food.

When *Listeria* is found in processed products, the contamination probably occurred after processing, rather than due to poor heating or pasteurizing.

Babies can be born with listeriosis if their mothers ate contaminated food during pregnancy. Pregnant women are 20 times more likely than other healthy adults to get the disease; about a third of all cases occur during pregnancy. However, it is newborns rather than their mothers who suffer the most serious effects of infection during the pregnancy.

Symptoms

If the fetus is affected early in the pregnancy, the baby will probably be born prematurely. Infants in this situation are usually quite ill, with low birth weight, breathing problems, blue skin, and low body temperature. If the baby survives, there may be a bloodstream infection or MENINGITIS. Half of these babies infected with *Listeria* die, even if treated.

Fetuses affected later in the pregnancy may be carried to term and be born at normal weight. If infected during delivery, the infants may develop meningitis; if so, 40 percent die. Some surviving babies who contract meningitis may have permanent brain damage or mental retardation.

Most normal, healthy children who become infected with the bacteria suffer few symptoms, or may experience a flu-like illness with fever, muscle aches, and nausea or diarrhea. If infection spreads to the nervous system, however, it can cause a type of meningitis.

Diagnosis

There is no routine screening test for susceptibility during pregnancy as there is for rubella and other infections. A blood or spinal fluid culture will reveal the infection.

Treatment

Antibiotics given to the pregnant mother can prevent disease in the fetus. Babies with listeriosis receive the same antibiotics as adults, although a combination of antibiotics may be used until diagnosis is certain. However, even with prompt treatment, some infections result in fetal death.

Prevention

In order to protect unborn children, pregnant women are advised to avoid deli counter foods and soft cheeses. There is no risk in hard cheese, processed slices, cottage cheese, or yogurt.

Those at risk should cook hot dogs to 160°F for several minutes to avoid contamination. Hot dogs at restaurants, ball parks, and so on, should be avoided, since cooking temperatures cannot be verified.

liver disorders   There are several problems with the liver that may affect children, including JAUNDICE, cholestasis, enlarged liver, portal hypertension, ascites or liver encephalopathy, and liver failure.

Diagnosis

When diagnosing liver disease, the pediatrician conducts a physical exam and checks the child's symptoms. In addition, a doctor may order a liver biopsy, liver enzyme tests, an ultrasound, or a computerized tomography (CT) scan.

Problems

Jaundice   This condition refers to a yellow discoloration of the skin and whites of the eyes due to an abnormally high level of bilirubin (bile pigment) in the blood. In newborns, jaundice is often caused by the breakdown of a large number of red blood cells, which can simply be treated by exposure to special lights and temporary bottle feeding. Otherwise, high levels of bilirubin may be caused by inflammation or other abnormalities of the liver cells, or blockage of the bile ducts. Jaundice is usually the first—and sometimes the only—sign of liver disease.

Cholestasis   This condition refers to reduced or blocked bile flow that may occur inside or outside the liver (or in both places). Symptoms of problems with bile flow may include jaundice, dark urine, pale stool, bone loss, easy bleeding, itching, spidery blood vessels in the skin, enlarged spleen, fluid in the abdominal cavity, chills, pain, or enlarged gallbladder. Cholestasis can be caused by HEPATITIS, metabolic liver diseases, drug effects, a stone in the bile duct, narrowed bile duct, biliary atresia, or inflamed pancreas.

Liver enlargement   An enlarged liver usually heralds some type of liver disease. While a slightly enlarged liver may cause no symptoms, a significant problem may trigger feelings of abdominal discomfort.

Portal hypertension Abnormally high blood pressure in the portal vein linking the intestine to the liver that may be due to higher blood pressure in the portal blood vessels or resistance to blood flow through the liver. Portal hypertension can trigger the growth of new blood vessels bypassing the liver, bringing blood from the intestine directly to the general circulation. When this occurs, substances that the liver normally would filter out instead pass into general circulation. Symptoms of portal hypertension may include a distended abdominal cavity, spider veins, and bleeding of the veins at the lower end of the esophagus and in the stomach lining.

Ascites This condition refers to fluid buildup in the abdominal cavity caused by fluid leaks from the vessels on the surface of the liver and intestine. Ascites due to liver disease usually accompanies other liver disease characteristics such as portal hypertension. Symptoms may include a distended abdomen, discomfort, and shortness of breath.

Liver encephalopathy This condition is caused by the deterioration of brain function due to toxic substances building up in the blood that are normally removed by the liver. Liver encephalopathy is also called portal-systemic encephalopathy, hepatic encephalopathy, or hepatic coma. Symptoms may include changes in mood, logical thinking, personality, and behavior; impaired judgment; drowsiness and confusion; sluggish speech and movement; disorientation; loss of consciousness and coma.

Liver failure This severe deterioration of liver function occurs when a large portion of the liver is damaged. Symptoms may include jaundice, bruising or bleeding, abdomen distention, impaired brain function, poor weight gain and growth, fatigue, weakness, nausea, and appetite loss.

lockjaw See TETANUS.

low birth weight See BIRTH RATE, LOW.

low blood sugar See HYPOGLYCEMIA.

lower respiratory tract infections See RESPIRATORY TRACT INFECTIONS.

lupus An autoimmune disease in which a person's immune system mistakenly works against the body's own tissues. Systemic lupus erythematosus (SLE), the most common type of lupus, typically develops during the 20s, 30s, or 40s—mbut about 15 percent to 17 percent of people with systemic lupus first notice symptoms during childhood or adolescence. Most of these are children 10 years or older; it is extremely rare in children under five. Experts estimate that between 5,000 and 10,000 children in the United States have SLE.

Children diagnosed with lupus often have been ill for a longer period and are more likely to have significant internal organ involvement than most adults with lupus. This may be because many children are not recognized as having early lupus until the disease has become worse. As a result children with lupus often are required to begin aggressive therapy soon after diagnosis. While lupus can be a severe and life-threatening disease, many children with lupus will do very well.

A healthy immune system produces proteins called antibodies that normally protect the body against bacterial and viral infections. In people with lupus, the immune system is unable to distinguish between foreign substances and the body's own cells, and it makes antibodies that target the patient's cells, sparking inflammation and pain. Systemic lupus, which can be mild or life-threatening, can affect many organs in the body.

Cause

The exact cause of lupus is unknown. Patients may have a genetic predisposition to the disease that is set in motion by an environmental factor such as an infection, medications, or extreme stress. Only about 10 percent to 12 percent of lupus patients have a family history of the disease. Estrogen may also play a role in lupus, which could help explain why more girls are diagnosed, most often during the childbearing years. Lupus also occurs more frequently in African Americans, Asian Americans, Latinos, and Native Americans than in Caucasians.

Drug-induced lupus occurs in about 10 percent of lupus patients who develop this form of the disease as a reaction to specific groups of medications. In children, antiseizure medications (such as phenytoin), thyroid medications, and minocycline (to treat acne) are the most common culprits. The symptoms of drug-induced lupus are similar to those of the systemic form, but they are usually milder.

Symptoms

Symptoms of SLE may increase or decrease unpredictably. Children with lupus often have fever, weakness, fatigue, or weight loss. They may experience muscle aches, loss of appetite, swollen glands, hair loss, or abdominal pain, which can be accompanied by nausea, diarrhea, and vomiting. Sometimes the child's fingers, toes, nose, or ears will be particularly sensitive to cold and will turn blue or white in cold temperatures.

The American College of Rheumatology has compiled a list of symptoms, including:

- malar rash across the cheeks and the bridge of the nose (also called a "butterfly" rash because it looks like a butterfly)
- photosensitivity to either sunlight or certain types of fluorescent light that causes a rash
- painless ulcers in the nose or mouth
- arthritis that does not destroy the bones around the joints
- inflammation of the lining around the heart, abdomen, or lungs
- kidney problems, either mild or severe
- neurological disorders such as seizures or psychosis
- blood problems, such as anemia, a low white blood cell count (leukopenia), or a low platelet count (thrombocytopenia)
- problems with the immune system
- positive test for antinuclear antibodies (ANA)

Diagnosis

Lupus can be difficult to diagnose because it can affect almost any organ in the body, and its symptoms vary so much from patient to patient. That variability is one of the greatest challenges of treating the disease for both doctors and their patients. Some children have obvious disease symptoms with fever, rash, and kidney involve-

ment, while others may only complain of not feeling well, being tired, and weight loss. Some children may look fine but may have blood in their urine or other unseen problems that require additional tests that will help the physician to make the diagnosis. Although a positive ANA test is generally required to make the diagnosis, there are many children with positive ANAs who do not have lupus.

Treatment

Lupus is a chronic disease with no known cure, but it can be controlled. Since lupus is different from person to person, the treatment program must be tailored to the needs of the individual patient. Living with lupus involves recognizing and managing symptoms as well as being able to control or modify a daily routine.

Almost all patients take medication to control inflammation and reduce the risk of flares. Corticosteroids are commonly prescribed, but their side effects (including a puffy round face) can be disturbing to children. Cytotoxic drugs are one alternative to high doses of corticosteroids and allow a dramatic reduction in the corticosteroid dosage, often to a level without obvious or severe side effects. This is often a major medical and psychological benefit to children. However, cytotoxic drugs also carry several risks.

Short-term cytotoxic drugs can damage bone marrow, causing bleeding or affecting immunity. Careful monitoring usually reduces these risks. Cytotoxic drugs also may increase a child's risk of developing certain forms of cancer. There is also evidence that cytotoxic drugs may interfere with the ability to bear children in the future. Doctors and parents must balance the risk of these future problems against the benefits of better control of the lupus and fewer corticosteroids.

Antimalarial drugs such as hydroxychloroquine are sometimes prescribed to ease skin and joint symptoms. For day-to-day muscle and joint pain, patients can take acetaminophen or any of a variety of nonsteroidal anti-inflammatory drugs (NSAIDs) such as ibuprofen or naproxen. Some children with kidney disease may require more aggressive treatment with the anticancer drug cyclophosphamide.

Preventive behavior can also help minimize lupus flares, so children should wear sunscreen and protective clothing when outside. Regular exercise can help prevent fatigue and joint stiffness. A balanced diet and sufficient rest are also important for maintaining general health and well-being. Children taking steroids may need extra calcium in their diet.

Despite these precautions and lifestyle changes, the progression of the disease often cannot be predicted. Living with lupus depends on respecting limits every day, and that can be a problem for teenagers. Teens also tend to spend more time in the sun and may not take their medications, or they may take on too many projects, all of which can trigger a lupus flare.

Children with lupus are prone to childhood illnesses such as a viral infection or diarrhea, but a fever, rash, or mouth sore may also indicate the beginning of a flare. Over time, as parents become more familiar with the child's disease, they may learn to recognize signs of an impending flare.

Call the Doctor

A doctor should be consulted immediately if the child experiences a flare or reports bloody stools, easy bruising (with or without nosebleeds), chest or abdominal pain, seizures, or new or high fever.

Prognosis

The prognosis of lupus in childhood depends on the severity of the internal organ involvement. Children with significant kidney or other internal organ disease require aggressive treatment. Outlook is poorest for children who develop serious kidney disease or persistent central nervous system disease. Children with mild rash and arthritis may be easily controlled, but lupus is unpredictable, and no one will be able to predict with certainty the long-term outcome for a specific child.

However, over the past three decades, better diagnostic tools and treatments have significantly improved the long-term prognosis for children with lupus. Recent advances leading to earlier diagnosis and more effective treatment have significantly improved the quality of life and life expectancy of children with lupus.

Lupus Foundation of America (LFA) The only nationwide voluntary health organization working exclusively on behalf of the 1.4 million Americans with lupus. The Lupus Foundation of America mission is to educate and support those affected by lupus and find the cure. In addition to sponsoring support groups, helping people find a doctor, and advocating for the cause, the LFA provides reliable and accurate information. The LFA has 25 brochures written by leading experts in the field of lupus, as well as approved literature that offers more in-depth information about the disease. A free packet is sent to anyone requesting information and includes a basic information pamphlet, a list of chapters, and details about available services. (For contact information, see Appendix I.)

Lyme disease A tick-borne illness whose hallmark symptom is a bull's-eye-shaped red rash surrounding a tick bite. Untreated Lyme disease can cause a host of problems, including arthritis and disorders of the heart and central nervous system. The disease is most commonly found in the northeast coastal states from Maine to Maryland, in the upper Midwest, and on the Pacific coast. It is usually contracted in the late spring or early summer, when ticks are abundant, although it may occur whenever the temperature is above 40°F for several consecutive days.

While the disease has been portrayed in sometimes frightening fashion, most of the time it is easily treated and does not progress to the chronic stages. It probably causes severe long-term effects in fewer than 10 percent of untreated children; moreover, recent studies indicate that many people who think they have Lyme disease actually have other conditions.

The number of new cases of Lyme disease has doubled in the United States since 1991, from more than 9,000 cases in 1991 to nearly 18,000 new cases in 2000. In 2000 Lyme disease cases increased by 8 percent compared to 1999, when 16,273 cases were reported. The increases in new cases may be partly due to better awareness and reporting of Lyme disease, but it also may be due to the fact that more people were exposed to ticks in densely populated areas.

Most of the new cases in 2000 were reported by 12 states in the northeastern, mid-Atlantic, and north-central United States, including Connecticut, Rhode Island, New Jersey, New York, and Delaware. The highest number of cases was reported by Columbia County, New York. Only six states reported no cases of Lyme disease in 2000: Colorado, Georgia, Hawaii, Montana, New Mexico, and South Dakota. Children aged five to nine are among the hardest hit groups, because they are more likely to be exposed to infected ticks and are less likely to use protective measures than other age groups.

History

In the United States, the disease was first recognized in Lyme, Connecticut, after two mothers were told in 1975 that their children had juvenile rheumatoid arthritis, a type of disabling arthritis of childhood characterized by swollen, painful joints. When the women discovered many others in the area had the same disease—which does not normally occur in clusters—they took their concerns to Yale University.

By the late 1970s Yale researchers discovered that many patients they studied were afflicted with a mysterious disease that produced a variety of symptoms in addition to joint swelling. They determined the cause was apparently a microorganism transmitted by at least one species of tick found widely in the woods around Lyme. In 1982 the bacteria was identified by Willy Burgdorfer in Montana, who discovered the spiral-shaped bacterial species that today bears his name: *Borrelia burgdorferi.*

Once scientists knew the cause, they confirmed that a group of skin conditions and neurological syndromes identified in Europe were also manifestations of Lyme disease. European patients suffer slightly different forms of the disease, probably because of differences in the strains of *B. burgdorferi* active in different parts of the world. Europeans experience long-term neurological complications, such as thinking problems and dementia; up to 10 percent of untreated Europeans also suffer for many years with a skin condition in which the affected areas of the skin become red, thin, and wrinkled. These symptoms

are rarely found among patients with Lyme disease in the United States. Researchers have now identified the disease throughout the world, including Australia, Africa, and Asia.

Cause

The spirochete form of the bacteria is transmitted primarily by the deer tick, the tiniest of which is about the size of the period at the end of this sentence. These ticks are found on deer, birds, field mice, and other rodents. The tick must be attached to its victim for between 36 to 48 hours before an infectious dose of spirochetes are transmitted. For this reason, simply by checking children often for ticks, most can avoid being infected.

Most children are diagnosed in the spring, summer or early fall. In the northern states, about half of all adult *Ixodes scapularis* ticks are infected. In some places, such as Block Island and Nantucket, the numbers are even higher. Even so, in most sections of the northeast, only between 1 percent and 3 percent of children have contracted Lyme disease.

The tick that transmits Lyme diseases in California relies on intermediate hosts, such as lizards, that are resistant to infection. For this reason, ticks (and, consequently, humans) are infected much less often in the state of California than in the states of the Northeast.

Symptoms

Most children who do become infected with lyme disease usually display one or more symptoms between three days and a month after becoming infected. About 60 percent of victims will notice a small red spot that expands over a period of days or weeks, forming a circular, triangular, or oval-shaped rash. Sometimes the rash resembles a red, raised bull's-eye with a clear center. The rash can range in size from a dime to the entire width of a child's body. As the infection spread, several rashes can appear at different places on the body. Without treatment, the rash begins to disappear within days or weeks.

As the spirochetes move through the body via the blood, other symptoms affecting other parts of the body may appear. These may include such flu-like symptoms as headache, stiff neck, appetite loss, body aches, and fatigue. Although these symptoms may resemble those of common viral infections, Lyme disease symptoms tend to persist or may occur intermittently.

About 20 percent of children may experience early neurological problems. Some children may have facial paralysis, MENINGITIS, ENCEPHALITIS, or numbness or tingling in other parts of the body.

Complications

After several months of being infected, slightly more than half of those children not treated with antibiotics develop recurrent attacks of painful and swollen joints that last a few days to a few months. The arthritis can shift from one joint to another; most often, the knee is infected. About 10 percent to 20 percent of untreated patients who experience temporary arthritic symptoms will go on to develop chronic Lyme arthritis. In contrast to many other forms of arthritis, Lyme arthritis typically is not symmetrical.

One out of 100 Lyme patients develop temporary heart problems (such as irregular heartbeat) several weeks after infection. Most children will not be aware of this problem unless their doctor detects it. Other nervous system complications include memory loss, concentration problems, and changes in mood or sleeping habits. Nervous system abnormalities usually develop several weeks, months, or even years after an untreated infection. These symptoms may last for weeks or months and may recur.

Diagnosis

Lyme disease is not easy to diagnose because its symptoms mimic those of many other diseases, such as viral infections or MONONUCLEOSIS. Joint pain can be misdiagnosed as inflammatory arthritis, and neurologic signs may be misidentified.

Diagnosis includes a history of exposure to ticks, typical symptoms, and blood tests revealing antibodies to Lyme bacteria. The tests are most useful in later stages.

Treatment

Antibiotics usually provide a complete recovery if given early enough. Most children who are treated in later stages of the disease also respond well. Unfortunately, cases that are not diagnosed

soon enough may resist antibiotic treatment. In a few children, symptoms of persistent infection may continue, or the disease may recur, so that doctors prescribe repeated long courses of antibiotics. The value of this approach remains controversial.

Children with chronic Lyme disease may exhibit varying degrees of permanent damage to joints or the nervous system. This usually occurs among children who were not diagnosed in the early stages of the disease, or for whom early treatment was not successful. Deaths from Lyme disease have been reported only rarely.

However, experts at the Centers for Disease Control and Prevention do not recommend automatic treatment with antibiotics after every tick bite. Instead, they say it is better to avoid ticks in the first place.

Prevention

Lyme vaccine Although a vaccine against Lyme disease (LYMErix) had been approved in 1998 for people aged 15 to 70 years, in, 2002 the manufacturer announced that the vaccine would no longer be commercially available, citing poor sales. LYMErix had caused controversy in recent years, as patients complained that they were sickened by the vaccine and asked the government to restrict sales; some filed lawsuits against maker GlaxoSmith Kline. Federal health officials insisted there was no evidence that the vaccine was dangerous.

When the vaccine was first approved, the Centers for Disease Control and Prevention (CDC) had urged that only people at high risk of Lyme disease get vaccinated because the expensive vaccine did not offer complete protection. Studies had showed it was 80 percent effective after people got all three required shots. After vaccinations began, however, some patients reported arthritis, muscle pain, and other symptoms similar to Lyme disease itself. Because 15 percent of the U.S. population has arthritis anyway, scientists found it difficult to determine how the symptoms were connected to LYMErix.

When the CDC reexamined 905 possible side effects reported to the government between 1998 and July 2000, they found no signs that LYMErix caused arthritis although they did find 22 cases of allergic reaction. Nevertheless, at least 60 patients are suing the manufacturer for monetary damages. Other class action suits also have been filed.

Other prevention Ticks do not hop, jump, fly, or descend from trees, although they may blow in a strong breeze. In the woods, children should walk only on trails and avoid brushing against low bushes or tall grass. To prevent tick bites, children should wear protective clothing, with long-sleeved shirts and pants tucked into boots or socks. Light-colored clothes allow ticks to be more easily spotted.

An insect repellent may be used on bare skin and clothing, but all insect repellents should be used with caution in children and should not be used on hands or face. Repellent should not be used at all on infants.

Ticks and their hosts (chipmunks, voles, mice, and other small mammals) need moisture, a place hidden from direct sun, and a place to hide. Therefore, the cleaner the area around a house, the less chance there will be of getting a tick bite. All leaf litter and brush should be removed as far as possible away from the house. Low-lying bushes should be pruned to let in more sun. Leaves should be raked up every fall, since ticks prefer to overwinter in fallen leaves. Woodpiles are favorite hiding places for mammals carrying ticks; to discourage mammal visitors, woodpiles should be neat, off the ground, in a sunny place, and under cover. Gardens should be cleaned up every fall; foliage left on the ground over the winter provides shelter for mammals that may harbor ticks. Stone walls on the property increase the potential for ticks as well. Shady lawns may support ticks in epidemic areas; lawns should be mowed and edged. Entire fields should be mowed in fall, preferably with a rotary mower. Bird feeders attract birds that carry infected ticks, so feeders should not be placed too close to the house. The ground should be cleaned under the feeder regularly. Bird feeding should be stopped during late spring and summer, when infected ticks are most active. Building eight-foot fences to keep out deer may significantly reduce the abundance of ticks on large land parcels. Pets allowed outside should be examined daily.

Lyme Disease Foundation (LDF) A nonprofit medical health care agency established in 1988 and dedicated to finding solutions to tick-borne disorders. The LDF is the first and largest organization, with strong ties in the international scientific community. (For contact information, see Appendix I.)

lymphangitis Inflammation of the lymph vessels seen most often as red streaks on the skin near a streptococcus-infected wound.

lymphocytic choriomeningitis virus (LCMV) A virus carried by hamsters and wild or lab mice that is not harmful to adults, but that can cause birth defects in unborn children whose mothers contract the virus. LCMV was first identified in 1933 in a woman who was thought to have a form of ENCEPHALITIS. In 1955 it was first recognized in the United Kingdom as a virus that could cause congenital disease. Since then, individual cases of congenital LCMV infection have been identified in Germany, France, Lithuania, and across the United States.

Mice and hamsters are the primary sources of LCMV infections. Humans acquire this virus by direct contact with infected rodents or by inhaling the virus. So far, more than 49 infants around the world have been diagnosed with congenital LCMV. However, experts really are not sure how many infants have been affected by LCMV before birth because doctors do not routinely look at LCMV as a possible cause of congenital blindness or retardation. In one instance, twin girls from Cochise County, Arizona, were born to a mother who had unknowingly contracted LCMV during pregnancy. One girl was born with vision problems and the other has seizures and severe developmental delays. More than 90 percent of the babies who have contracted the LCMV virus before birth have had adverse effects, the most common of which were vision problems. Other problems include neurological conditions such as CEREBRAL PALSY, MENTAL RETARDATION, SEIZURES, and decreased visual acuity.

A pregnant woman with a pet hamster should have someone else take care of it during the pregnancy. If cleaning up after wild mice, pregnant women should wear gloves and spray the area with water to avoid the possibility of wafting the virus into the air. Pregnant women who work with mice in a laboratory setting should have the mice tested for LCMV.